Physiologic Anchorage Control

Tian Min Xu
Editor

Physiologic Anchorage Control

A New Orthodontic Concept and its Clinical Application

Springer

Editor
Tian Min Xu
Department of Orthodontics
Peking University School and Hospital of Stomatology
Beijing
China

ISBN 978-3-319-48331-3 ISBN 978-3-319-48333-7 (eBook)
DOI 10.1007/978-3-319-48333-7

Library of Congress Control Number: 2017932924

Printed on acid-free paper

This Springer imprint is published by Springer Nature
The registered company is Springer International Publishing AG
The registered company address is: Gewerbestrasse 11, 6330 Cham, Switzerland

Foreword

During my orthodontic residency in 1965, one of the requirements was to complete a publishable thesis. At the time, I thought that this would be my last academic experience. At the Oregon Health and Sciences University, it was possible for me to explore the current situation in molecular biology. Just before I had started my residency, I had just audited an upper division course taught by Professor Daniel Mazia at UC Berkeley called "Physical Chemical Basis of Biology." That was just 9 years after the critical publication of Watson and Crick and 2 years after Jacob and Monod's publication on DNA coding of proteins.

Dr. Ernest Hixon, Department Chair in Orthodontics at the University of Oregon School of Dentistry, urged me to do a study linked to the work of Kaare Reitan on fundamental changes in the periodontal ligament associated with initial orthodontic tooth movement. During my residency, I had access to the lab of Dr. Adam Lis, professor in the School of Medicine, who had himself been a student of one of my former patients at the University of California, Berkeley.

Dr. Lis and I set up a very ambitious study on changes in cell replication and protein synthesis in the PDL associated with orthodontic-type forces. We would track the effects of forces to move teeth in Sprague-Dawley rats as a stimulus for changes in cell replication and protein synthesis using the model of Waldo and Yen. The experimental sample consisted of three groups of 24 60 g Sprague-Dawley rats each plus an untreated control group of 24 animals. Each group included 24 rats that had rubber wedges inserted between their lower first and second mandibular molars and 24 Sprague-Dawley rats were injected with tritiated versions of thymidine, a precursor to thymine, essential for nucleic acid. The next 24 rats were injected with tritiated uridine, a precursor to messenger RNA; and the last 24 experimental animals were injected with tritiated hydroxyproline to measure protein synthesis in the extracellular matrix. The control group of 24 rats remained untreated.

I worked in the animal lab every night from 6:30 to 12, a minimum of 6 days a week, and I remember the head of the lab telling me if I didn't go home earlier he would have to charge me rack rent. At the end of the schedule, the animals were killed and the appropriate teeth for each animal were prepared autoradiographically. During the first 2 years of my orthodontic practice, I spent all my down time counting silver grains on photomicrographs with a Coulter counter. I did cell counts on the lower first molars of all the thymidine rats on both sides of each animal. (Molar separation had been introduced unilaterally within nonseparated side being used as in-animal controls.) But by the time we got to the uridine animals, I had spoken to Dr. Mazia at Berkeley and he had assured me uridine incorporation was not a completely valid way of tracking messenger RNA formation. I had my first look at the hydroxyproline slides and there was evidence of incorporation throughout the cellular matrix, which at my level of nonknowledge indicated contamination, so I was left to focus on the thymidine cells, which I did.

The study resulted in two papers published in the AJO. One paper was on cell replication and the other was on bone bending. They were both read more seriously by periodontal residents than by our own residents. I went back to building a practice in orthodontics in Berkeley and teaching an introductory course in statistics at UCSF. To my great satisfaction, Dr. Eugene West, then the Chair of Orthodontics at UCSF and a leading person in the field, urged me to speak to the residents on my observations, with himself in attendance. After my presentation, Chuck Ware, one of the residents asked, "Has your experience with that experience caused you to treat your own patients differently?" "Absolutely not," I said. "I don't think that a controlled experiment on 100 rats would tell me more about tooth movement than a one hour discussion with an experienced orthodontic clinician."

To my great surprise, Dr. West and others in attendance seemed quite irritated by this response. I had answered naively, thinking that orthodontists would be happy to have their diagnostic prowess recognized. But Dr. West, a highly skilled diagnostician, was looking to fundamental science for direct answers to clinical questions that had baffled orthodontic practitioners since before Angle. I thought about Dr. West's reply to my response for a long time, and realized that I could not be both a fundamental biologist and an orthodontist. Since I was interested in clinically useful answers, I decided to change my area of interest within orthodontic research and turned to the measurement and interpretation of orthodontic images, which has remained my main area of research.

This brings us to the larger question of how one should view the problems of fundamental biology from the perspective of the orthodontist: Should our approach be bottom-up or top-down? My own decision reflects the development during the past two decades of a defined field called translational research, which seeks to bring to top-down research the rigor and organizational character of the best bottom-up approaches of fundamental biologists. With very little hesitation I decided that the best contributions I would make as an orthodontist were top-down, leaving bottom-up approaches to research scientists in the several fields of development and genetics.

Dr. Xu's systematic approach to clinical translational research is precisely in line with the idea of rigorous investigation of the outcome of well-documented routine orthodontic treatment. In introducing the PASS method, he outlines a system by means of which comprehensive systematic 3D data on routine clinical treatment can be captured and applied to the study of tissue response to therapeutic orthodontic interventions. Dr. Xu's lab has already established a laudable record of systematic data acquisition in orthodontics. New treatment modalities like XBT tube and MLF brackets, in addition to the popular TADs and self-ligating brackets, can now be investigated using 3D CBCT x-ray records integrated with scanned data from study casts. We can expect future editions of this very volume to reach new levels of scientific accuracy and precision. In addition, these records will make it possible to study the greatest problem raised by orthodontic treatment – the problem of relapse and of developing techniques for minimizing it.

There are many ways to look at the world of orthodontics from top-down. Here I will outline my own. The largest area of orthodontic research should be the subject of relapses – Why is it that some patients maintain the results of treatment relatively intact for the remainder of their lives, while others regress toward the antecedent condition soon after the end of treatment? I attempt to answer this question from the perspective of a physical scientist. When a patient presents for orthodontic treatment, the clinician examines him/her carefully. Regardless of whether or not treatment is desirable, the patient at presentation presents with the dentition at equilibrium. We may find that relationship satisfactory, or alternatively, we may find it compromised either physiologically or aesthetically. If we find it compromised, we initiate treatment aimed at aligning the dentition more appropriately.

Equilibrium in the absence of external inputs will tend to maintain itself indefinitely with a minimum of external energy investment. If treatment has not reached a state of equilibrium, the dentition will regress toward conditions with lower energy input requirements. This is what we call "relapse." In practice, orthodontic treatment terminates with the placement of a "retainer" that becomes part of the new occlusal system. If an equilibrium has not been achieved during treatment, then no matter how long the retainer is used its removal will result in regression toward a lower energy state.

Unfortunately, we do not yet know with precision how to measure or characterize the state of equilibrium of the teeth in orthodontic patients. We have only a few rules of thumb. We know, for example, that orthodontic forces do not of themselves move teeth. Rather, they cause signals to the local muscles and nerves, which produce movement among anatomical structures to minimize forces and move the entire physiological system toward new equilibriums at lower force levels. The study of these forces and movements is the role of translational research. It incorporates the principles of fundamental biology but is more specifically concerning with factors that can be altered by clinical intervention. We know that there are true changes in the positions of the teeth through time in all active individuals. We know that advancing teeth or over-expanding the arches is not stable. Most important, we know that accumulation and analysis of data bases using hypothesis testing approaches are most likely to produce new information.

This is the strength of Dr. Xu's new volume. Malocclusions occur through time. Their treatment takes place through time, and the outcomes must be measured and tested through time. This volume is a product of the work of dedicated expert clinicians, each employing treatment modality which he or she believes to be an efficient and effective method of treating a specific type of malocclusion. The records of antecedent state, course of treatment, and post-treatment history have been recorded into a database and are amenable to rigorous and systematic analysis.

Dr. Xu and his associates have developed a research laboratory strongly focused on translational orthodontic research. They are developing a well-organized clinical database containing an integrated series of projects seeking rigorous answers to clinical problems. The goal is to develop clinically meaningful results by evaluating the clinical beliefs of experienced orthodontists in hypothesis testing studies of treatment outcomes through time. Their studies are conducted in collaboration with other concerned investigators throughout the world. The continuing task of Dr. Xu and his colleagues is the development of methods for gathering and analyzing clinical data in a blinded and unbiased fashion. The studies reported in this volume constitute input to Dr. Xu's records base. He and his associates are to be congratulated for their dedicated contributions to systematic development of meaningful translational research in orthodontics.

California, USA Sheldon Baumrind

Preface

Orthodontics is a discipline of experience, as are most other disciplines in clinical medicine. Most orthodontic techniques have been invented by outstanding expert clinicians with keen insight; few such techniques have been invented by orthodontic scholars who research orthodontics full time at university. Since evidence-based medicine has been introduced into orthodontics, high-quality clinical studies have been emphasized, and more discoveries have been made than what we can observe directly from the clinic. Should these endeavors serve orthodontic practice or are they just for publication? And how can we apply these academic achievements to improve orthodontic treatment?

To bridge clinical studies and orthodontic practice, this book joins contributions from many leading figures in the field. An iconic figure in the technique school, Professor James Vaden from the Tweed International Foundation, introduces the art "from Farrar, through Angle, Tweed, and into the present day", and highlights the importance of anchorage preparation in the classical Edgewise Appliance. An authority figure in academia, Professor Lysle Johnston, a former chair of the Department of Orthodontics and Pediatric Dentistry at the University of Michigan and the Orthodontic Department of Case Western Reserve University, and St. Louis University, summarizes the intrinsic character of orthodontic treatment, defining the treatment of malocclusion as "a prevention, reduction, or reversal of maxillary dentoalveolar compensation" through his thorough and critical evaluation of various treatment strategies, "regardless of label – fixed or functional; early or late", and his longitudinal study of craniofacial growth samples, which sustains the philosophy of physiological anchorage control. An orthodontist with an engineering background, Dr. Ching-Chang Ko, Fred Hale distinguished professor and program director of the Orthodontic Department at the University of North Carolina, Chapel Hill, has studied the mechanical properties of various archwires in Cross(X) Buccal Tube (XBT) and Multi-level Low Friction (MLF) brackets. A group of Chinese orthodontists from Peking University School and Hospital of Stomatology, who devote themselves to rigorous clinical studies under the influence of the distinguished scientist in orthodontic clinical study – Professor Sheldon Baumrind from the University of The Pacific, Arthur A. Dugoni School of Dentistry, share their experience with the clinical application of the Physiologic Anchorage Spee-wire System (PASS) technique.

The new concepts and treatment measures introduced in this book are mostly based on the best available evidence obtained through studies on craniofacial growth, occlusion development, biomechanics and materials, orognathic function, and current prospective or retrospective clinical trials. As Professor Baumrind writes in the Foreword, we are just getting on the road of translational orthodontic research to solve clinical problems. Although we have overcome some common weaknesses in contemporary fixed appliances, we are still far away from the last goal. Ongoing studies in this direction will certainly enrich our knowledge in this field. It is hoped that the more physiological orthodontic approach may help the results of treatment to become more stable and function better.

Parts of the studies presented in this book are funded by NIH/NIDCR R01DE022816-01; National Natural Science Foundation of China No.81371192; International Science & Technology Cooperation Program of China No. 2014DFA31800; and Beijing Municipal Science & Technology Commission No. Z141107002514054. I appreciate this support and all the efforts the researchers and authors have made in each chapter, and I acknowledge the copyright permission we have been granted from the original publishers for all the figures we quote in the book. Finally, we thank all the patients whose details are presented in the clinical application chapters for their help in developing our specialty.

Beijing, China Tian Min Xu

Contents

Part I

Fundamental Theory of Physiologic Anchorage Control

Classical Orthodontic Anchorage: A Century of Progress

1

James L. Vaden

Abstract

Anchorage preparation is a vital part of orthodontic treatment. Without anchorage, teeth cannot be placed into their proper positions and facial imbalance cannot be corrected. Anchorage has been discussed and studied since the days when orthodontics began as a specialty. This chapter will discuss the issues and the personalities involved in the drama. It discusses classical anchorage preparation from Farrar, through Angle, Tweed, and into the present day. The journey that anchorage preparation has taken has been very interesting and very colorful. Its history is discussed in the chapter via direct quotations from the participants. The comments made by Angle, and later by Tweed, are particularly interesting.

Anchorage is a tooth movement issue that has been discussed and subjected to study after study. Without anchorage, teeth cannot be moved. The American Heritage College Dictionary [1] defines anchorage as "a means of securing or stabilizing." This definition implies that the source of attachment, the anchorage unit, is stable and rigid or, in other words, immovable. When dental units or teeth are used as anchorage to move other teeth, Newton's law "for every action, there is an equal and opposite reaction" must not be forgotten.

There is no such thing as absolute anchorage when teeth are pitted against teeth. Intraoral anchorage has, therefore, been a source of study and of great concern since the very first attempts at tooth movement. One of the first people to discuss anchorage in an orthodontic textbook was John Nutting Farrar. In his Vol. 2 text, he has a topic on anchorage, "Proper and Improper" [2]. Dr. Farrar discussed the first molar and how much it can be moved if premolars are to be retracted. In discussing the

J.L. Vaden
Private Practice 308 East First Street, Cookeville, Tennessee, USA
e-mail: jvaden@uthsc.edu

T.M. Xu (ed.), *Physiologic Anchorage Control*,
DOI 10.1007/978-3-319-48333-7_1

molars, he states, "It should not be inferred from this, however, that the starting forward only a short distance is dangerous to these teeth, as all anchor teeth are liable and even expected to be moved somewhat by the draught. The question to decide is, how long such started anchor teeth can be safely used to further the operation?" Dr. Farrar also discussed the fact that teeth are sometimes elevated when they are used for anchorage. He cautioned the practitioner against grinding on these teeth to reduce the occlusion until the teeth settle back into a normal occlusion.

Edward Angle's Sixth Edition [3] was published in 1900. In Chapter X of this edition he discussed principles of anchorage. Angle stated, "In accordance with laws of physics their movement into harmony with the line of occlusion can only be accomplished by the application of force from a fixed base of anchorage in one of three ways, pulling, pushing, or twisting. As 'for every action there is an equal and opposite reaction' that must follow. The same amount of force will be exerted upon the anchorage as upon the tooth to be moved, and if the anchorage offers no greater resistance than that offered by the tooth to be moved, equal displacement of both must follow. There must be two principle sources of anchorage; one, the anchorage that can be derived from the teeth themselves, or two, anchorage gained from attachments to the top and back of the head. The clinician must have a knowledge of the form and surface of the teeth, the occlusion, the surfaces of the teeth, the lengths, etc. in order to make an intelligent and comprehensive judgment of anchorage requirements and possibilities. The resistance offered by different teeth varies greatly according to their position, size, length and number of roots, the direction from which force is exerted and also the manner of mechanical attachment. Ideal anchorage would be accomplished from an immovable base. This immovable base idea is probably never fully possible in the mouth owing to the fact that teeth move and that the periodontium and the alveolus have a cushion like function." He talked about simple anchorage and stationary anchorage; simple anchorage was merely tipping teeth which required a minimal amount of force on the anchor teeth. (Fig. 1.1) He discussed stationary anchorage which is bodily movement of teeth (Fig. 1.2) and stated that "In no uncertain terms skill and judgment are necessary in the use of this form of anchorage. For its success depends, first on the absolute rigidity of the attachment and second, upon care that the force exerted be not at any time so great as to strain or injure it. This is of vital importance for any loosening or straining of it would change it to ordinary anchorage." In his Sixth Edition Angle stated that he introduced this concept of anchorage in 1887 in the First Edition of his book. He gave a dentist named Dr. Barrett credit for employing a form of stationary anchorage by the use of a vulcanite plate which entirely covered the molars.

In his Seventh Edition Angle [4] added one great new form of anchorage. This new method of anchorage that he discussed was intermaxillary anchorage. He defined it by stating that, "Intermaxillary anchorage is that form in which anchorage is secured by attachments to teeth in the opposite arch." He goes on to state, "I introduced it in an article in Dental Cosmos in September 1891 on page 743." Angle used intermaxillary anchorage from one arch to another to forcefully erupt cuspids which had not erupted. In the Seventh Edition he discussed this new intermaxillary anchorage by writing: "One of the most valuable modifications of this anchorage is

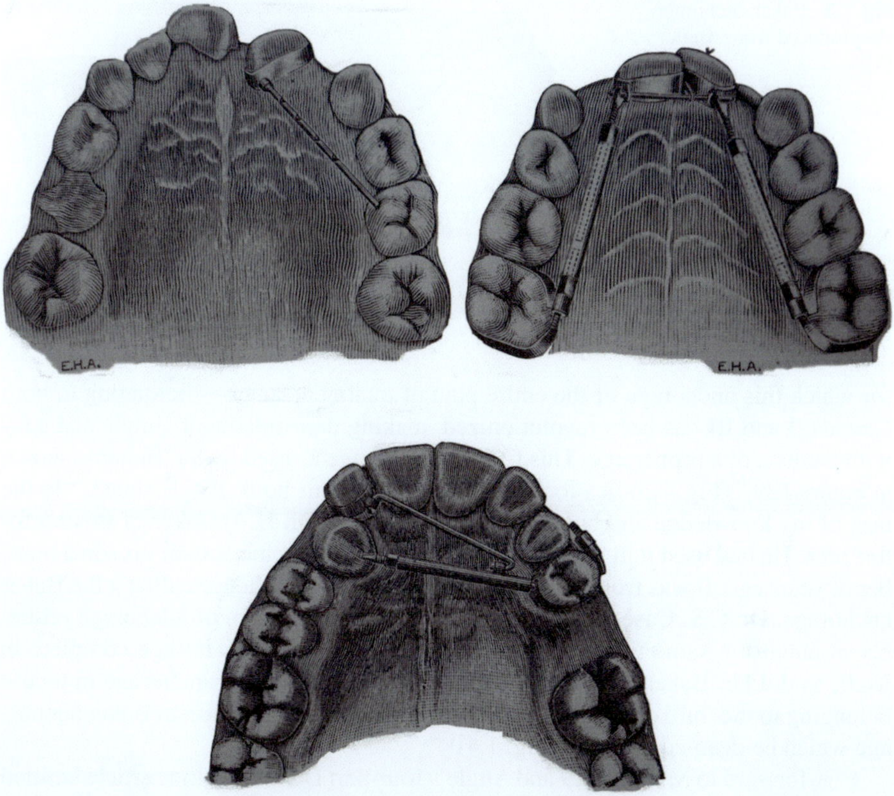

Fig. 1.1 Simple anchorage (Reproduced from Angle [3])

Fig. 1.2 Stationary anchorage (Reproduced from Angle [3])

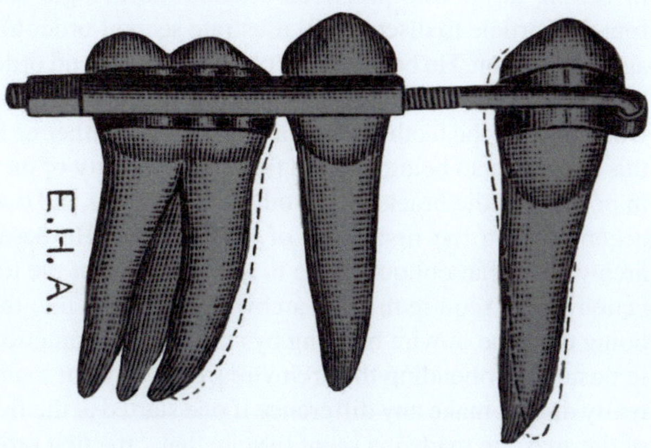

what is now known as the Baker anchorage by means of which the teeth of opposite arches may be reciprocally moved collectively, the uppers distally and the lowers mesially or vice versa. This marks an important step in the progress of orthodontia

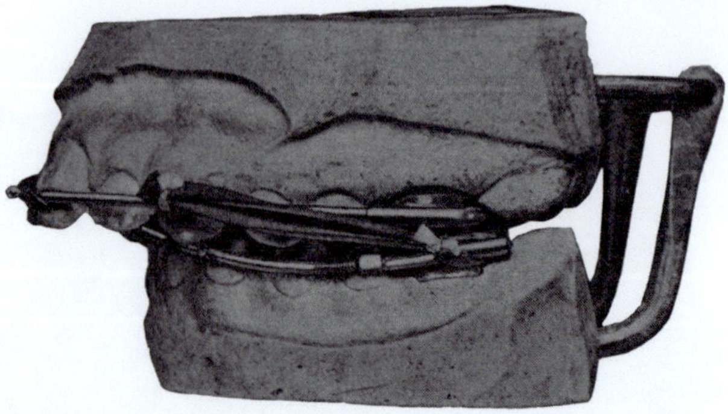

Fig. 1.3 Baker anchorage (Reproduced from Angle [4])

for which this anchorage of the entire plan of treatment of cases belonging to both Classes II and III has been revolutionized, making their treatment simple and easy with patients of a proper age. This form of anchorage as used by Dr. Baker is shown at Figure 189." (Fig. 1.3) In a footnote to a section of his book, Angle stated, "To the best of my knowledge and belief, we are indebted to Dr. H.A. Baker of Boston for this idea. He had used it in the retraction of the protruding incisors of his son a number of years ago. It was from him I received the idea. I have hence called it the Baker anchorage. Dr. C.S. Case of Chicago also employed this form of anchorage probably at about the same time as Dr. Baker not, however, as anchorage complete in itself, as did Dr. Baker but only as auxiliary to intermaxillary anchorage in a case belonging to the third class." Of course Angle made a modification to Baker anchorage which he deemed superior (Fig. 1.4)!

Fast-forward to March 1929 and Angle's four-part Dental Cosmos article entitled "The Latest and Best in Orthodontic Mechanism" [5]. With the Dental Cosmos article, Angle attempted to "sell" the edgewise appliance, his latest, best, and last invention, to all who practiced orthodontics. Angle used an entire section of this four-part article to discuss and illustrate second-order tooth movement, i.e., anchorage preparation. He began his explanation of second order by stating, "We shall now consider the second order of tooth movements or the simultaneous tipping backward of all of the teeth on one or both sides of either or both dental arches, force for this purpose also being derived from the elasticity of the delicate metal arch already in position in the brackets and other attachments and operating at the same time for accomplishing the first order of movements." He described placing his "delicate archwires" at an oblique angle to the long axes of the tooth and contended that this action would require that the archwire be sprung into the brackets. He talked about doing this type of wire bending by starting at the anterior and bending from anterior to posterior or bending the archwire from posterior to anterior. He contended that it really did not make any difference if one started at the front of the arch or at the back of the arch. He made it a point to state that, "the first order of movement and second order movement should be done at the same time." When he discussed his "uprighting" bends that accomplished second-order tooth movement, he stated that, "I would, therefore, emphasize the fact that these uprighting bends should always be slight, never greater than will permit the arch to be readily seated into the brackets

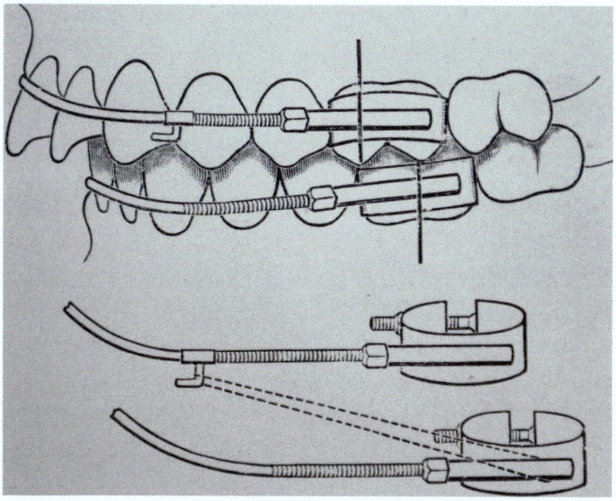

Fig. 1.4 Angle's modification to Baker anchorage. (Reproduced from Angle [4])

with the fingers, when not more than a slightly snug feeling on the tooth should be caused. In uprighting the buccal teeth en phalanx into their correct axial relations, I would emphasize the great importance of so making the bends in the metal arch that *equal force* will be exerted on each tooth. It should be very clear that otherwise the forces will conflict and the full, free, equal tipping of the teeth be obstructed." (Fig. 1.5) Angle stated that there should be no upward spring in the metal arch that was placed into the brackets and that there should be no elevation of the anchored teeth. He wanted only the distal tipping of these teeth and contended that the distal tipping of the teeth should be done *en phalanx* – all together or en masse. He maintained that the force on the teeth should remain active without interruption for 2–3 weeks and that one should then remove the archwire, increase the bends, and reinsert the archwire. This was Angle's way of preparing anchorage. An interesting side note that can be found in this Dental Cosmos article is the following statement; "Another excellent way of causing the arch to bind within the brackets and anchor sheaths and thus to enlist force for the uprighting or distal tipping of the crowns of teeth is to change the positions of the brackets on the bands, thus changing the angles of relation of the slots of the brackets to the long axes of the teeth as shown in Figure 38, instead of making the vertical bends in the arch as in the manner just described. This permits the use of the arch in its simplest form, or that freest from bends which, of course, has advantages." (Fig. 1.6) Interesting that Angle discussed a pre-adjusted appliance in 1928!

Dr. Angle, in the Dental Cosmos article, spent a lot of time discussing the stabilization of anchorage. After discussing types of anchorage, he made the following statement about stabilization. "This is something of such importance that all will appreciate it. Orthodontists have often felt this need, especially in the treatment of cases belonging to Class II. The modern, correct treatment of these cases demands the pronounced distal movement en phalanx of the teeth of the upper arch in order that they may be in normal cusp relationship with those of the lower arch. This

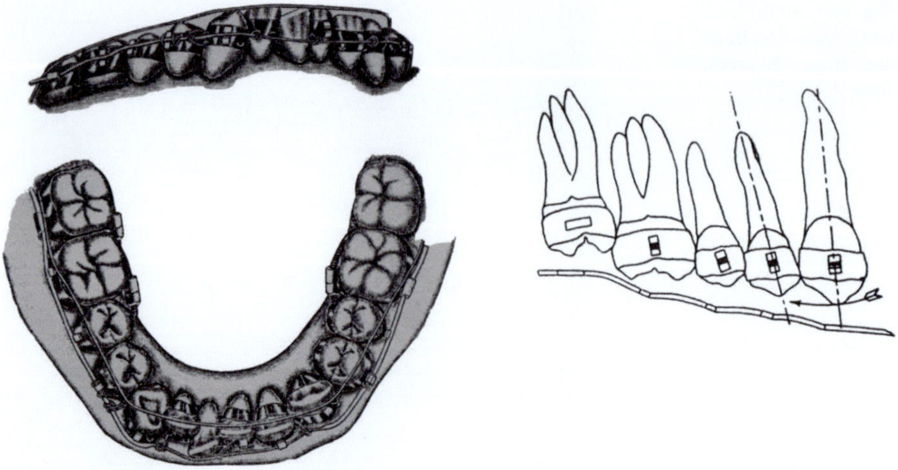

Fig. 1.5 Angle's drawing of mesially inclined teeth and the second-order archwire (Reproduced from Angle [5])

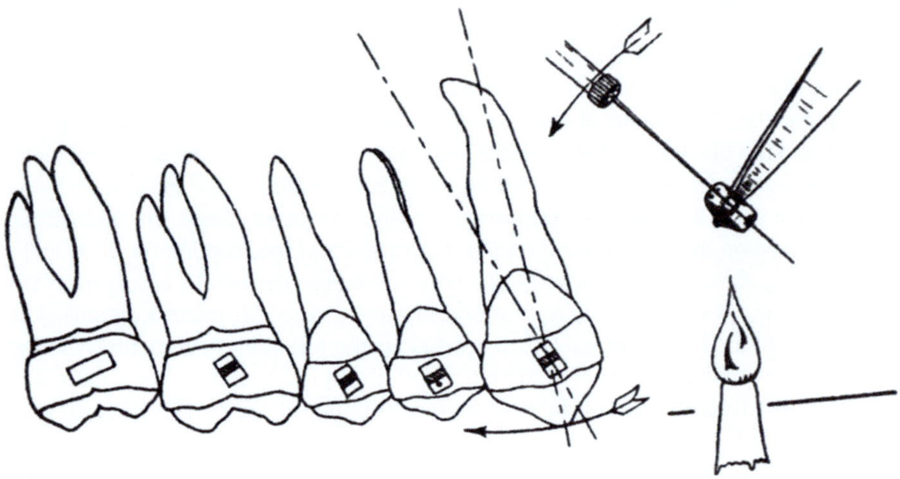

Fig. 1.6 Angle's illustration of pre-angulated brackets (Reproduced from Angle [5])

should be done without mesial movement of the lower teeth (even though intermaxillary anchorage be employed), and without mesial displacement of the mandible from the normal, habitual relations of its condyles in the glenoid fossa as manifest in the act of swallowing. The importance of avoiding mesial displacement of the mandible in the treatment of these cases has been ably emphasized by Dr. Cecil Steiner in a paper recently read before this society and soon to be published. If I have made clear the technique of the use of this mechanism for uprighting teeth, you will readily comprehend that not only may upper teeth be thus moved in these cases (Class II), but that lower teeth, used as anchorage through intermaxillary attachments, may be prevented from moving mesially and even themselves tipped backwardly and upwardly at the same time that the upper teeth are being so moved, as is often required."

In his textbook entitled "Principles of Orthodontics" [6], J.A. Salzman discussed anchorage and stated that resistance to orthodontic forces can come from the following areas:

1. The bone in which the teeth are situated.
2. Root area of the teeth. Resistance is directly proportional to root area, all other factors being equal.
3. Teeth undergoing active growth offer increased resistance to movement opposite the direction of natural growth.
4. Muscular pressure can offer active resistance to orthodontic tooth movement.
5. The manner of interlocking of the cusps can act as resistance to orthodontic tooth movement.

Dr. Salzman described four types of intermaxillary anchorage. He classified them as:

(a) Simple (single): A tooth of greater support in the alveolar process is used to move another tooth of lesser support, i.e., a molar used to move an incisor.
(b) Simple (compound): A number of teeth of greater support are used to move groups of teeth of lesser support.
(c) Stationary: The appliance is constructed so that no tipping force is exerted on the anchor teeth. The anchor teeth would have to be moved bodily when used as stationary anchorage.
(d) Reciprocal: This term connotes a reciprocal force exerted between the teeth or teeth to be moved, i.e., squeezing the posterior teeth against the anterior teeth.

RHW Strang, for the first time in the literature [7], mentioned an issue that has plagued orthodontics since the beginnings of tooth movement. He stated, "It is also undoubtedly true that the ability of operators to conserve the sources of anchorage and to obtain the best possible advantage from such dental units varies to a marked degree. This places some men at a decided disadvantage. For the successful treatment of complicated cases of malocclusion depends, most emphatically, upon conservation of anchorage areas." Strang disputed Angle's claim that the maxillary crowns tipped distally during Class II treatment with intermaxillary elastics. He stated, "Distal crown tipping bends were placed in the first molar/premolar and canine areas of the archwire which when the archwire was locked in the brackets of all the maxillary teeth, set in action a series of double levers consisting of four anterior levers and three posterior levers, and these very effectively tipped the teeth in the buccal segments and depressed the incisors, a reciprocal action that was very desirable. However, these levers produced a minimum amount of distal action upon the crowns. Rather did they tend to tip the roots of the buccal teeth forward. In order to obtain a definite backward thrust upon these teeth, it was necessary to bring into action a distinctly distally propelling force from an entirely new source of anchorage. This, of course, was intermaxillary elastic force acting from the mandibular base. In the use of this intermaxillary force, it was essential to consider its reciprocal action and to stabilize the anchorage units from which this force was applied or a reciprocal movement would result." Strang discussed many ways of attempting to prepare mandibular anchorage. In his textbook he introduced the reader to a "force" who had come into the orthodontic picture – Charles Tweed. He stated, "Dr. Tweed lays great emphasis upon primarily reorienting every tooth in the anchorage section of the denture to an axial position wherein it is best able to mechanically resist the force that will eventually be used in producing the tooth movements required in treatment."

Charles Tweed first discussed anchorage in a paper [8] read before the tenth meeting of the Edward H. Angle Society of Orthodontia in Del Monte, California, April 10, 1936. In this paper, he stated, "Anchorage – one of the biggest words in orthodontia – is not being utilized to its utmost in applying the principles of the edgewise arch mechanism in the treatment of Class II division I malocclusions, with the result that we are causing more double protrusions than are necessary. This is not the fault of the mechanism. The fault lies in our inability to master its potentialities. Try kicking those lower molars up and back, gaining toe hold, and then with second order bends do the same to all the bicuspids and cuspids so that you have toe hold all around, and all the lower teeth are vertical and stand up like a row of little soldiers ready to work for you without faltering. Keep them in that position, and every time the patient comes in thoroughly examine the mouth to make sure that none of them are slipping. If you keep them in this position throughout treatment, which is usually possible, you will, when the upper teeth have been moved back to normal cuspal relations, find that you have built a good old chin and that you will have no difficulty in determining which photograph was taken before and which after the treatment of your Class II division I malocclusions." Tweed gave a very detailed description of his concept of anchorage which can be found in Vol. 1 of his two-volume text [9]. In Chap. 2 Tweed stated, "Anchorage preparation, in my opinion, is the most important step in clinical orthodontics. Although, highly controversial, this procedure is lightly dwelt upon by a great many clinical orthodontists. I am of the opinion that this is true only because its meaning and purposes are not understood by all. Simply stated: Anchorage preparation is mechanical in nature. If we position the teeth in the buccal segments of the mandibular denture in upright positions, with the terminal molars tipped back like tent stakes so that the pull of the intermaxillary elastics, when related to the long axes of the terminal molars, does not exceed 90° when the mouth is functioning, the entire mandibular denture will be more stable and better able to resist forward displacement. If movement does occur, it will be slow mesial bodily movement of the entire mandibular denture. On the other hand, when we fail to prepare mandibular anchorage or leave the anchor molars in their mesially inclined, undisturbed positions, the action of the intermaxillary elastic Class II pull is upward and forward. This condition will result in the elevation and uprooting of the terminal anchor molars. When such reaction is allowed to occur, it is followed by excessive depression of the mandibular incisors, with a drastic and unnecessary alteration of the occlusal plane. The FMA will open up and point B will drop downward and backward as the entire mandibular denture is tipped and displaced forward into protrusion."

Mandibular anchorage preparation was essentially prepared in the following manner by Charles Tweed. First, a stabilizing archwire was bent for the maxillary arch along with a working archwire for the mandibular arch. All mandibular second-order bends were placed at one time into the archwire (Fig. 1.7) [10]. In order to control these second-order bends, Tweed used Class III elastics and intermediate headgear to the maxillary arch and vertical up and down elastic force. After en masse mandibular anchorage had been prepared, the mandibular arch was stabilized with a 0.215 × 0.28 archwire that was continuously tied in the posterior segments. This stabilizing archwire was an exact duplicate of the previously used working archwire, only larger. It had the same second-order bends as the working archwire. The maxillary archwire was then changed to a smaller dimension maxillary working archwire. Tweed then distalized the maxillary arch if the treatment was nonextraction or retracted the maxillary anterior teeth if the patient had extraction space mesial to the distalized maxillary canines. The patient generally wore Class II elastics, anterior vertical elastics, and again, a headgear. The final step of treatment was to finish the correction of the malocclusion. This step required the use of 0.215 × 0.28 rectangular archwires with soldered spurs and vertical elastics. This treatment protocol, which initially started with anchorage preparation in the mandibular arch, proved to be very successful. After anchorage preparation, there was en masse movement to correct jaw relationships. The third step was to detail tooth position preparatory to retention. Tweed firmly believed that anchorage preparation in the mandibular arch should be the first step in the treatment of all Class II malocclusions. Tweed's method was conventional anchorage at its finest hour. The big problem with Tweed's approach was patient cooperation. A patient who did not exhibit explicit cooperation would have problems with the first step of treatment – anchorage preparation. Tweed's methods also required ten to twelve sets of archwires, and this was quite cumbersome to the orthodontic clinician.

In 1970, L. Levern Merrifield (Fig. 1.8) of Ponca City, Oklahoma, became the Tweed Study Course Director. He and Tweed had worked closely together and discussed many, many things about the edgewise appliance and, particularly, about anchorage preparation. Merrifield was the Co-Director of the Tweed Study with Tweed from 1960 until 1970. At Tweed's death, Merrifield was determined to make the use of the appliance more efficient but remain true to Tweed's concepts of anchorage preparation with vertical control during protrusion reduction. After years of study and experimentation, Merrifield introduced a totally new concept of conventional anchorage preparation. He called this concept "edgewise sequential directional force technology" [11]. This system would streamline the use of Angle's appliance and of Tweed's anchorage preparation technique. Merrifield's concepts remained true to Tweed's philosophy but made anchorage preparation more reliable and more predictable. Since Merrifield's original efforts, Herb Klontz [12, 13] and

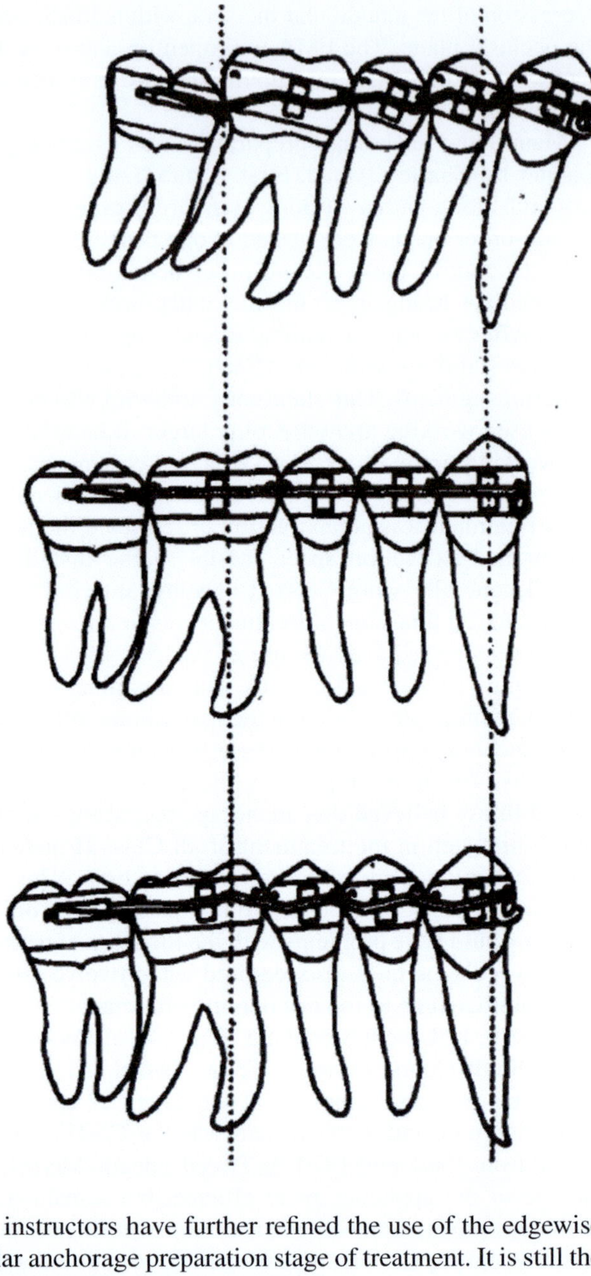

Fig. 1.7 En Masse anchorage preparation (Reproduced from Tweed [10])

other Tweed Study Course instructors have further refined the use of the edgewise appliance and the mandibular anchorage preparation stage of treatment. It is still the hallmark of Tweed-Merrifield directional forces treatment.

The maxillary and the mandibular arches are treated independently when Merrifield's directional forces system is used. If the malocclusion correction requires premolar extraction, the canines are simultaneously retracted in both arches. Space mesial to the canines is closed with closing loops. While canine

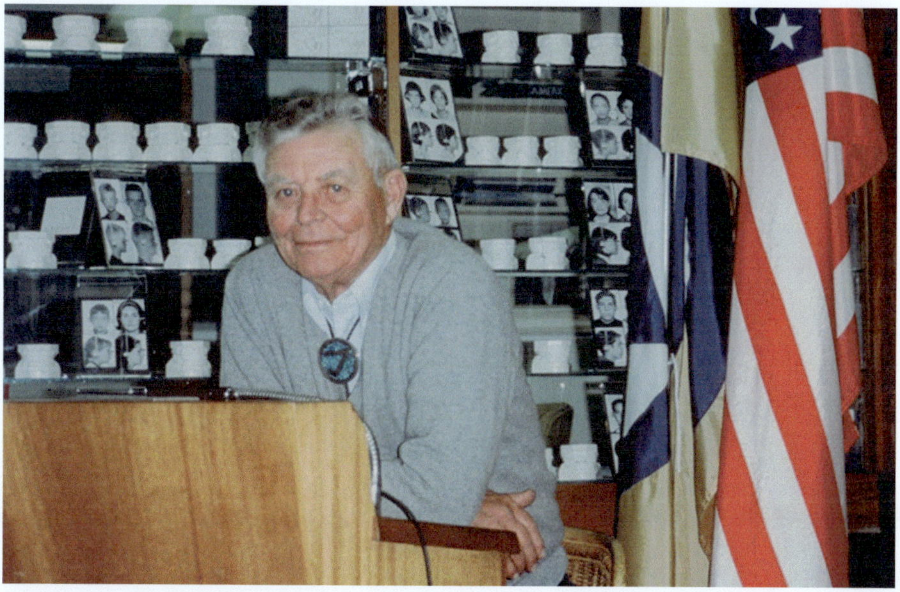

Fig. 1.8 L. Levern Merrifield

retraction and space closure are being accomplished in the maxillary arch, an exaggerated curve of occlusion is placed into the maxillary archwire. The second molars receive a distal tip of 20°, the first molars receive a distal tip of 10°, and the second premolars receive a distal tip of 5° in both the initial leveling archwire and in the closing loop archwire. This exaggerated curve of occlusion prevents the extrusion of the maxillary posterior teeth during treatment. This curve of occlusion has an anchorage "effect" because it gives the maxillary posterior teeth a distal inclination that facilitates their resistance to the mesial force placed on them when the closing loop is activated. The primary purpose of the curve of occlusion, however, is to control vertical dimension by not allowing the maxillary posterior teeth to supra-erupt. After space closure in both arches, mandibular anchorage preparation is accomplished.

Mandibular anchorage preparation is done sequentially. The anchorage preparation archwire produces an active force on only two teeth while remaining passive to the other teeth in the arch. Therefore, the remaining teeth act as stabilizing or anchorage units as two teeth are tipped. The method is referred to as the "10–2" (ten teeth versus two teeth) anchorage system, and it allows a quickly controlled response without serious adverse reaction. The mandibular anchorage preparation system is supported by anterior vertical elastics attached to spurs that are soldered to the mandibular archwire distal and gingival to the mandibular lateral incisors. The elastics are hooked to the closing loops of the maxillary archwire. They are supported by a high-pull headgear that is attached to hooks soldered to the maxillary archwire.

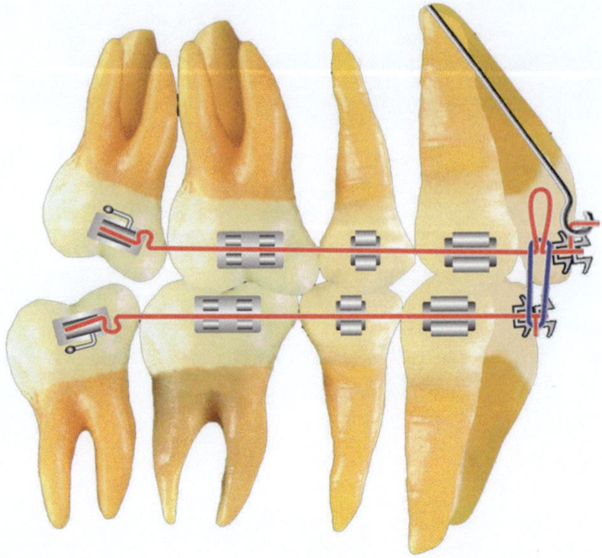

Fig. 1.9 Mandibular anchorage preparation. The second molar is tipped to its anchorage prepared position

When all space in the mandibular arch is closed and the arch is level, the first step of sequential mandibular anchorage preparation, second molar anchorage, is initiated. A 0.19 × 0.25 in. archwire with the omega loop stops bent flush against the second molar tubes is fabricated. First- and third-order bends are ideal. Gingival spurs for anterior vertical elastics are soldered to the archwire distal to the lateral incisors.

In order to tip the mandibular second molars to an anchorage prepared position, a 15° tip is placed distal to the omega loop stop. The second molar is tipped to an anchorage prepared position. It should have a distal inclination of 10°–15° (Fig. 1.9).

After the second molar has been tipped, the first molar is tipped to its anchorage prepared position by placing a 10° distal tip 1 mm mesial to the first molar bracket. When this first molar tip is placed in the archwire, a compensating bend that maintains the 15° second molar inclination must be placed mesial to the omega loop stop (Fig. 1.10).

The archwire is now passive to the second molar and crosses the twin brackets of the first molar at a 10° bias. The second molars are now part of the ten stabilizing units, and the first molars are the two teeth that receive the action of the directional forces and the archwire. After 1 month the archwire is removed and a readout should show a 5°–8° distal inclination of the first molars. The second molars should continue to readout at 15°. Mandibular anchorage prepared in this sequential manner can be done easily and with great predictability.

The denture correction step of treatment should now be complete for the Class I malocclusion. The objectives of the denture correction step are (1) complete space closure in both arches if the treatment plan required extraction, (2) sequential anchorage preparation in the mandibular arch, (3) an enhanced curve of occlusion in the maxillary arch, and (4) a Class I intercuspation of the canines and premolars.

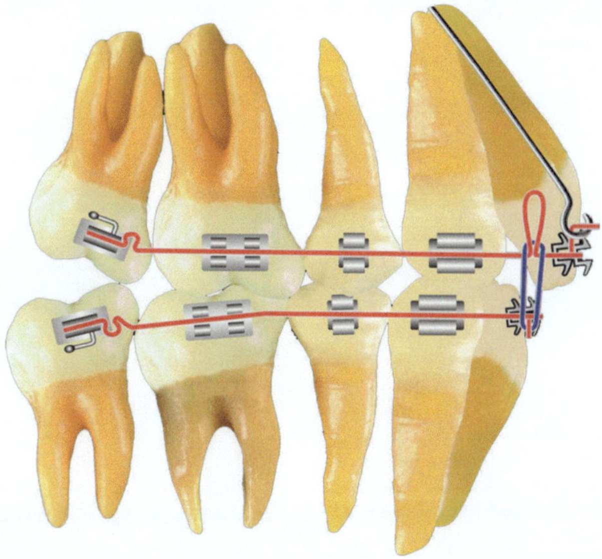

Fig. 1.10 Mandibular anchorage preparation. The first molar is tipped to its anchorage prepared position

Class II Force System

For patients with and "end-on" Class II dental relationship of the buccal segments at the conclusion of space closure, a new and different force system must be used to complete the denture correction stage of treatment. The Class II force system *must not* be used unless mandibular anchorage has been adequately and thoroughly prepared. Mandibular anchorage makes Class II correction possible.

At the end of sequential mandibular anchorage preparation, a mandibular 0.215 × 0.28 in. stabilizing archwire is fabricated. Ideal first-, second-, and third-order bends are incorporated into the archwire. The omega loop stop must be 0.5 mm short of the molar tubes, and the archwire must be passive to all the brackets. Gingival spurs are soldered distal to the mandibular lateral incisors. The archwire is seated and ligated, and the second molar is cinched tightly to the loop stop.

An 0.20 × 0.25 in. maxillary archwire with 7.5 mm closed helical bulbous loops bent flush against the second molar tubes is fabricated. This archwire has ideal first- and second-order bends. A gingival spur is attached to the archwire immediately distal to the maxillary second premolar bracket. Gingival high-pull headgear hooks are soldered distal to the central incisors. Class II "lay on" hooks with a gingival extension for anterior vertical elastics are soldered distal to the lateral incisors. Prior to archwire insertion, the closed helical bulbous loops are opened 1 mm on each side. Class II elastics are worn from the hooks on the mandibular second molar tubes to the Class II hooks on the maxillary archwire. Anterior vertical elastics are worn from the spurs on the mandibular archwire to the gingival extension hooks on the maxillary archwire. The high-pull headgear is worn on the maxillary headgear hooks (Fig. 1.11).

Fig. 1.11 Class II force system

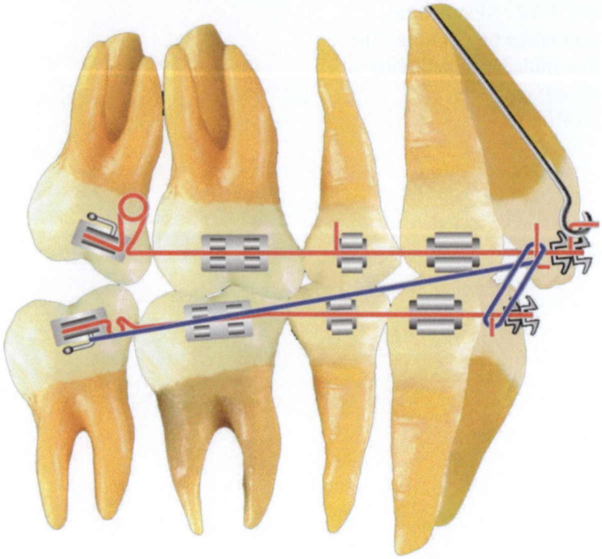

This force system is used to sequentially move the maxillary second molars distally. The activation of the maxillary archwire is repeated until the second molars have a Class I dental relationship (Fig. 1.12). When the Class I relationship of the second molars has been established, a closed coil spring is "wound" distal to the second premolar spur and compressed between the spur and the first molar bracket when the maxillary archwire is inserted. (The coil spring length should be 1.5 times the space between the second premolar and the first molar brackets.) An elastic chain is stretched from the second molar to the distal bracket of the first molar. The spring and the elastic chain create a distal force on the maxillary first molar. Additionally, a Class II elastic is continuously worn from the mandibular second molar hook to the Class II hook on the maxillary archwire. An anterior vertical elastic is worn 12 h each day (Fig. 1.13). The high-pull headgear is worn 14 h per day on the spurs soldered to the maxillary archwire.

After the first molars have been moved distally into an overcorrected Class I dental relationship (Fig. 1.14), the spur that was attached distal to the second premolar bracket is removed. The coil spring is moved mesially so that it is compressed between the lay on hook and the canine bracket. Subsequently, the maxillary second premolars and the maxillary canines are moved distally with elastic chain and headgear force (Fig. 1.15).

After correction of the Class II dental relationship, a 0.20 × 0.25 in. maxillary archwire with 7.5 mm closing loops distal to the lateral incisors is fabricated. Gingival headgear hooks are soldered distal to the central brachets. Class II elastics, anterior vertical elastics, and the maxillary high-pull headgear are used. The maxillary anterior teeth are retracted (Fig. 1.16).

The Class II correction force system that has been described makes use of mandibular anchorage that has been prepared as well as anchorage provided by the maxillary teeth that are not being moved. When only two teeth are moved at any

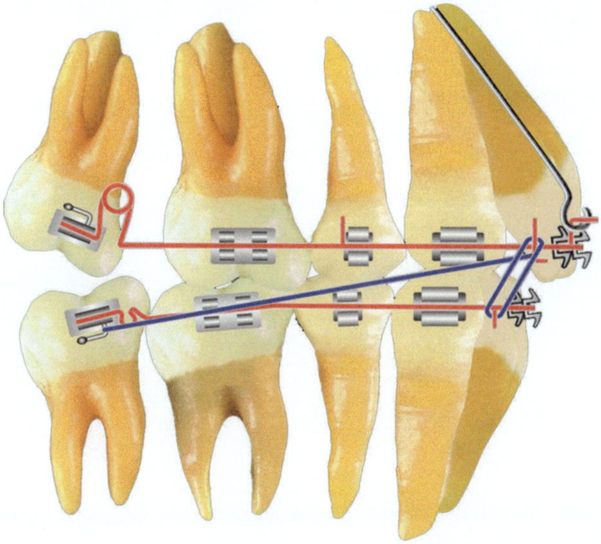

Fig. 1.12 Class II force system. Denture correction: The helical bulbous loop pushes the maxillary molar distally

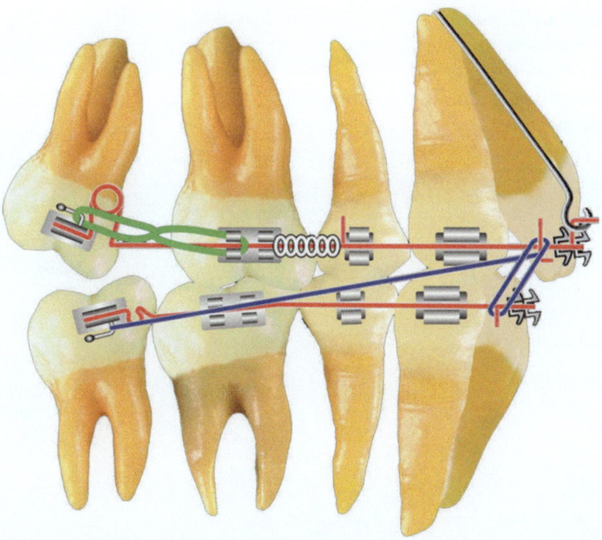

Fig. 1.13 Class II force system. Denture correction: a coil spring is trapped mesial to the first molar

given time, all the other teeth in the arch act as anchorage units. Class II correction, therefore, utilizes anchorage provided by teeth in both arches.

Denture Completion

The third step of treatment is identified as denture completion. Ideal first-, second-, and third-order bends are placed in finishing mandibular and maxillary 0.215 × 0.28 resilient archwires. The mandibular archwire duplicates the

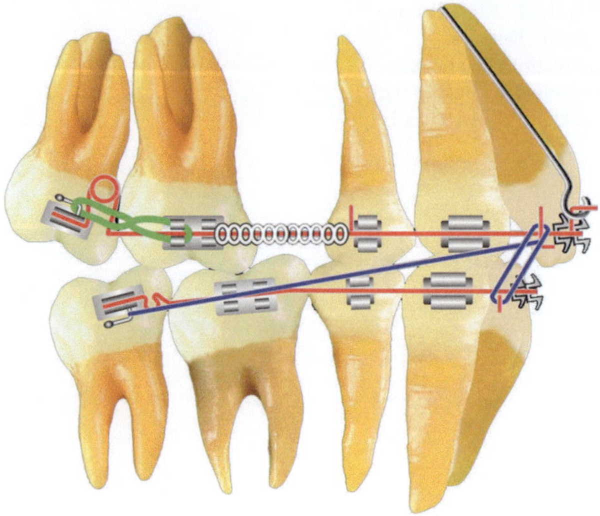

Fig. 1.14 Class II force system. Denture correction: maxillary first molar distalization

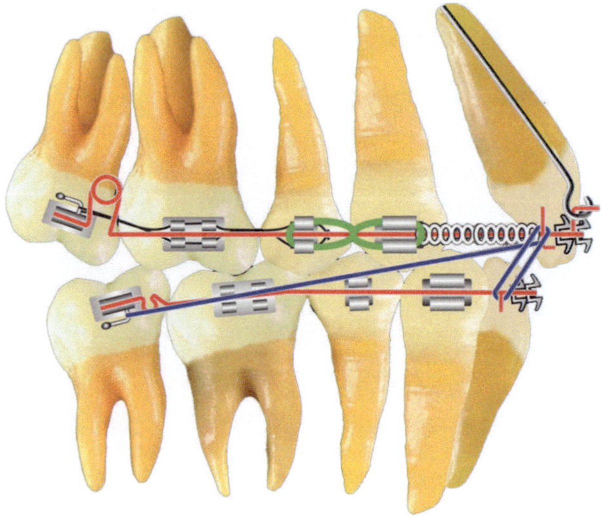

Fig. 1.15 Class II force system. Denture correction: maxillary second premolar and maxillary canine distalization

previously used mandibular stabilizing archwire. The maxillary archwire has artistic bends and hooks for the high-pull headgear, anterior vertical elastics, and Class II elastics. Supplemental hooks for vertical elastics are soldered as needed (Fig. 1.17).

The forces used during denture completion are based on a careful study of the arrangement of each tooth in each arch. The orthodontist must also study the relationship of one arch to the other and the relationship of the arches to their environment. Denture completion can be considered as minitreatment of the malocclusion. During this treatment step, the orthodontist uses the forces that are necessary until the original malocclusion is overcorrected.

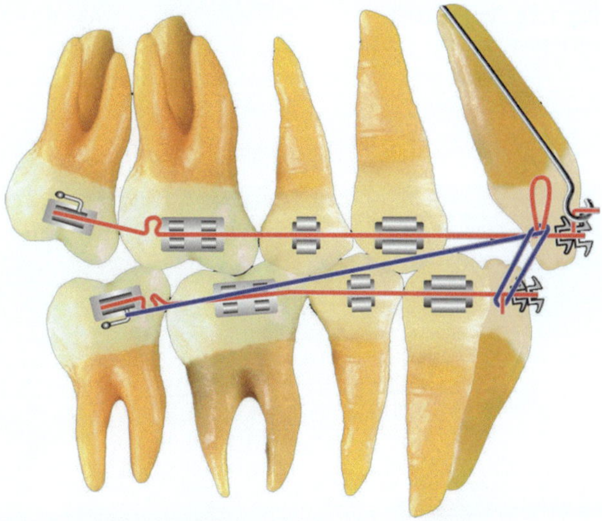

Fig. 1.16 Class II force system. Denture correction: maxillary anterior space closure

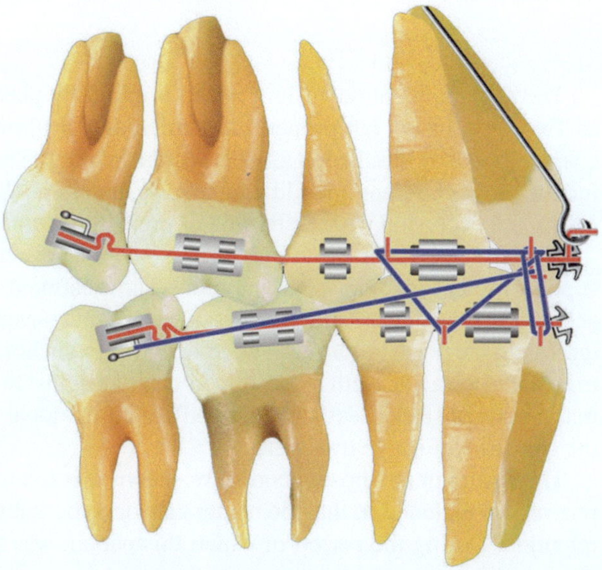

Fig. 1.17 Denture completion. Maxillary and mandibular stabilizing wires, along with the proper elastics and headgear force, are used to complete the orthodontic treatment

Denture Recovery

An ideal occlusion will be present only after all treatment mechanics are discontinued and uninhibited function and other environmental influences active in the post-treatment period stabilize and finalize the position of the total dentition. When all appliances are removed and the retainers are placed, a most crucial "recovery" phase occurs. During this recovery period, the forces involved are those of the surrounding environment, primarily the muscles and the periodontium.

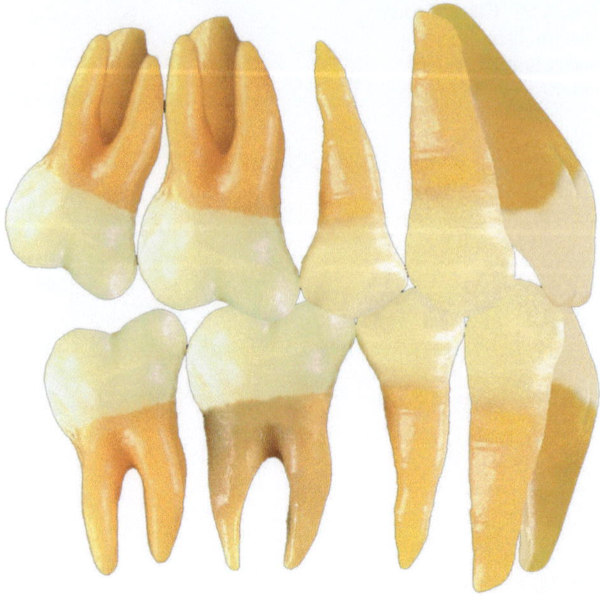

Fig. 1.18 Transitional occlusion

The posttreatment occlusion, which is carefully planned, sometimes referred to as Tweed occlusion but properly identified as transitional occlusion (Fig. 1.18), is characterized by disclusion of the second molars. The slightly intruded distally inclined maxillary and mandibular second molars now can “re-erupt” to a healthy functional occlusion without trauma or premature contact (Fig. 1.19).

The two case reports that follow illustrate the sequential directional forces concept as well as anchorage preparation. The treatment of both these patients was accomplished using essentially the same steps that have been described in this chapter. Mandibular posterior teeth were tipped into anchorage prepared positions, and maxillary posterior teeth were tipped out of occlusion. The tipped maxillary and mandibular posterior teeth “re-erupted” to a functional and healthy occlusion after the cessation of active treatment.

The first patient whose records are shown was treated in the 1970s. Thirty-year records are included so that the reader can view the stability that has existed without retention. During the period in which this patient was treated, it was believed that the maxillary curve of occlusion in the archwire was needed to be more than the 20°, 10°, and 5° that is now used, and the mandibular molar anchorage was more than the 15° and 10° that is taught today. Records of this patient illustrate the concepts that were used in the late 1970s and early 1980s when Merrifield initially introduced the sequential anchorage preparation concepts. This patient’s posttreatment occlusion was the type of posttreatment occlusion for which Dr. Tweed strived. Today’s patients do not have this degree of mandibular anchorage or curve of occlusion.

The second case report illustrates the changes that have been made over the last 20 years. Neither present-day mandibular anchorage preparation nor the maxillary curve of occlusion is as pronounced as in Tweed’s day and in Merrifield’s earlier

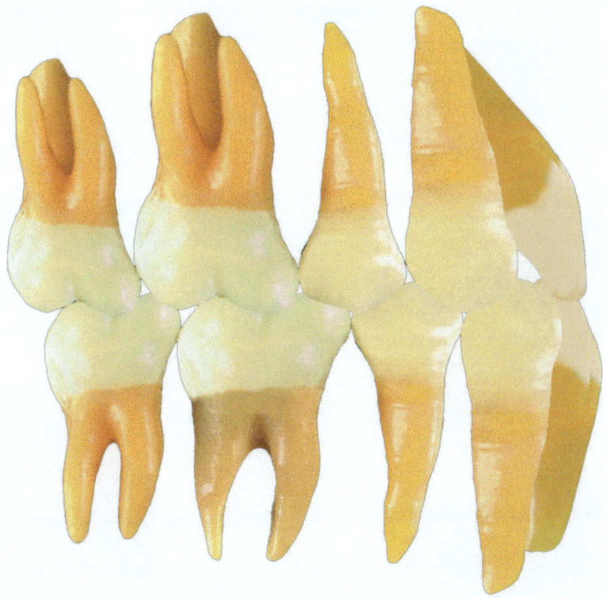

Fig. 1.19 Final occlusion is characterized by the teeth settling into their most efficient, healthy, and stable positions

10–2 system days. These two case reports are shown to illustrate the progression of classical anchorage preparation from Tweed's day and the early Merrifield days to the present time.

Case 1

This 12-year-old young lady presented for correction of a Class II division I malocclusion. Medical history was negative. The etiology of the malocclusion was heredity. The facial photographs (Fig. 1.20) exhibit an unbalanced face with a recessive mandibular position. The mandibular lip has an outward curl. The casts (Fig. 1.21) confirm a Class II malocclusion with a deep impinging overbite, 8 mm of overjet, irregular mandibular anterior teeth, and a deep curve of Spee. The pretreatment cephalogram and its tracing (Fig. 1.22) confirm the Class II skeletal pattern, the procumbent mandibular incisors, and the poor facial esthetics. The treatment plan was designed to correct the Class II dentition, upright the mandibular incisors a small amount, and reduce the overjet. Of course, the leveling of the curve of Spee, correction of the Class II dental relationship, and alignment of the mandibular anterior teeth required space. Maxillary first premolars and mandibular second premolars were removed. The posttreatment facial photographs (Fig. 1.23) confirm much more balance and harmony of the face. The mandible is in a better relationship with the maxilla. The curl of the maxillary lip has been maintained. The eversion of the lower lip is not as pronounced. The face has pleasing balance and harmony. The immediate posttreatment casts (Fig. 1.24) confirm correction of the Class II dental relationship, reduction of the overjet, leveling of the curve of Spee, the anchorage that was prepared in the mandibular arch, and the curve of occlusion in the

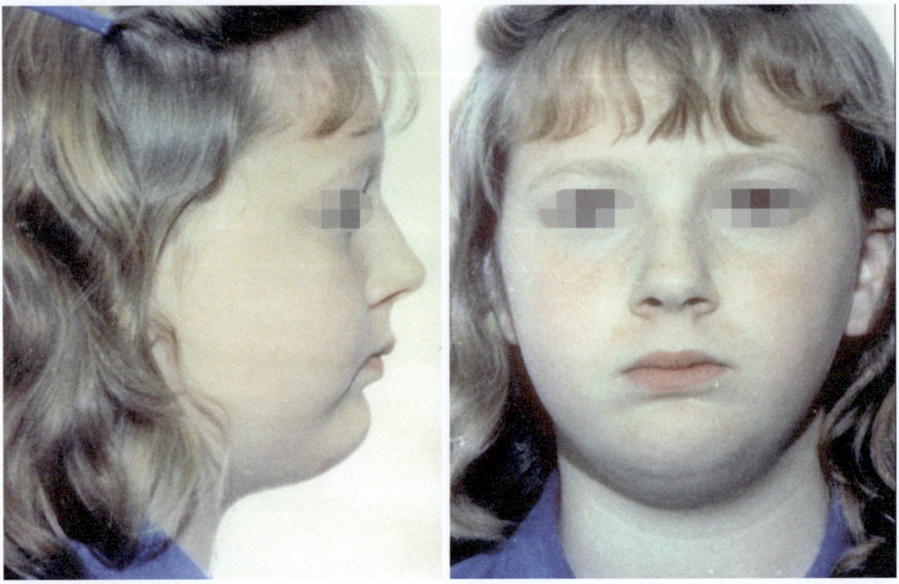

Fig. 1.20 Pretreatment facial photographs

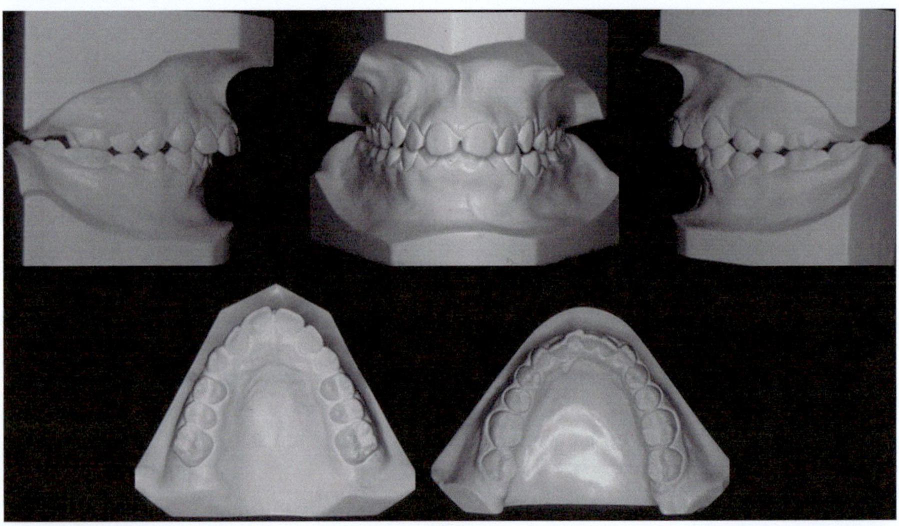

Fig. 1.21 Pretreatment casts

maxillary arch. This patient was treated when it was desired to have a 30° angulation of the maxillary second molars and a 20° angulation of the mandibular second molars. Arch form was maintained. Mandibular incisors were aligned. The posttreatment cephalogram and its tracing (Fig. 1.25) confirm uprighting of the mandibular incisors, correction of the Class II dental relationship, and reduction of the overjet. The pretreatment/posttreatment superimpositions (Fig. 1.26) illustrate

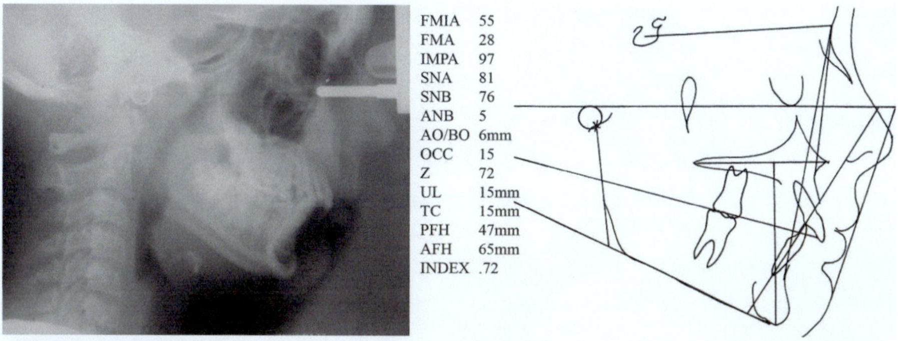

Fig. 1.22 Pretreatment cephalogram and tracing

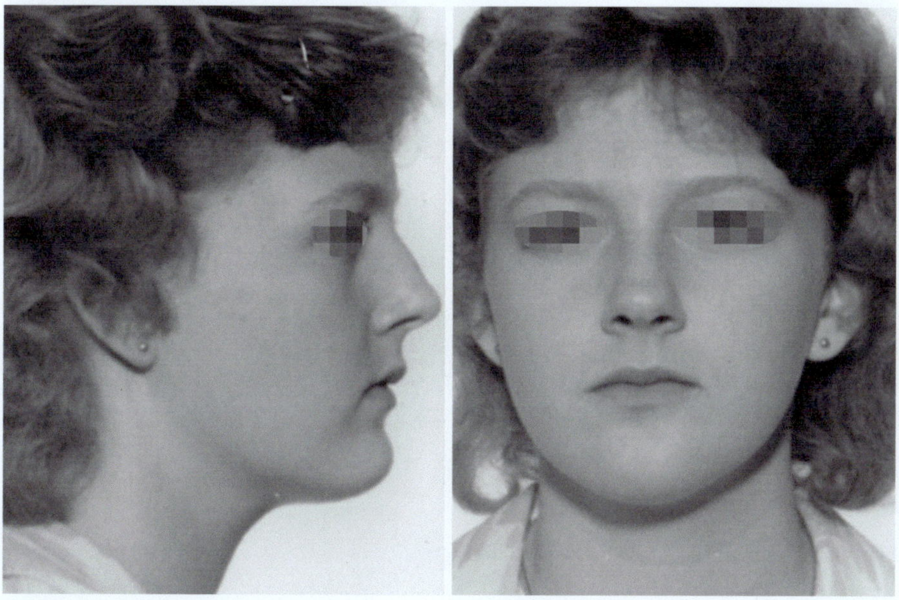

Fig. 1.23 Posttreatment facial photographs

vertical dimension control of the posterior part of the arch, upward and distal movement of the maxillary incisors, uprighting of the mandibular incisors, and the favorable change in the facial profile. The patient was recalled approximately 30 years after the completion of orthodontic treatment. Facial esthetics 30 years after treatment (Fig. 1.27) remains pleasing. There is balance and harmony of the face with good lip posture and nice curl of both maxillary and mandibular lip structures. The 30-year recall casts (Fig. 1.28) illustrate a well-interdigitated occlusion with occlusal contacts throughout the arch. The teeth that were tipped out of occlusion in both maxillary and mandibular arches have settled into an excellent functional occlusion. The mandibular casts exhibit a very small amount of mandibular crowding. No spaces have reopened. All in all the dentition is in excellent shape. The recall

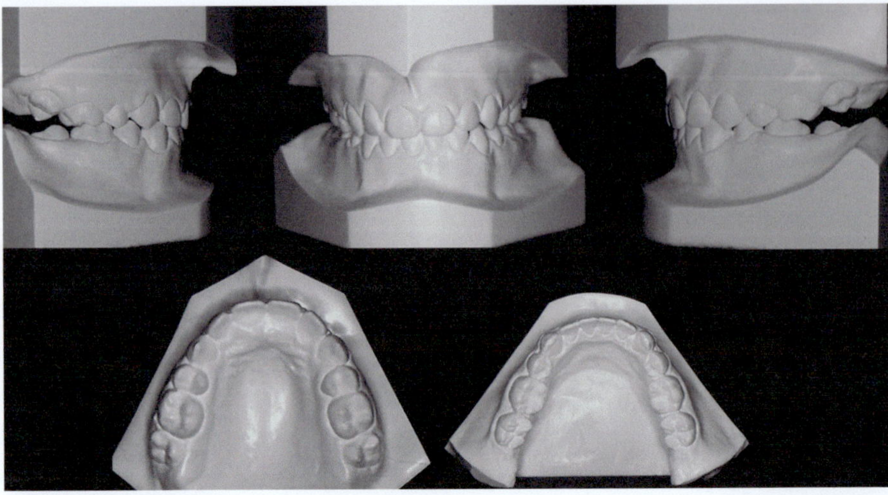

Fig. 1.24 Posttreatment cast

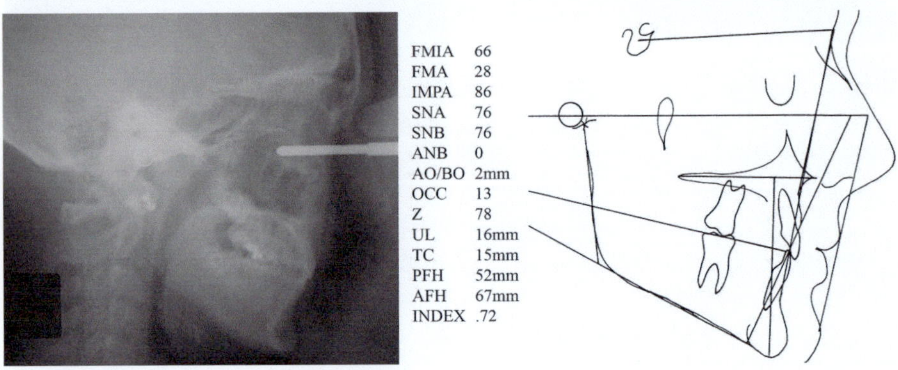

Fig. 1.25 Posttreatment cephalogram and tracing

cephalogram and its tracing (Fig. 1.29) confirm the stability of the correction. The pretreatment/posttreatment recovery superimpositions (Fig. 1.30) confirm the stability of the tooth positions as well as good downward and forward change in the relationship of the mandible to the maxilla over time. The records of this patient reflect classical anchorage preparation and the transitional dentition that recovers nicely over time to give the patient a stable, esthetic, healthy, and functional result.

Case 2

This 13-year-old boy presented with a mild facial imbalance (Fig. 1.31). There is some lower lip aversion, but the patient would not be treated unless he had a dental malocclusion. The casts (Fig. 1.32) confirm an Angle's Class II malocclusion with a deep impinging overbite, an excessive cure of Spree, and a full step Angle's Class

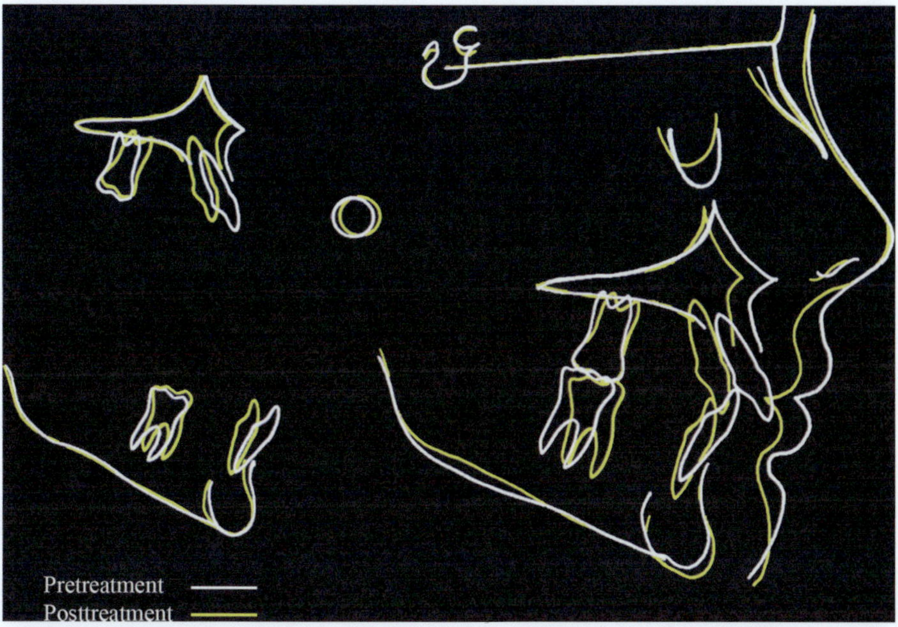

Fig. 1.26 Pretreatment/posttreatment superimpositions

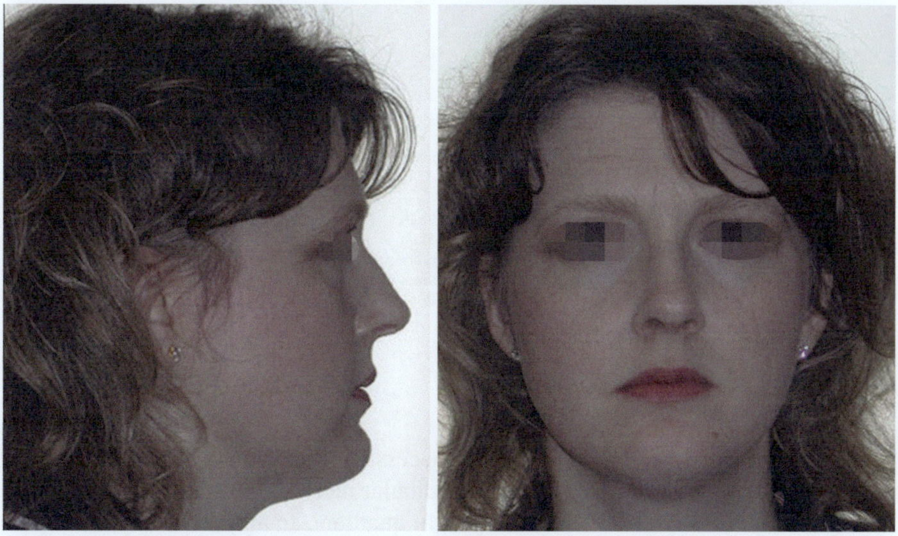

Fig. 1.27 Recall facial photographs – 30 years after treatment

II dental relationship on the patient's right side. The pretreatment cephalogram and its tracing (Fig. 1.33) reflect good values of the Tweed triangle with an ANB of 6° and an SNB of 75°. After careful thought, the patient was treatment planned for the removal of only the third molars. Third molar removal would take place during the

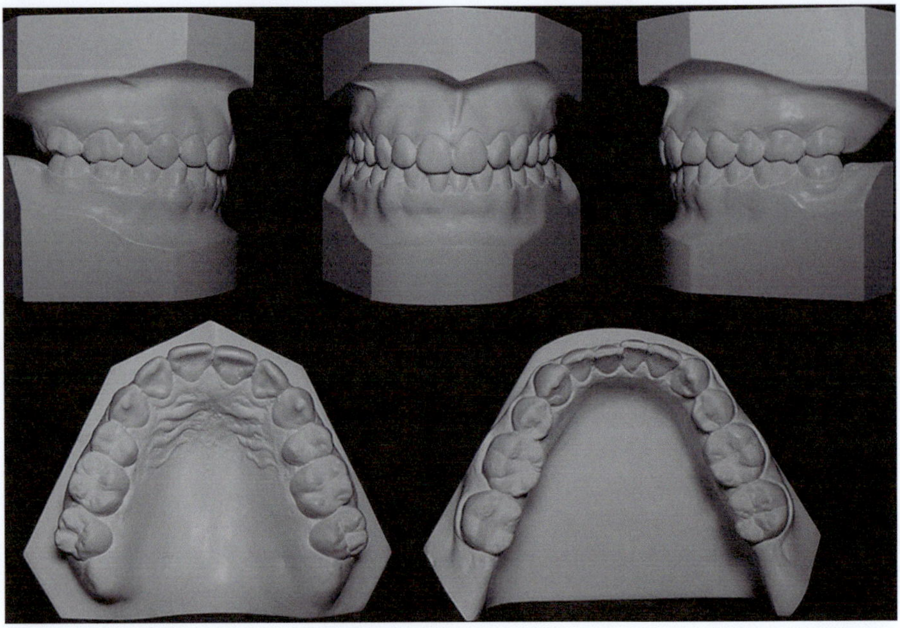

Fig. 1.28 Recall cast – 30 years after treatment

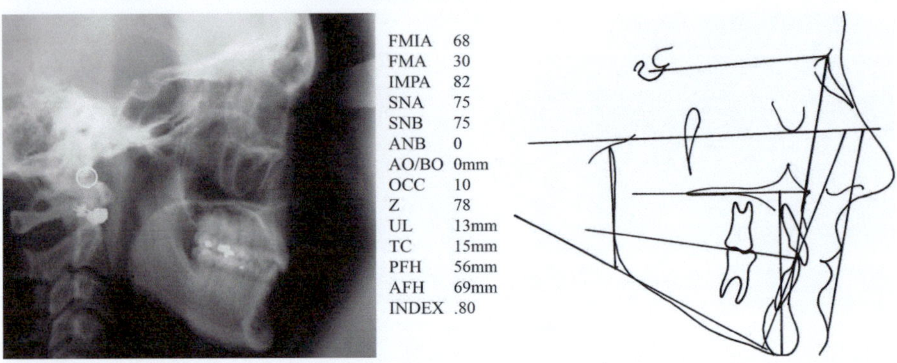

Fig. 1.29 Recall cephalogram and its tracing

course of treatment. This treatment plan necessitated that the mandibular arch be leveled and that it be stabilized so that mandibular incisors were not moved forward during the distalization of the maxillary right quadrant. In all probability, a nonpremolar extraction patient has greater anchorage requirements than a premolar extraction patient. For this reason, this patient's malocclusion is being used to illustrate the current classical anchorage preparation concept. The patient was treated, the mandibular arch was leveled with a mandibular headgear, and the mandibular second molars were tipped to approximately a 12° distal inclination. The first molars had a 3° distal inclination. The maxillary arch was treated with a curve of occlusion

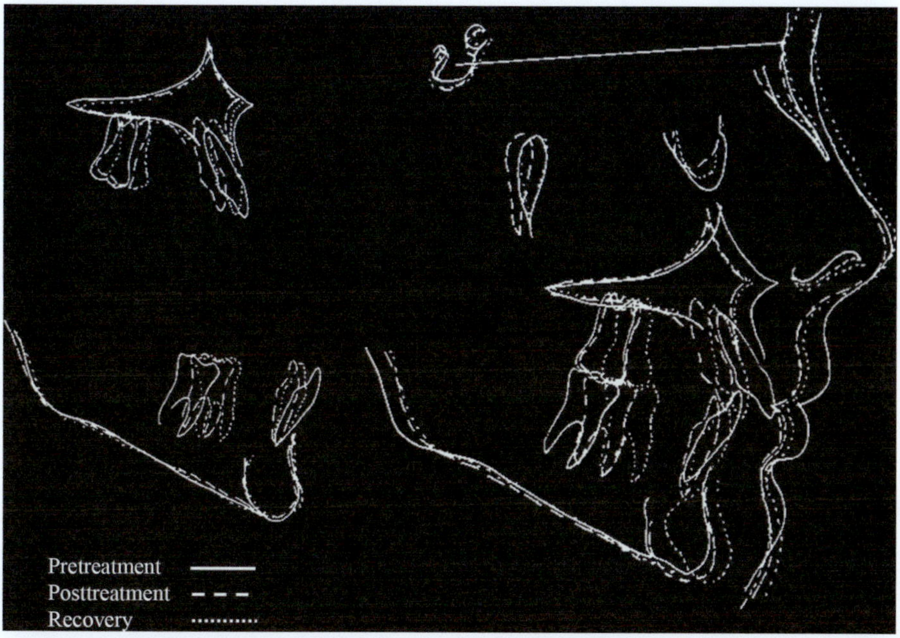

Fig. 1.30 Pretreatment/posttreatment/recovery superimpositions

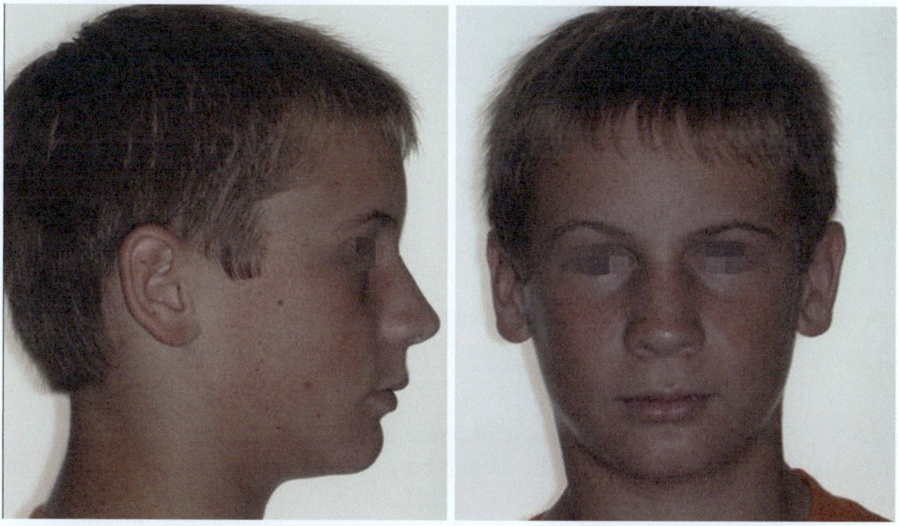

Fig. 1.31 Pretreatment facial photographs

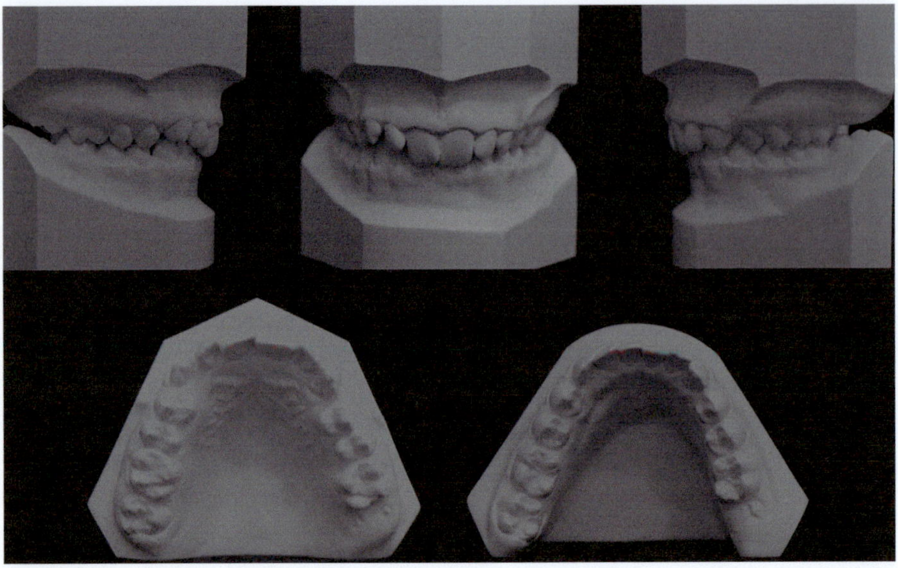

Fig. 1.32 Pretreatment casts

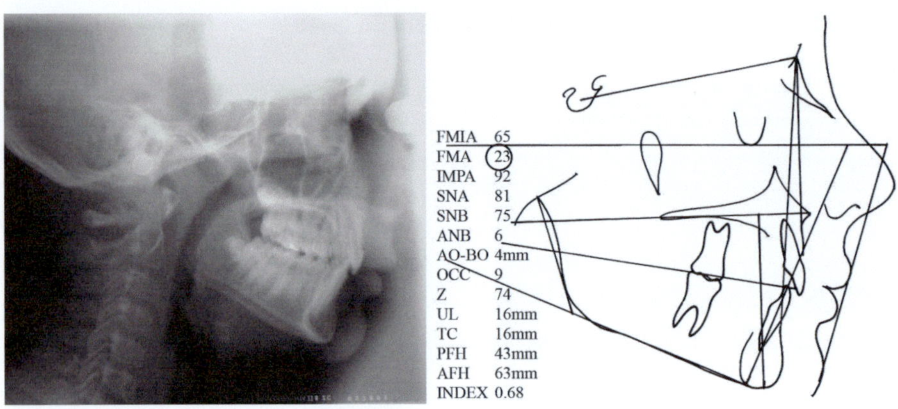

Fig. 1.33 Pretreatment cephalogram and tracing

of 5°, 10°, and 20°. The posttreatment photographs (Fig. 1.34) reflect a very balanced and harmonious face. Chin projection is better than it was at the outset of treatment. The posttreatment casts (Fig. 1.35) confirm distalization of the maxillary right side. One can see that the mandibular molars have been tipped distally as the curve of Spee has been leveled. The maxillary molars, though out of occlusion, are not out of occlusion near as much as the molars of a patient who was treated in the 1970s and 1980s. Arch form and arch width have been preserved. The posttreatment cephalogram and its tracing (Fig. 1.36) confirm control of the mandibular anterior teeth. They even uprighted 3°! The ANB has been reduced to 2°. The profile/nose

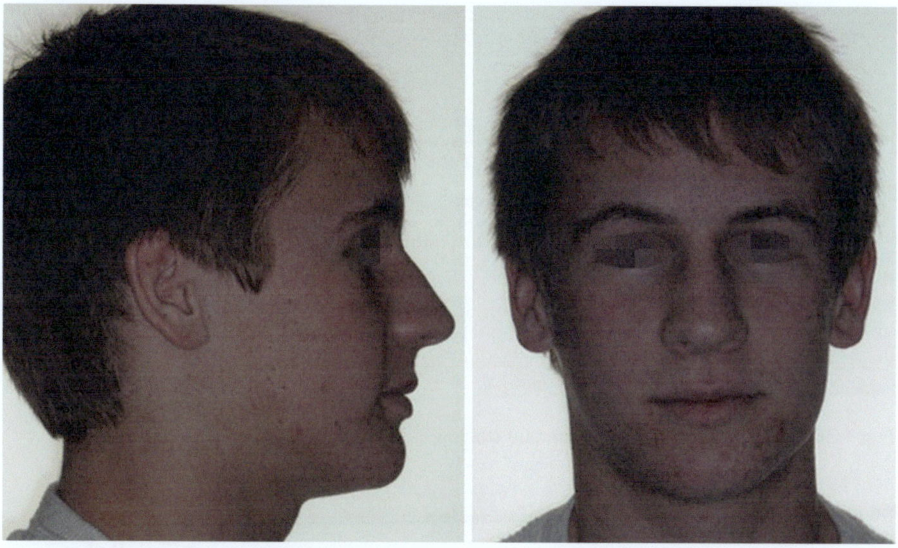

Fig. 1.34 Posttreatment facial photographs

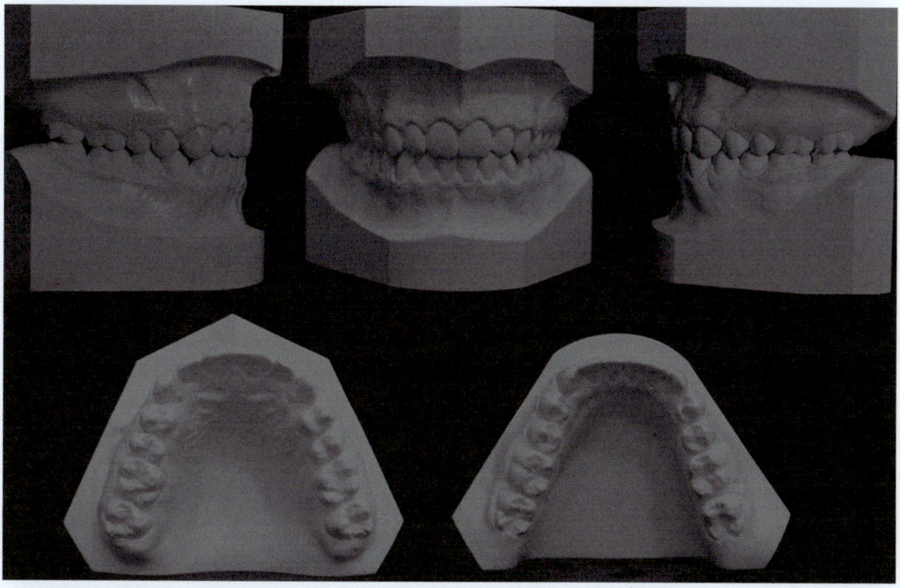

Fig. 1.35 Posttreatment cast

relationship is ideal. The superimpositions (Fig. 1.37) reflect control of the vertical dimension, retraction, and third-order control of the maxillary incisors and control of mandibular incisor position in a nonextraction mandibular arch. The change in the relationship of the mandible to the maxilla was excellent during the time of

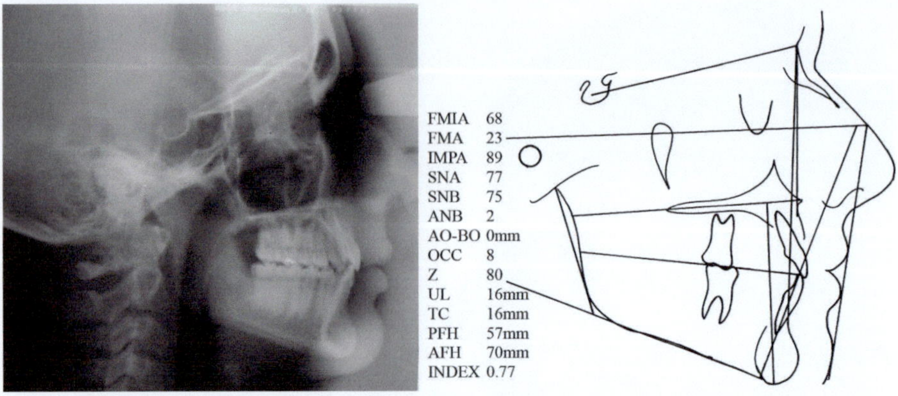

Fig. 1.36 Posttreatment cephalogram and tracing

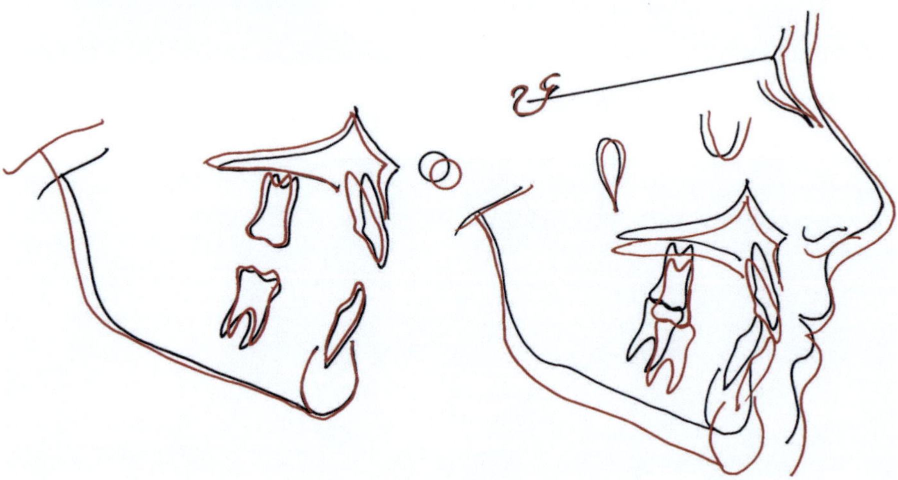

Fig. 1.37 Pretreatment/posttreatment superimpositions

treatment. The patient was recalled 3 years later. The facial photographs (Fig. 1.38) reflect the continued balance and harmony of the face. The 3-year posttreatment casts (Fig. 1.39) confirm total settling of the dentition into a very ideal Class I dental relationship. Arch form and arch width have remained the same. Mandibular incisor position is excellent. The recall cephalogram and tracing (Fig. 1.40) illustrate the continued maintenance of the ANB correction and incisor position. The pretreatment/posttreatment superimpositions (Fig. 1.41) confirm a continued downward and forward change in the spatial relationship of the mandible to the maxilla which increases the prominence of the chin and improves facial balance and harmony. The patient's dentition settled within 6 months of the time of appliance removal.

The records of these two patients have been included to illustrate classical anchorage. The transitional dentition that is created by classical anchorage settles

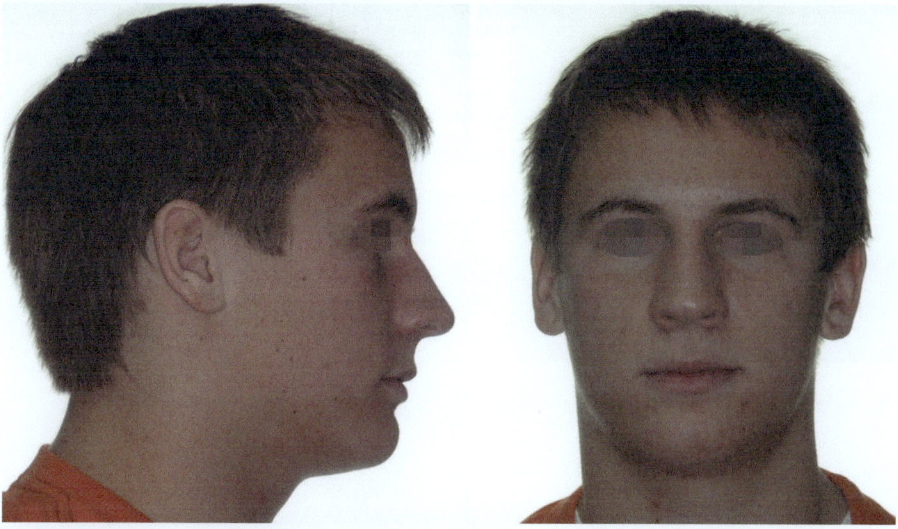

Fig. 1.38 Three year posttreatment facial photographs

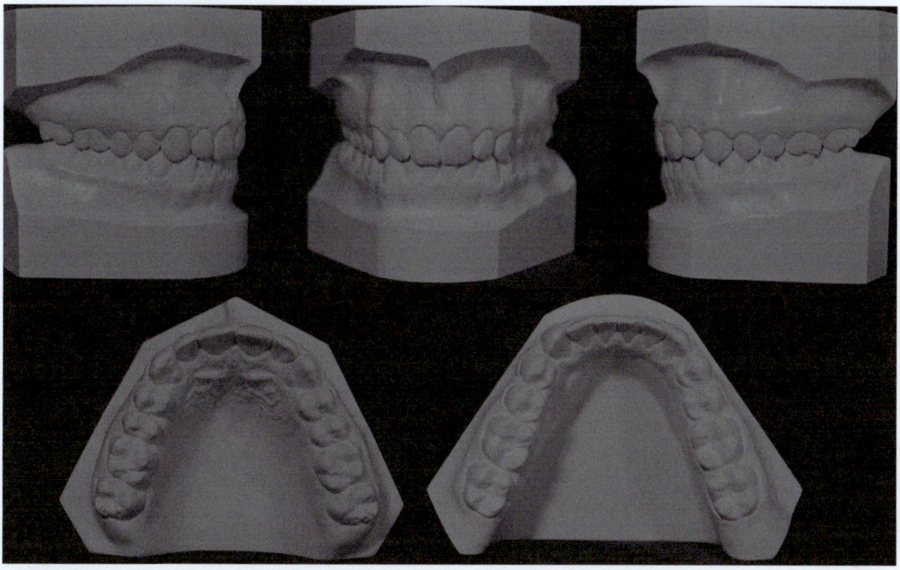

Fig. 1.39 Three year posttreatment casts

well into an excellent interdigitation of the teeth, functional occlusion that is characterized by a canine-protected occlusion with no balancing or working prematurities. The pretreatment/posttreatment/recall smiles of both patients (Fig. 1.42) illustrate the type of treatment outcome that classical anchorage preparation can help generate for patients.

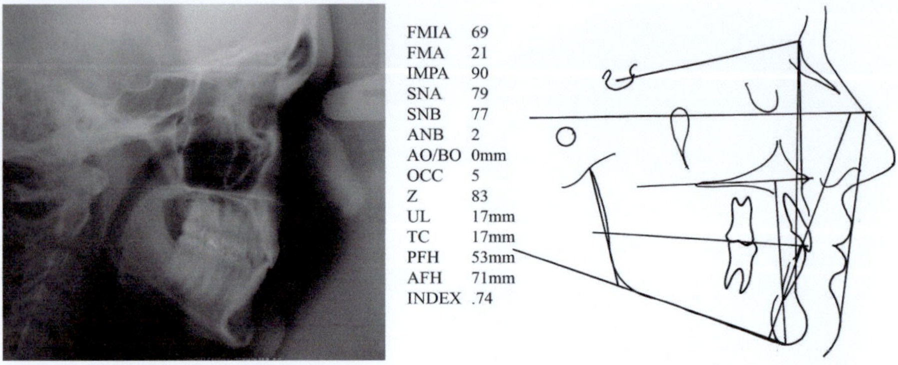

Fig. 1.40 Recall cephalogram and tracing

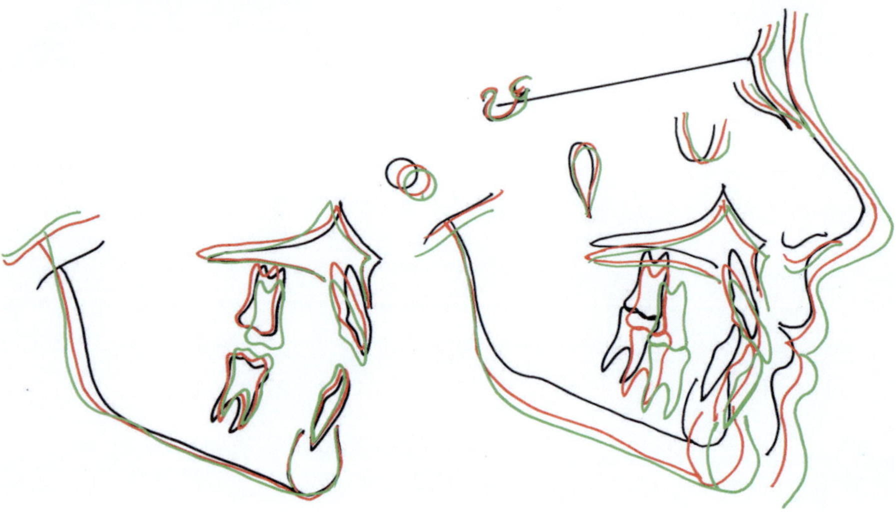

Fig. 1.41 Pretreatment/posttreatment superimpositions

Angle was very interested in mandibular anchorage preparation. He understood how important it was for the axial inclination of the mandibular posterior teeth to resist the force of Class II elastic pull. Yet, he did not devise a method to successfully make it happen. That remained for Charles Tweed to accomplish. Tweed used Angle's appliance and a few of Angle's ideas. He made them work with extra oral forces. The problem Tweed had with en masse anchorage was, of course, patient cooperation. Tweed placed all the second-order bends in the mandibular archwire and at one time. This method would work if the patient followed directions explicitly. Merrifield understood the problems with his mentor's approach. He set out to devise a way to prepare conventional mandibular anchorage in a more predictable manner and with a system that required not as much patient cooperation. He did so by developing his sequential mandibular anchorage concepts. Conventional

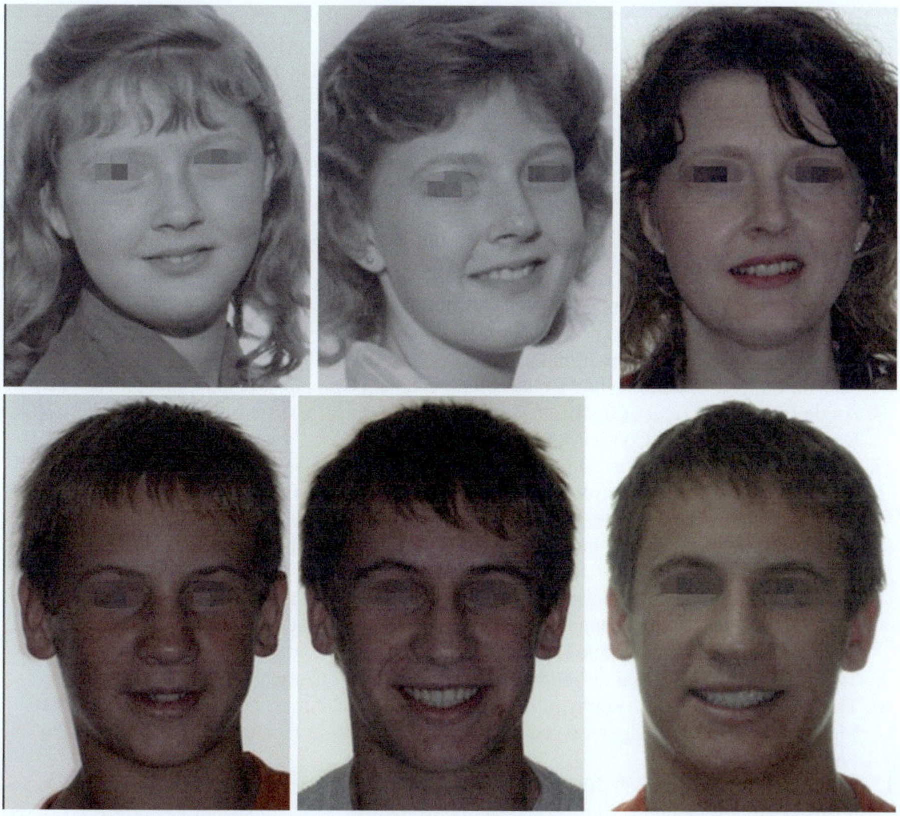

Fig. 1.42 Pretreatment/posttreatment/recall smiles of both patients

mandibular anchorage is now prepared efficiently and predictably for each and every patient who needs it. Mandibular anchorage preparation, as it is done at the present time, has two essential purposes.

1. It contributes to the control of the vertical dimension of the posterior segments of the malocclusion. Anchorage prevents the opening of the Frankfort mandibular plane angle. Vertical control is a vital function of mandibular anchorage preparation.
2. The mandibular posterior teeth are placed in positions that resist the forward and upward pull of Class II elastic force. This was the original intent of Angle and of Tweed. It still remains as one of the primary purposes of mandibular anchorage preparation.

Mandibular anchorage preparation is the most important step that must be accomplished during the routine correction of most malocclusions. It must be done carefully. The present method that is used to prepare mandibular anchorage, sequential mandibular anchorage preparation, enjoys great predictability and resounding success.

Acknowledgment Figures 1.8, 1.9, 1.10, 1.11, 1.12, 1.13, 1.14, 1.15, 1.16, 1.17, 1.18, and 1.19 are used with permission of Tweed Study Course. The images which illustrate the force systems (Figs. 1.9, 1.10, 1.11, 1.12, 1.13, 1.14, 1.15, 1.16, 1.17, 1.18, and 1.19) that are described in this chapter were created by Sergio Cardiel Rios, Morelia, Michoacan, Mexico.

References

1. The American Heritage College Dictionary (1993) 3rd edn. Houghton Mifflin Co., Boston/New York, p 49
2. Farrar JN (1889) A treatise on irregularities of the teeth and their correction. The International News Company, New York, p 771–774
3. Angle EH (1900) Treatment of malocclusion of the teeth and fractures of the Maxillae, Angle's system. 6th edn The S.S. White Dental Manufacturing Company, Philadelphia, p 109–116
4. Angle EH (1907) Treat of malocclusion of the teeth, Angle's system, 7th edn. The S.S. White Dental Manufacturing Company, Philadelphia
5. Angle EH (1929) The latest and best in orthodontic mechanism. Dental Cosmos 70:260–268
6. Salzman JA (1943) Principles of orthodontics. J.B. Lippincott Company, Philadelphia, p 546–547
7. Strang RHW (1943) Text book of orthodontia, 2nd edn Lea and Febiger, Philadelphia, p 398–413
8. Tweed CH (1936) The application of the principles of the edgewise arch in the treatment of class II, division I malocclusion, part II: a discussion of extraction in the treatment of marked double protrusion cases. Angle Orthod 6(4):255–257
9. Tweed CH (1966) Clinical orthodontics. The C.V. Mosby Company, St. Louis
10. Tweed CH (1945) A philosophy of orthodontic treatment. Am J Orthod Oral Surg 31(2):19
11. Merrifield LL (1986) Edgewise sequential directional force technology. J Charles Tweed Int Foundation 14:22–37
12. Vaden JL, Klontz HA, Dale JG (2012) Standard edgewise: Tweed-Merrifield philosophy, diagnosis, treatment planning and force systems. In: Graber TM, Vanarsdall RL, Vig KWL (eds) Orthodontics: current principles and techniques, 5th edn. Elsevier, Philadelphia, p 517–559
13. Klontz HA, Vaden JL (2016) Tweed study course syllabus. Tweed Memorial Center, Tucson

Paradigm Shift by Straight Wire Appliance and Its Impact on Anchorage Control

2

Tian Min Xu

Abstract

Classical anchorage like in Tweed Edgewise and Begg technique all includes tip back bends on molars. With the development of straight wire appliance, especially the wide spread of NiTi wire that makes bending tip backs impractical if not impossible, orthodontists then gradually discard tip back bend and look for other anchorage methods. We then see a lot of TPA, Nance bar, headgear, and more and more TAD. Our recent study showed the conventional headgear can't prevent upper molar from forward tipping on straight wire technique probably because it can't resist 24 hours tip forward moment exerted by a straight wire on conventional molar tube when the dental arch was not straight before treatment. TAD is absolute anchorage; it won't yield at all when pitting with other teeth. Then we see a lot of alveolar defects or root resorption of anterior teeth especially with the application of CBCT imaging technology. The emergence of TAD represents the end of the time of ever looking for stronger anchorage and meanwhile the advent of a new time of looking for more individualized and more physiologic anchorage.

One of the driven force for technological progress is believed from one of the human nature—do-nothingism—or making things as simple as possible. Being tired of wire bending, smart orthodontists start to put the first-, second-, and third-order bends into brackets. The most received idea is Andrews's Straight Wire Appliance. By measuring the study casts of 120 optimal nature occlusion in adulthood, Andrews set up six keys as the treatment goal and created his original straight wire brackets

T.M. Xu
Department of Orthodontics, Peking University School and Hospital of Stomatology, Beijing, China
e-mail: tmxuortho@163.com

T.M. Xu (ed.), *Physiologic Anchorage Control*,
DOI 10.1007/978-3-319-48333-7_2

based on it [1]. To reach this goal, he even made 11 sets of bracket prescription by adding various anti-tipping, anti-rotation angles according to the amount of different teeth movements. When orthodontists see that all three-order bends can be put into brackets, more and more of them gradually give up wire bending. Especially with the wide application of NiTi wires, bending wire becomes impractical if not impossible. However, a group of orthodontists—Tweed people—still insists on wire bending. And they teach wire bending technique 2–3 times a year in Tucson to students from all over the world. A lot of orthodontic programs in the USA send their residents to Tucson to learn this technique. And the Tweed teachers from different countries also teach Tweed technique in their own countries. If straight wire appliance can substitute classical Edgewise completely, why Tweed people working so hard on wire bending?

Let's look at how straight wire appliance determines bracket prescription first. Andrews prescribed his original straight wire brackets based on the data he measured from 120 optimal nature occlusions in adulthood. The basic idea is to avoid or at least minimize wire bending in the last stainless steel rectangular wire. Although putting the goal data into brackets may serve this purpose well in the last treatment stage, it does not validate using straight wire in the initial treatment stage when teeth are in malocclusion. Not all wire bending in Edgewise appliance is for detailing in the last stage, some of them are for other purpose. For example, anchorage bend, do we really know how to put an anchorage bend into bracket? Anchorage bend is a simplest V bend. Although it's easy to bend a 10° tip back bend like in Fig. 2.1a, transferring this 10° into buccal tube or bracket is not that simple. Can we just put this 10° angle to buccal tube as in Fig. 2.1b and conceive they are equal?

Orthodontists are familiar with V bend mechanics. We all know when we put a V bend in the center of the span between two teeth, for example, between upper second premolar and canine as in Fig. 2.2, both teeth get equal and opposite moments. The net moment is zero; therefore, the force system meets static equilibrium condition. When V bend deviates from the center toward second premolar (Fig. 2.3), the moment on second premolar increases while the moment on canine decreases. The net moment is no more zero; therefore, canine will get intrusion force and second premolar will get extrusion force, which compose a couple; the magnitude must be equal to the difference between the moments on premolar and canine to reach static equilibrium. When V bend locates at about 1/3 of the inter-bracket distance (Fig. 2.4) closer to second premolar, the wire-slot angulation on canine may become zero, so there will be no moment on canine, a pair of larger forces on premolar and canine is needed to meet static equilibrium condition. When V bend locates very close to premolar, less than 1/4 of the inter-bracket distance (Fig. 2.5), the wire-slot angulation on canine may become opposite to that in Figs. 2.2 and 2.3. The moment direction on canine becomes the same as on premolar. A pair of even larger forces on premolar and canine is needed to reach static equilibrium status. From the above four situations, we have learned even with the same angle V bend, as long as they are put in different positions, the force system will be different (Fig. 2.6). It was called

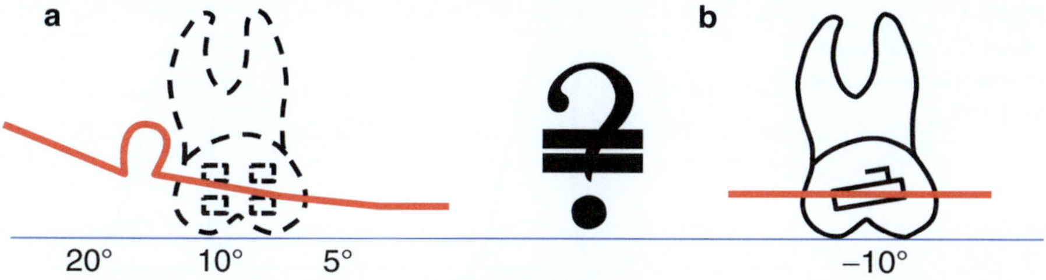

Fig. 2.1 10° tip back bend **(a)** vs. 10° tip back tube **(b)**

Fig. 2.2 V bend in the center of upper second premolar and canine

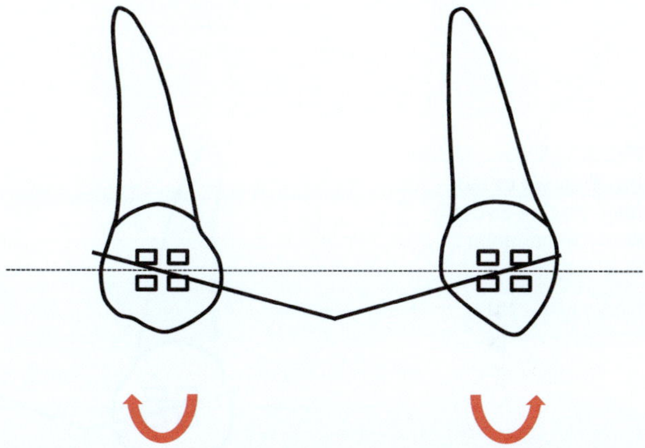

Fig. 2.3 V bend deviates from the center toward second premolar

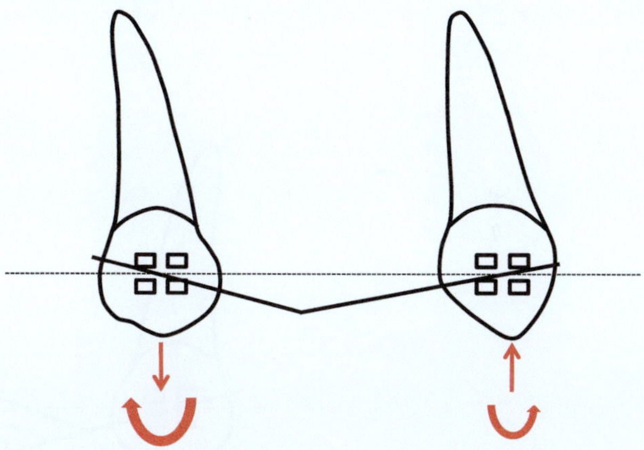

differential torque or differential moment by Mulligan [2]. So orthodontic force system is not just determined by wire bending angle, but also affected by its location. Therefore, in clinic, "put a 10° tip back on molar" does not always mean the same force system if you don't define where to put it. So how to transfer a V bend angle from an arch wire to a bracket is far more difficult than we expected.

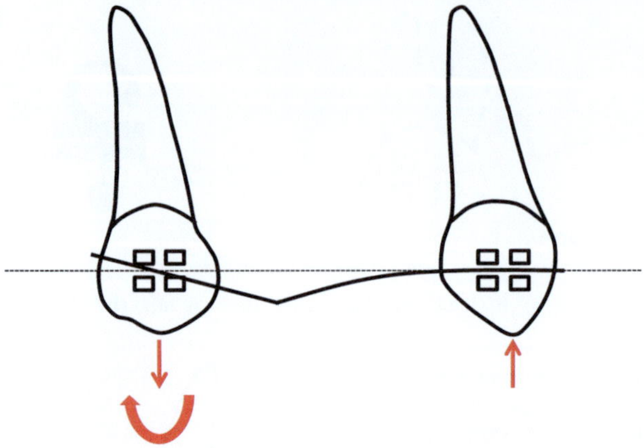

Fig. 2.4 V bend locates at about 1/3 of the inter-bracket distance closer to premolar

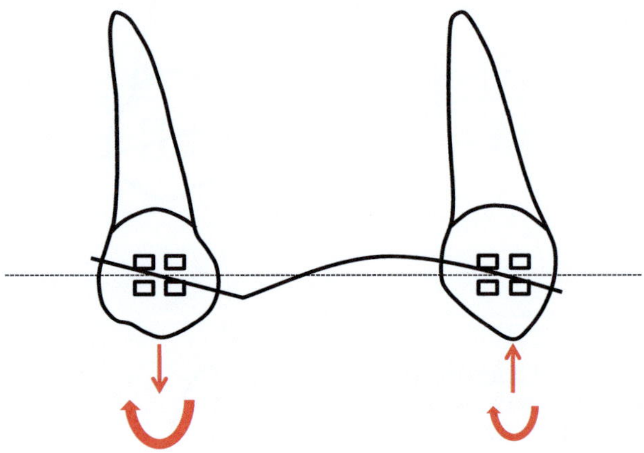

Fig. 2.5 V bend locates less than 1/4 of the inter-bracket distance closer to premolar

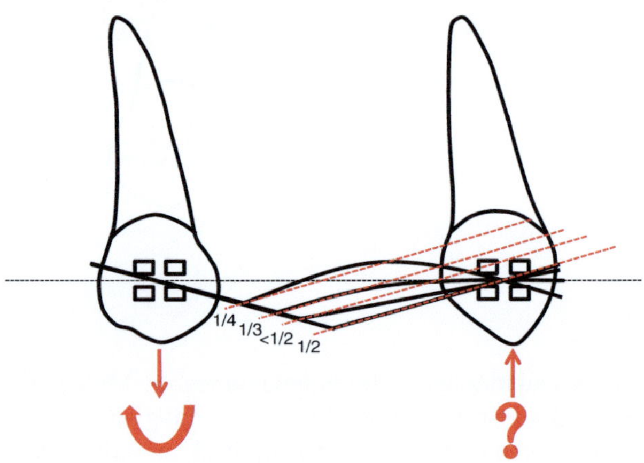

Fig. 2.6 Same V bend angle at different locations creates different force system

Then can we transfer V bend position information into straight wire appliance? To answer this question, let's look at what the V bend position really affect. From Figs. 2.2, 2.3, 2.4, and 2.5, we see when V bend moves toward a tooth, the wire-slot angle on that tooth increases and the wire-slot angle on the other tooth decreases. If we compare the relationship between wire-slot angulation and the moment, we can see the larger the wire-slot angle on second premolar, the larger the moment it creates on it, and the moment keeps the same direction on second premolar in all four situations. When the wire-slot angle is smaller on canine, the moment is smaller, and when the V bend displaces toward premolar, the moment on canine changes from the opposite direction as premolar to zero to the same direction. And the net moment direction of the system is always the same as the larger one on premolar; moreover, the net moment dictates the magnitude and direction of balancing force on the two teeth in this system. So the larger moment dominates the two-tooth force system, we call it dominant moment. From the above analysis, we now know the V bend position actually determines the wire-slot angulation, and it then determines which tooth dominates the system moment. Translating this knowledge into straight wire appliance, we can now judge which tooth dominates the system moment. For example, if canine is in forward tipping position like in Fig. 2.7, engaging a straight wire, the wire-slot angle is larger on canine than on premolar, then canine will dominate the moment and the system moment is in clockwise direction. If canine is in backward tipping position like in Fig. 2.8, engaging a straight wire, the wire-slot angle is also larger on canine, but in opposite direction, so the system moment will be in counterclockwise direction.

In these two situations, the second premolar may get opposite moments even if it's in normal angulation at the beginning. These two examples tell us, if we use straight NiTi wire to align teeth, the most malpositioned tooth will dominate the system moment, and it may tip normal positioned teeth to abnormal angulation.

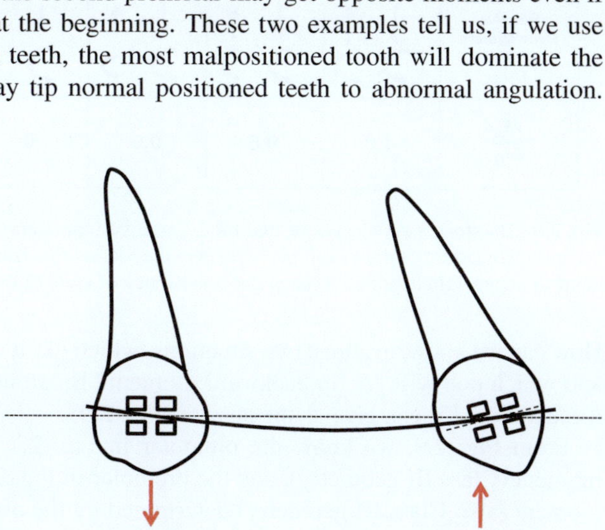

Fig. 2.7 Force system when engaging a straight wire in a forward tipping canine and an upright premolar

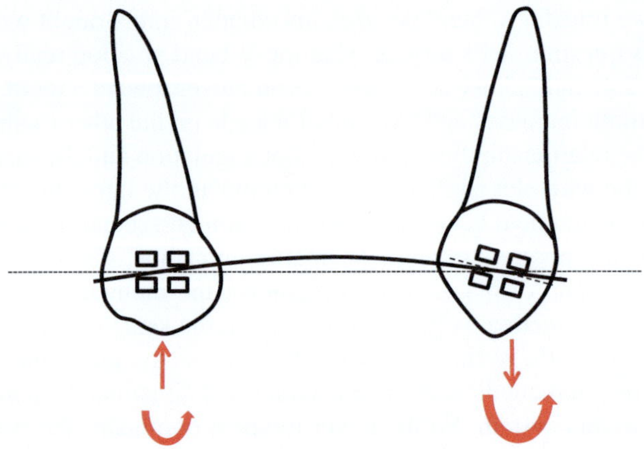

Fig. 2.8 Force system when engaging a straight wire in a backward tipping canine and an upright premolar

CLASS:	I	II	III	IV	V	VI
$\frac{\theta_A}{\theta_B}$	1.0	0.5	0	–0.5	–0.75	–1.0
Upper right quadrant	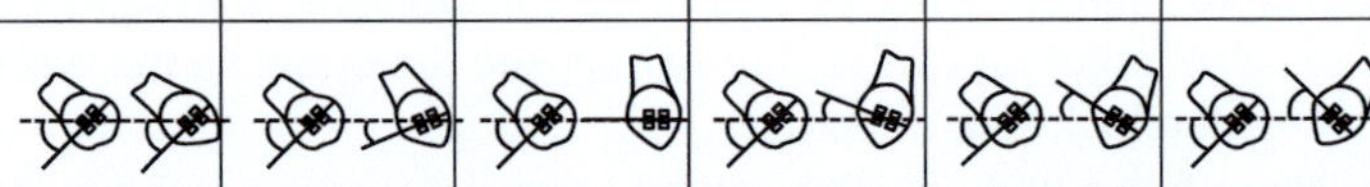					
Relative force system on teeth L = 7	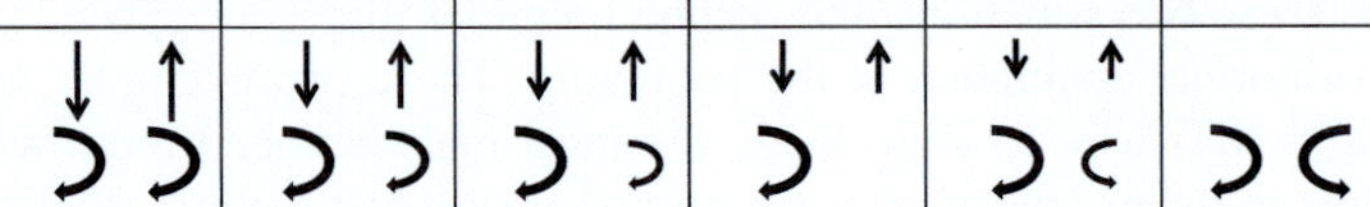					
$\frac{M_A}{M_B}$	1.0	0.8	0.5	0	–0.4	–1.0

Fig. 2.9 Burstone's six classes of two-tooth force system (Reproduced from Burstone et al. [3]. We just changed Burstone's example of teeth in the second row from lower left quadrant of original chart to upper right quadrant to keep the consistency of style of this chapter)

How can we know, in above two situations, which tooth will get tip forward moment and which one will get tip backward moment? Burstone's six classes of two-tooth force system [3] can give us the answer (Fig. 2.9).

From Fig. 2.9, we know the premolar in Fig. 2.7 will get backward tipping moment (Class III geometry), and the premolar in Fig. 2.8 will get forward tipping moment (also Class III geometry) determined by the dominant moment on canine. Although it's difficult for orthodontists to remember the classification of the six basic two-tooth geometries, it really gives important clues to understand force system in straight wire appliance.

Firstly, let's look at the relationship between V bend mechanics and the six classes of two-tooth force system. We will notice the Class VI is equivalent to a centered V bend in two-tooth span (Fig. 2.10); Class V is equivalent to an off-centered V bend (Fig. 2.11); Class IV is equivalent to a V bend located around 1/3 of inter-bracket span (Fig. 2.12); Class III is equivalent to a V bend located within 1/4 of the span (Fig. 2.13). Class I and Class II cannot be realized by simple V bend. Class I is actually equivalent to a standard step bend (Fig. 2.14), and Class II is equivalent to the step bend with unparalleled legs (Fig. 2.15).

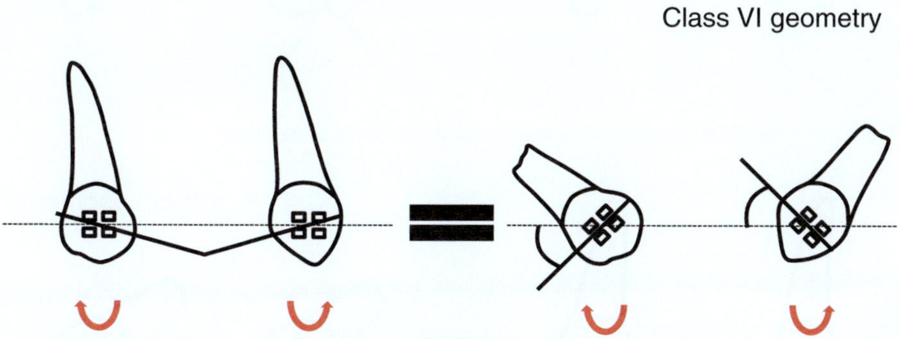

Fig. 2.10 Class VI equivalent to a centered V bend

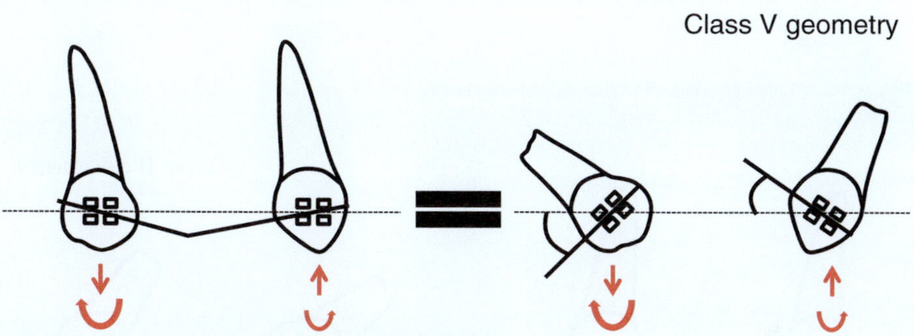

Fig. 2.11 Class V equivalent to an off-centered V bend

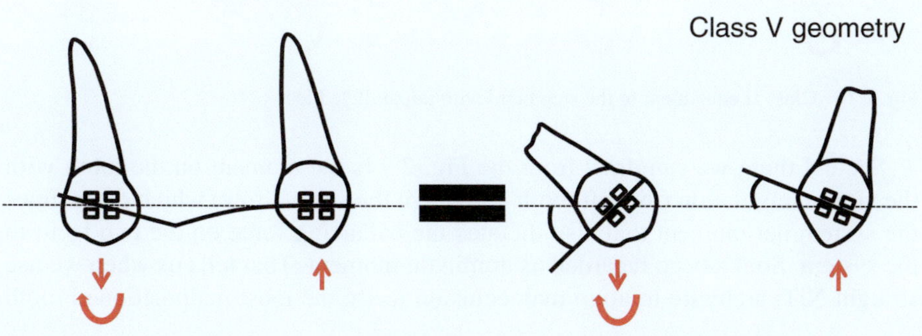

Fig. 2.12 Class IV equivalent to a V bend locates around 1/3 of the inter-bracket span

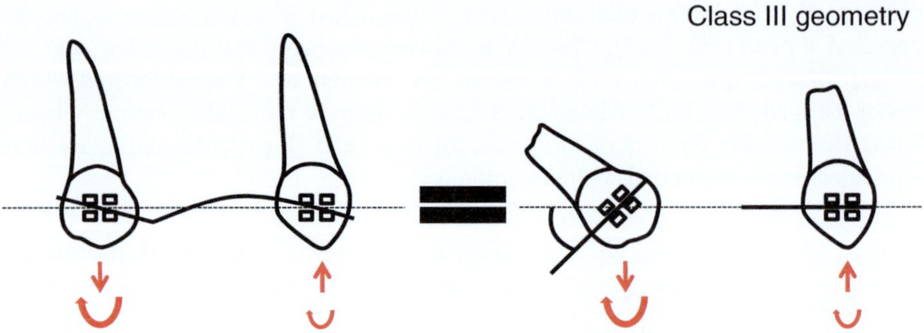

Fig. 2.13 Class III equivalent to a V bend located within 1/4 of the span

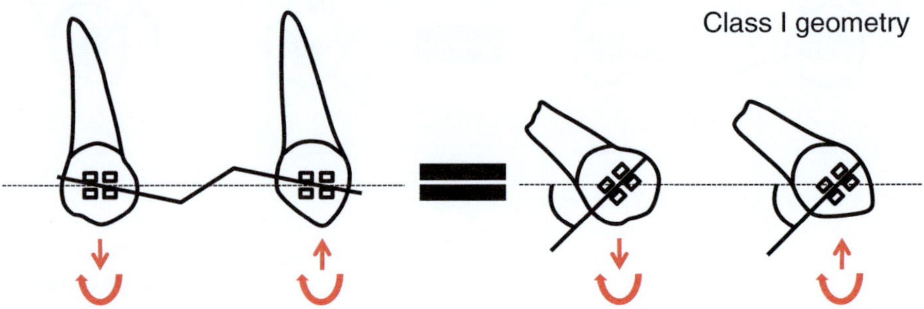

Fig. 2.14 Class I equivalent to a standard step bend

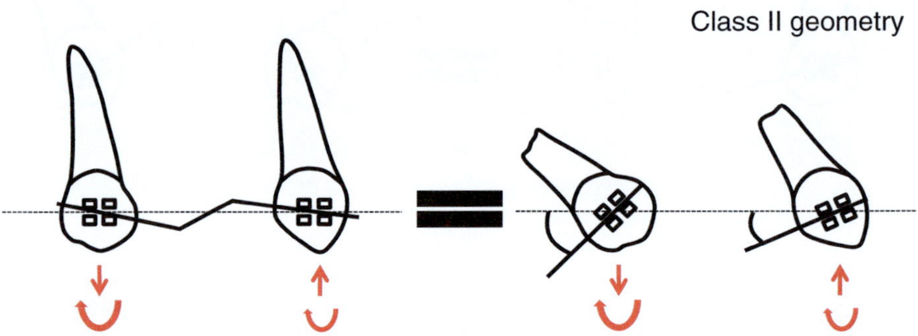

Fig. 2.15 Class II equivalent to the step bend with unparalleled legs

Second thing we can draw from the Fig. 2.9 is the moment on the tooth with the largest angulation (the left tooth with θ_B in the second row) which determines the system net moment that also dictates the balancing force on the two teeth in the system. So it's been regarded as dominant moment. That tells us when we use straight NiTi archwire to align malocclusion teeth; the most malpositioned tooth

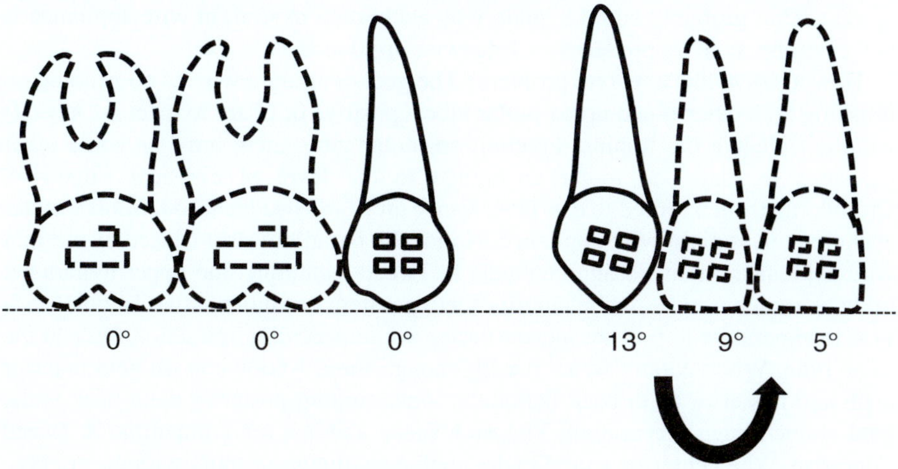

Fig. 2.16 In straight wire prescription, all anterior teeth are giving forward tipping angle, while all posterior upper teeth are giving 0°or forward tipping angle, making anterior teeth a better chance to occupy dominant moment

may dominate the force system and tip the relatively normally positioned teeth to abnormal angulation. From anchorage control perspective, in extraction treatment, the teeth posterior to extraction space are usually considered anchorage segment, and teeth anterior to it are considered to be corrected segment. In straight wire appliance, posterior teeth are given 0° or positive degree while all anterior teeth are given positive degree (Fig. 2.16). So if taking upper arch as a whole, the system moment will have greater chance to be in counterclockwise direction. If considering upper arch as two segments, anchorage segment posterior to extraction space and malocclusion segment anterior to extraction space, the dominant moment will have greater chance to be in malocclusion segment because clinical impression tells us that anterior teeth are more prone to be malpositioned or inclined more than posterior teeth, in addition to the preadjusted angles in brackets. We can then imagine in most situations, when engaging a straight wire, anterior teeth dominate the system moment while posterior teeth will get either anterior or posterior tipping moments depending on their geometric relationship with anterior teeth. From mechanical point of view, changing preadjusted angle on posterior teeth from 0° or positive angle to negative degree will help anchorage preservation. Classical Edgewise put a wire bending angle −5°, −10°, and −20°on the second premolar, first molar, and second molar, which certainly has more chance to get dominant moment on posterior teeth segment. And from Burstone force system classification, we know only dominant moment can keep consistent direction, or unaffected by moments on malocclusion teeth. In other words, in Edgewise time, orthodontists control force system by wire bending, while in straight wire time, the most malpositioned tooth grabs the control power of force system. That probably could explain why anchorage in straight wire appliance is not as strong as in its predecessor Edgewise appliance.

How to solve this apparent problem? The goal of straight wire of no bending on finishing arch determined upper molar tube a positive or 0° tip to meet six keys. If we don't change the tipping direction on molar tube, there must be some other measures to make up molar anchorage to the level of classical Edgewise. Orthodontists then turned to use TPA, Nance arch, and headgear to reinforce molar anchorage in straight wire appliance. Notice the paradigm shift caused by straight wire appliance on anchorage methods. In Tweed technique, the upper molars get tip back moment, meanwhile anterior teeth get flare out moment, so J-hook headgear is imperative to prevent incisor flaring while providing retraction force at the same time. When patient wears it with enough time, J-hook can tip both anterior teeth and posterior teeth back definitely. Since tipping posterior teeth back is the goal of anchorage preparation, TPA and Nance arch are not compatible in Tweed Edgewise. When entering straight wire appliance time, especially with the application of NiTi wire, orthodontists are giving up wire bending. If no tip back bend, anterior teeth will not receive flaring out force. J-hook is no more necessary in early stage of treatment although it still can be used in retraction stage with stainless steel rectangular wire. From aforementioned Burstone's six classes of force system, the relative straight-up molar is difficult to get dominant moment; it therefore has big chance to be tipped forward by malocclusion teeth anterior to it in straight wire appliance. To deal with this, orthodontists apply headgear force directly to molar, and TPA or Nance arch are also believed helpful in stabilizing anchor molar. So straight wire appliance actually changed the feature of anchorage control in fixed appliance dramatically. Among headgear, TPA, and Nance arch, the strongest anchorage is certainly headgear. Conventional headgear applies backward force to molar directly; can this force resist molar forward tipping moment just like molar tip back bend on rectangular arch with J-hook in Tweed technique? Unfortunately, our prospective randomized clinical trial showed upper molar tipped forward 7.2° on average in maximum anchorage extraction cases treated with MBT prescription appliance even though all patients in that sample wore headgear [4]. Why is that?

If we look at a real case with straight wire appliance in place, we may understand why upper molar tipped forward with our contemporary fixed appliance. Figure 2.17 is a common Class II[1] case; when we put a 0° buccal tube on, engaging a straight wire will give upper molar a forward tipping moment. Although headgear can provide a backward force against the tipping moment, it is usually worn less than 8 hours only at night, while archwire works 24 h a day. Comparing with untreated sample in Burlington growth center [5], 7.2° forward tipping in our sample during 2.5 years' orthodontic treatment is much larger than 2.8°

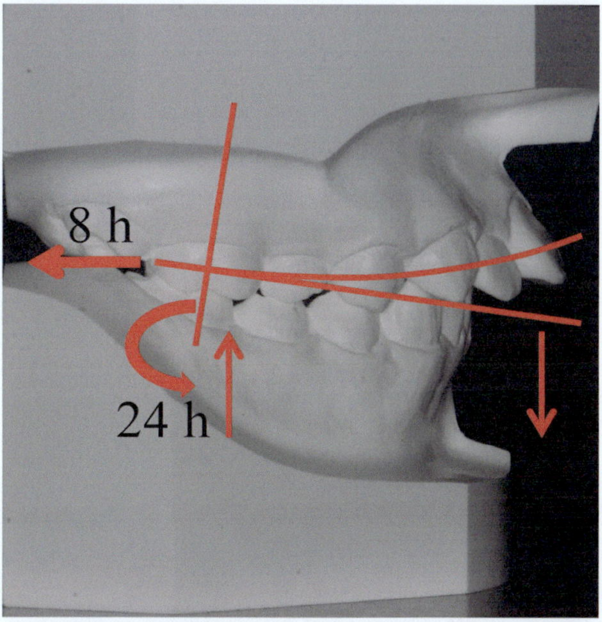

Fig. 2.17 A typical Class II[1] case shows a curved upper arch, when a straight NiTi wire engaged in, molar will get forward tipping moment to lose anchorage even with 8h headgear

nature forward tipping in their Class II sample observed in 2 years during 12–14 years of age. It seems to tell us contemporary straight wire appliance cannot control molar forward tipping in extraction treatment as effective as its predecessor—Tweed Edgewise appliance. When orthodontists find headgear anchorage is not strong enough, implant anchorage or TAD is invented and getting popular nowadays. By bypassing molar, implant anchorage can make 0 mm molar anchorage loss theoretically. Then orthodontists can move teeth to anywhere they want without worrying about anchorage. The problem is: is that good for incisor root and alveolar health?

Figure 2.18 is an adult bimaxillary protrusion case. To reduce her protrusive lips, we extracted her four first premolars and retracted the anterior teeth with implant anchorage. After both the patient and doctor were satisfied with her profile, we stopped retraction and took impression and CBCT as stage records. Superimposing digital study casts on unloaded mini-screw implants, we can see upper molars have not moved mesially at all, and upper incisors were retracted apparently.

Since her upper molars did not move mesially at all, we can call this case an absolute anchorage case. Then we were wondering where would be the roots. Checking her CBCT image, we can see apparent root resorption of upper central

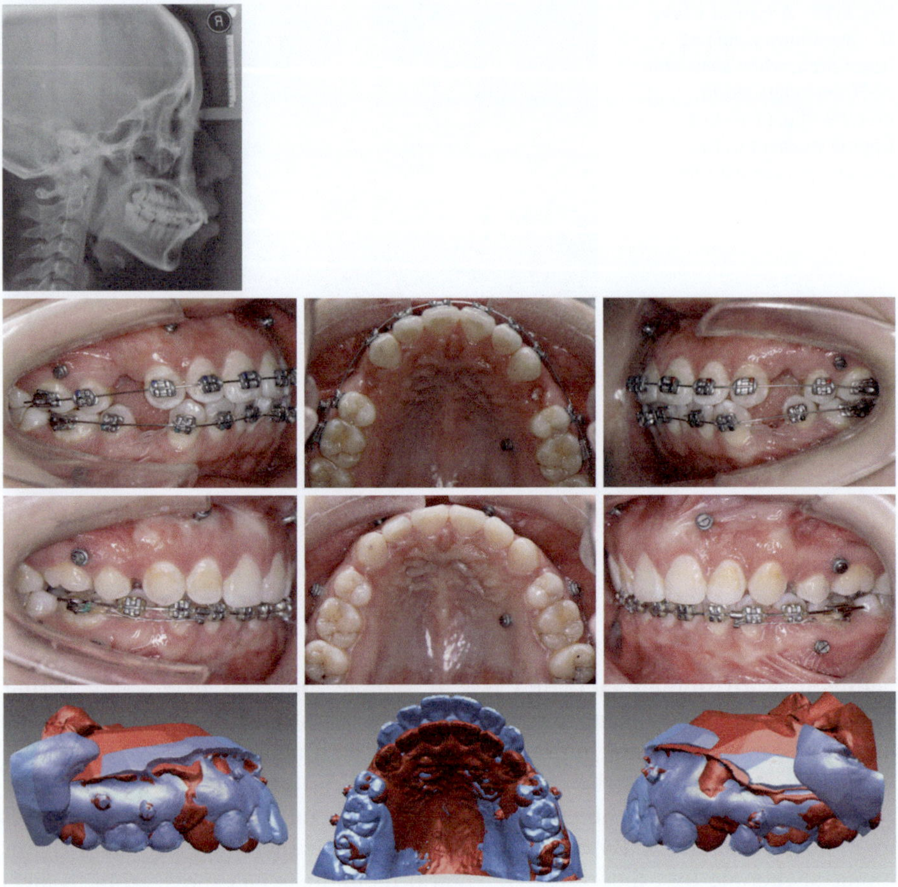

Fig. 2.18 An adult bimaxillary protrusion case, treated with four premolars extraction and using mini-screw implants as anchorage. Superimposition on unloaded mini-screws showed upper incisors retracted apparently and anchor molars no mesial movement at all (Reproduced from Xu [7])

incisors and alveolar defect on lingual side (Fig. 2.19). We can also see alveolar fenestration of upper left lateral incisor apex on labial side (Fig. 2.20). If we check her lower incisor, more than half of the root on lingual side is out of alveolar bone (Fig. 2.19). More than 70 years ago, Dr. Tweed, considering labial limits, advocated extraction treatment [6]. Today when we have absolute anchorage tools, shouldn't we consider the lingual limits?

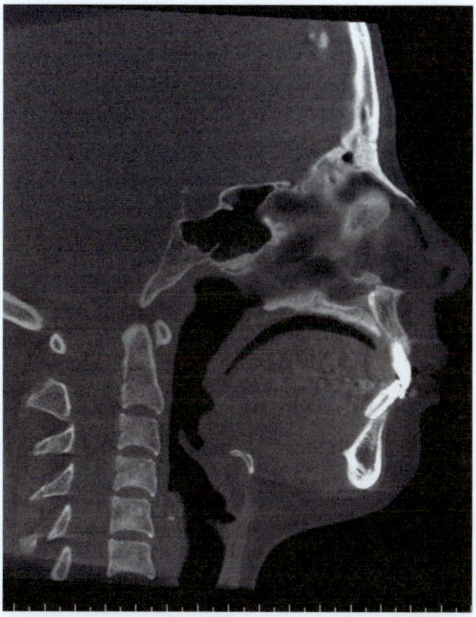

Fig. 2.19 After retraction of incisors with mini-screw implant, alveolar bone of both upper and lower central incisors lost on lingual sides and upper central incisor root apex resorbed (Reproduced from Xu [7])

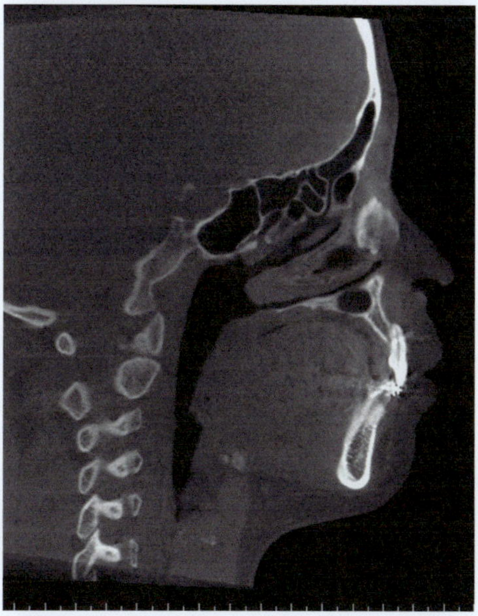

Fig. 2.20 Root apex of upper lateral incisor stick out of labial alveolar bone—alveolar fenestration (Reproduced from Xu [7])

As the strongest anchorage, the emergence of implant anchorage symbolizes the end of the time of ever looking for stronger anchorage and meanwhile the advent of a new time of looking for more individualized and more physiologic anchorage.

Acknowledgment The work was supported, in part, by National Natural Science Foundation of China No. 81371192.

References

1. Andrews LF (1972) The six keys to normal occlusion. Am J Orthod 62(3):296–309
2. Mulligan TF (1982) Common sense mechanics. 2122 East Kaler Drive, Phoenix, AZ 85020
3. Burstone CJ, Koenig HA (1974) Force systems from an ideal arch. Am J Orthod 65(3): 270–289
4. Xu TM, Zhang X, Oh HS et al (2010) Randomized clinical trial comparing control of maxillary anchorage with 2 retraction techniques. Am J Orthod Dentofacial Orthop 138(5):544.e1–9
5. Martinelli FL, de Oliveira Ruellas AC, de Lima EM, Bolognese AM (2010) Natural changes of the maxillary first molars in adolescents with skeletal Class II malocclusion. Am J Orthod Dentofacial Orthop 137(6):775–781
6. Tweed CH (1966) Clinical orthodontics. Mosby, St. Louis
7. Xu TM (2015) New concept of physiologic anchorage control. APOS Trends Orthod 5:250–254

Craniofacial Growth and Its Interaction with the Maxillary Anchor Molars

3

Lysle E. Johnston Jr

Abstract

In the orthodontics of the twenty-first century, many clinicians look to the mandible, both as a cause of Class II malocclusion and a cure, presumably by way of some sort of "growth modification." Indeed, some go so far as to say that the maxilla is the "wrong" jaw. In truth, there is little evidence that mandibular growth can be modified. No matter: the long-term pattern of mandibular growth is usually favorable in both Class I and Class II subjects. Unfortunately, whether normal or therapeutically augmented, maxillary dentoalveolar compensation would prevent any mandibular excess from changing the occlusion. Thus, in view of the ways that Class II malocclusions develop and are corrected, it is clear that control of maxillary anchorage is an important, rational component of both processes. This short chapter argues that regardless of label—fixed or functional; early or late—the final expression at the occlusion is in large measure a prevention, reduction, or reversal of maxillary dentoalveolar compensation. All roads lead to Rome; all roads to a normal molar relationship lead to the midface by way of maxillary anchorage control.

In an examination of the relationship between facial growth and maxillary anchorage loss in the prevention and treatment of Class II malocclusion, it must first be noted that the usual growth pattern features a mandibular excess relative to the midface. This pattern is seen both in Class II and Class I/Normal occlusions [1–3]. The fact that this presumably favorable growth pattern commonly has little effect on an established occlusion brings up a second salient mechanism: dentoalveolar

L.E. Johnston Jr
University of Michigan, Saint Louis University,
Saint Louis, USA
e-mail: lejjr@umich.edu

T.M. Xu (ed.), *Physiologic Anchorage Control*,
DOI 10.1007/978-3-319-48333-7_3

compensation [4]. Given a maxillo-mandibular growth differential and an intercuspated occlusion, the dentitions will shift so as to maintain the occlusion. The effect of this phenomenon can be seen in the range of Steiner's "acceptable compromises" going from Class II to Class III [5, 6] and is obvious when the first step in preparing for Class III surgery is to "remove the compensations." In passing, it must be noted that some argue that occlusal contact of only a few minutes a day is not enough to move teeth. Alternatively, one could argue that the mesial movement of the upper dentition is due to the anterior component of occlusal force [7, 8], in which case the mesial movement of the mandible relative to the maxilla might be the rate-limiting factor and thus would serve to match upper buccal-segment displacement to the increment of excess mandibular growth. Whatever the mechanism, it is clear that there is positional interaction between the maxillary dentition and the extent to which the mandible outgrows the maxilla. Accordingly, the important findings by Prof. Xu's group [9, 10]—increased maxillary anchorage loss in adolescents and males—can be interpreted as dentoalveolar compensations in subjects who can be expected to grow the most. (The increased anchorage loss seen in Class II subject and those who had the extraction of two upper bicuspids is a by-product of space closure.) His emphasis on the upper jaw is important: I will argue that all Class II treatments do much of what they do by controlling the *upper* buccal segments.

For a variety of reasons, many influential clinicians (e.g., McNamara [11]) argue that the upper jaw and its dentition are usually normal in terms of size and position and thus should not be the object of treatment, especially Class II treatment. McNamara's conclusions were based on an analysis of young children, who tend to have retrusive mandibles, not to mention a short stature and an inability to solve algebraic equations. As the normal pattern of growth and development unfolds during adolescence, the size and position of the maxilla and its teeth can be expected to change along with a probable improvement in both stature and mathematical ability. With respect to the face, one would expect the maxillary dentition to become more protrusive and the mandible to become more prominent. The supposed need to attack only the mandible, rather than the maxilla, is a mischievous canard that conflicts with therapeutic reality.

With respect to the correction of a Class II malocclusion, it is clear that there are only four possibilities. Above the occlusal plane, the molar relationship would be normalized if the maxilla or the maxillary dentition were to be driven distally. Conversely, below the occlusal plane, forward growth of the mandible or mesial movement of the lower buccal segments would tend to correct the distoclusion. These options are not equally desirable, effective, or possible. Ponderable distal movement of the maxilla is unlikely, and anchorage loss in the mandible is in many cases undesirable. Although it probably cannot be augmented by "functional therapy," mandibular growth is usually favorable, both in Class I and II malocclusions. As has been noted, the problem is that dentoalveolar compensation would prevent any excess—normal or even if in some way augmented—from having an effect on the molar relationship. This analysis argues that the key to occlusal development and to therapeutic correction is the upper dentition. It is the only realistic therapeutic opportunity. It is for this reason that Prof. Xu's research on anchorage loss serves once again to focus our attention on the maxillary dentition.

Occlusal Development

In populations that retain their cusps during the whole of occlusal development, first molars commonly are directed into an end-to-end relationship by a so-called "flush terminal plane" created by the distal surfaces of the deciduous second molars. It commonly is thought that this unstable molar relationship is resolved by a "late mesial shift," mesial molar movement into the newly liberated leeway/E spaces. Because, on average, the lower leeway space is bigger than the upper, the differential mesial drift that would result is thought to bias the occlusion toward a "Class I" [12]. This difference, however, is not enough to explain the correction of a half-cusp differential, especially if some of the leeway space has already been used to accommodate the "incisor liability." Recent evidence argues that other events and conditions are much more important.

Tsourakis and Johnston [13] conducted a longitudinal cephalometric study—10–12 years in length—of occlusal development in 39 young subjects. Their study quantified movement of the molars relative to basal bone and the movement of the jaws relative to each other, all measured relative to a common functional occlusal plane [14, 15]. The first molars in those who had a mesial or distal step at age 5 or 6 erupted immediately into a stable "Class I" or Class II molar relationship, maintained, presumably by dentoalveolar compensation (Figs. 3.1 and 3.2). In contrast, 24 of the 39 started the study with a flush terminal plane, an occlusion that would produce an initial end-to-end first-molar relationship. For these subjects, the final occlusion seemed to be the result of a race

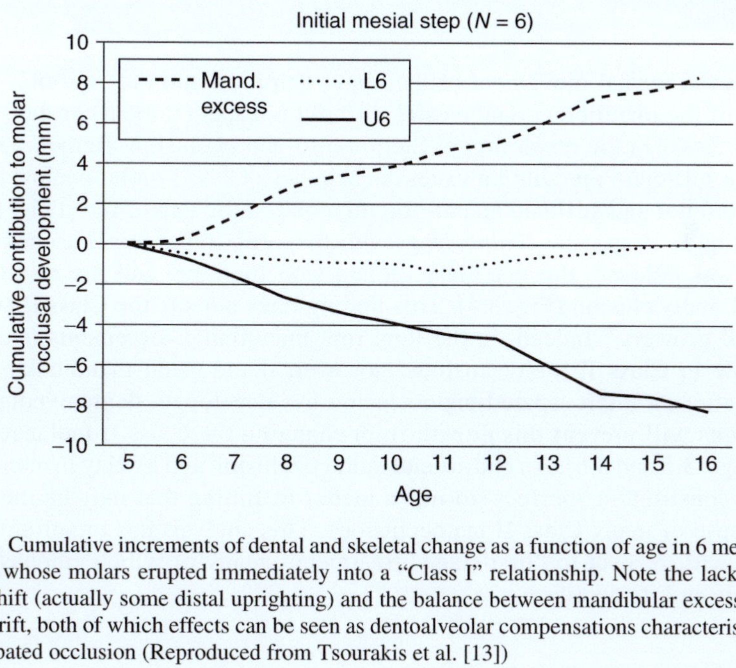

Fig. 3.1 Cumulative increments of dental and skeletal change as a function of age in 6 mesial-step subjects whose molars erupted immediately into a "Class I" relationship. Note the lack of a L6 mesial shift (actually some distal uprighting) and the balance between mandibular excess and U6 mesial drift, both of which effects can be seen as dentoalveolar compensations characteristic of an intercuspated occlusion (Reproduced from Tsourakis et al. [13])

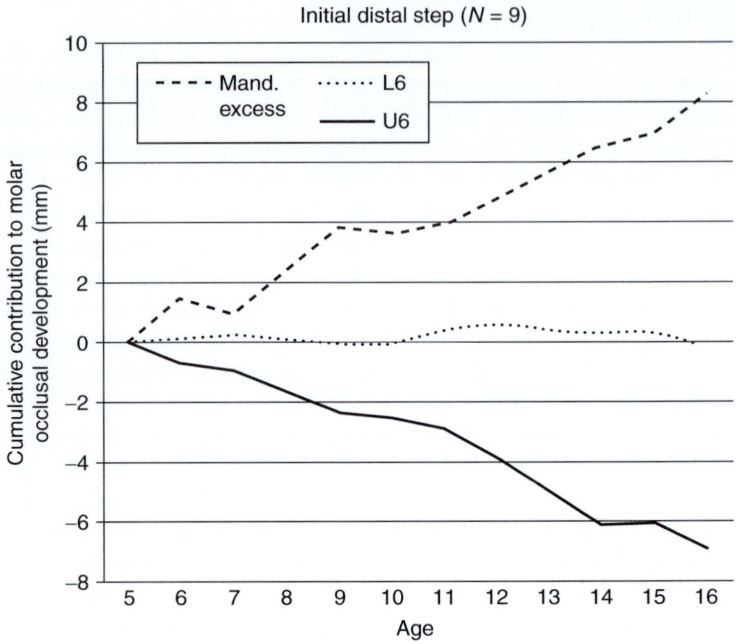

Fig. 3.2 Cumulative increments of mandibular excess and upper and lower first-molar mesial movement in 9 distal-step subjects. On average, there may be a slight, temporary mesial shift of about 1 mm at age 10. As with the mesial-step subjects, an initial "socked in" occlusion led subsequently to a balance between molar movement and mandibular excess (Reproduced from Tsourakis et al. [13])

between the mesial movement of the upper dentition and the "normal" excess growth of the mandible; a late mesial shift did not seem to be a constant or significant factor in the resolution of their end-to-end occlusion. Rather, 13 of the 24 had a sufficient mandibular excess to achieve a Class I molar occlusion (Fig. 3.3); 6 did not and still had an end-to-end molar at the end of the study. For the remaining 5, it was the *timing* of growth that was important: the mandibular excess was delayed, the maxillary molars won the race, and the result was a Class II malocclusion (Fig. 3.4). This finding does not say the Class II subjects are "bad growers." Indeed, in the long run, mandibular increments tend to be favorable in Class II malocclusions; however, if the usual mandibular excess occurs after an intercuspated malocclusion has developed, dentoalveolar compensations will prevent this growth from changing the Class II molar relationship (Figs. 3.5 and 3.6). An end-to-end molar occlusion and a delay in mandibular growth constitute a "perfect storm," a matter of timing that may be the proximate cause of many Class II malocclusions. This analysis has important implications with respect to "first-stage" treatments, many of which emphasize the mandible and its dentition.

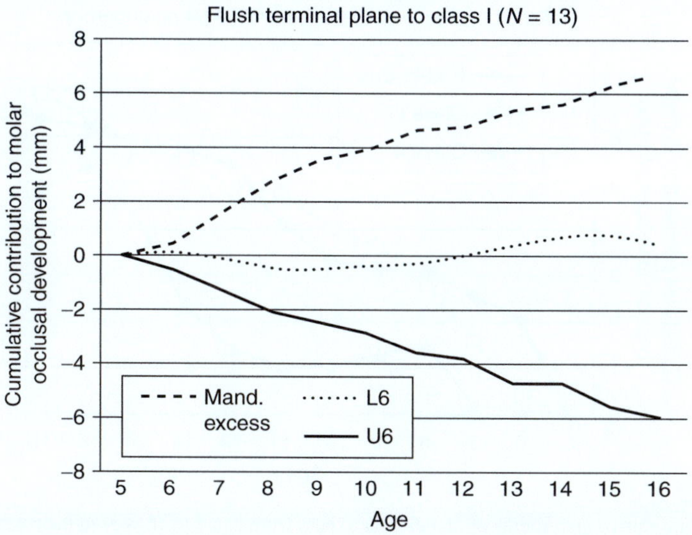

Fig. 3.3 Cumulative increments of change in 13 flush-terminal-plane subjects who progressed to a Class I molar relationship. Note that the mandibular excess was approximately 2 mm greater than the mesial drift of the upper molars, a "disconnect" that seems to suggest that dentoalveolar compensation comes into play only when a fully intercuspated dentition has developed. On average, there was no obvious late mesial shift until about age 12 and then only about 1 mm (Reproduced from Tsourakis et al. [13])

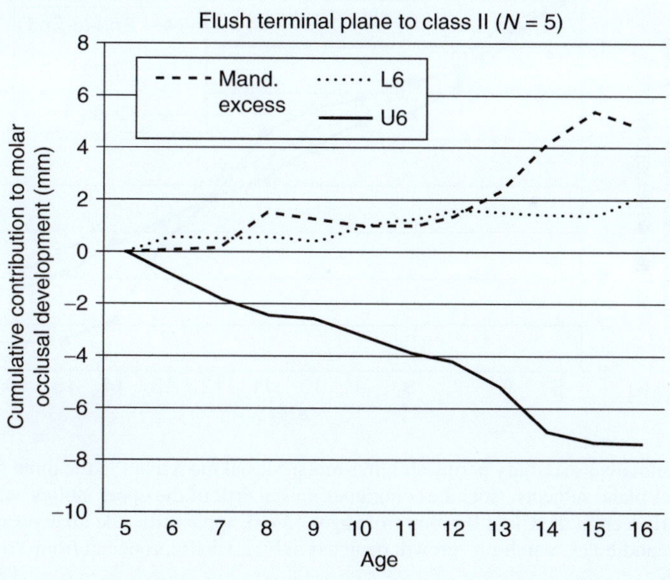

Fig. 3.4 Cumulative mandibular excess and U6 and L6 mesial movement in the 5 flush-terminal-plane subjects who settled into a molar Class II relationship. Note that there was a prolonged mandibular growth deficit up to age 12–13, during which time, the upper molars, not yet constrained by an occlusal lock, continued to drift forward into a Class II relationship (Reproduced from Tsourakis et al. [13])

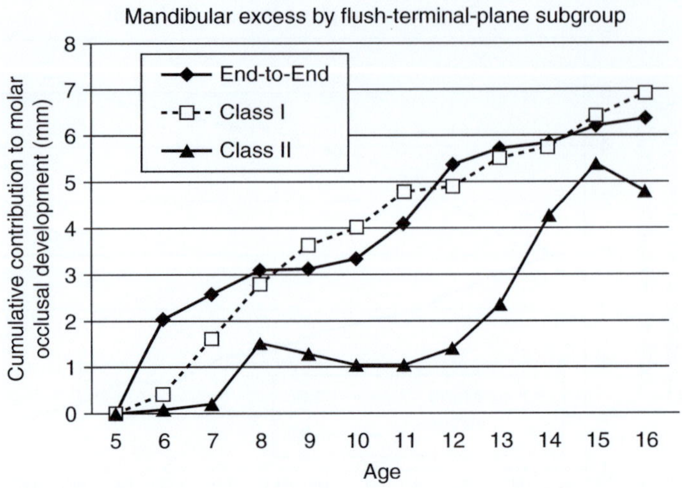

Fig. 3.5 Cumulative increments of mandibular excess from age 5 to 16 year in the three subgroups of the flush-terminal-plane group. Note the early (8–12 year) deficit in the mandibular excess for the Class II subgroup. This deficit is followed by what appears to be "catch-up" growth from ages 12–16. In the end, there were no significant among-groups differences in mandibular excess; the only difference was the timing (Reproduced from Tsourakis et al. [13])

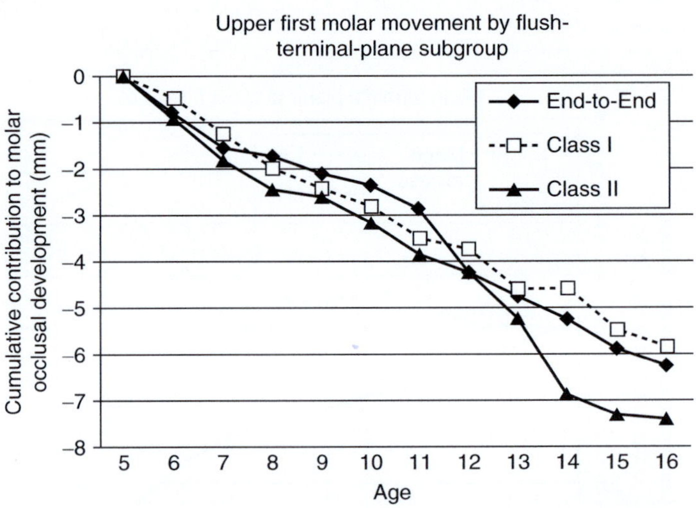

Fig. 3.6 Cumulative maxillary permanent first-molar mesial movement in the three subgroups of flush-terminal-plane subjects. Note the continuous mesial drift of the upper molars, with the greatest mesial drift seen in the Class II group from ages 13–16, apparently a dentoalveolar compensation for the mandibular "catch-up" growth depicted in Fig. 3.5 (Reproduced from Tsourakis et al. [13])

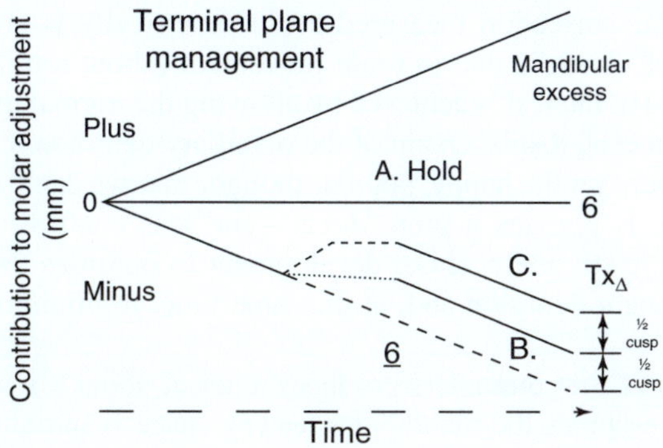

Fig. 3.7 Terminal plane management. In this diagrammatic summary of the present findings, mandibular excess and upper molar movement are depicted as being equal (presumably due to dentoalveolar compensation). *A*. Given any terminal plane, a major concern might be the preservation of lower leeway space by preventing mesial movement of the lower molars. Flush and distal-step terminal planes, however, require additional steps to achieve a Class I molar relationship. *B*. Flush terminal plane—the effect of a maxillary holding device (Nance button, pendulum, NiTi coils, Distal Jet, headgear, etc.) to produce a one-half cusp change by preventing maxillary dentoalveolar compensation. *C*. Distal step—U6 "distalization" (one-half cusp), plus a period in which the upper molars are prevented from compensating for an additional one-half cusp of normal mandibular excess. The total of *B* and *C* would produce a Class I/normal molar relationship (Reproduced from Tsourakis et al. [13])

Early Treatment

There are a host of so-called "early" treatments that jostle for attention in today's clinical marketplace. For many of these, there is no proof of efficacy beyond their impact on a practice's "bottom line." Perhaps the most popular treatment is a first phase of treatment by way of some sort of "functional" appliance. "Function" had meaning to Viggo Andresen; however, it is doubtful whether today's functional appliances are predicated on any particular concept or definition of function. Instead, all share one feature: they produce an instantaneous functional shift, but, in the long run, no "extra" growth. Given that the normal pattern of growth is favorable, this failure is no real problem. In the absence of a functional appliance, the excess mandibular growth will be rendered impotent by maxillary dentoalveolar compensation. Accordingly, by jumping the bite, a functional appliance would allow the usual mandibular excess to grow the condyles back into the fossae, thereby making the functional shift permanent [16]. By controlling the maxillary dentition, the long-term effect is seen in the midface, not the mandible (Fig. 3.7) [17, 18]. Those who have given up on growth modification now claim that a functional appliance correction is "dentoalveolar." Whereas growth modification seems to be wishful thinking, this alternative "explanation" is merely a substitute for evidence and careful thought.

The average molar correction measured cephalometrically is about 4 mm, only about a quarter of which is due to tooth movement (about a millimeter of lower anchorage loss [14]); the rest is achieved by allowing the normal mandibular excess to occur without mesial displacement of the maxillary dentition. Clearly, this interpretation casts doubt on the happy, popular thought that we can "grow mandibles." Fortunately, there is perhaps a more direct—and less controversial—method of interacting with growth and occlusal development to optimize the molar relationship in the permanent dentition and, at the same time, to minimize lower anterior crowing [19–22].

The extraction of first premolars produces a net of about 8 mm of space in the mandible. If one assumes the mandibular leeway space is initially about 6 mm, a lower lingual might be as much as 75 % efficient compared to later extraction. Given this approach, the importance of controlling the upper molars once again comes into play. For flush-terminal-plane and distal-step occlusions, the upper dentition must be held or "distalized" to permit the usual mandibular excess, no matter what its source, to produce a Cl I/Normal occlusion (Fig. 3.8). How? The options are almost endless: TADs, pendulum appliances, Nance buttons, HG, Distal Jets, etc. It is a practice management decision. Interestingly enough, countering or controlling upper dentoalveolar compensation also is a key feature of fixed-appliance Class II therapy in growing adolescents.

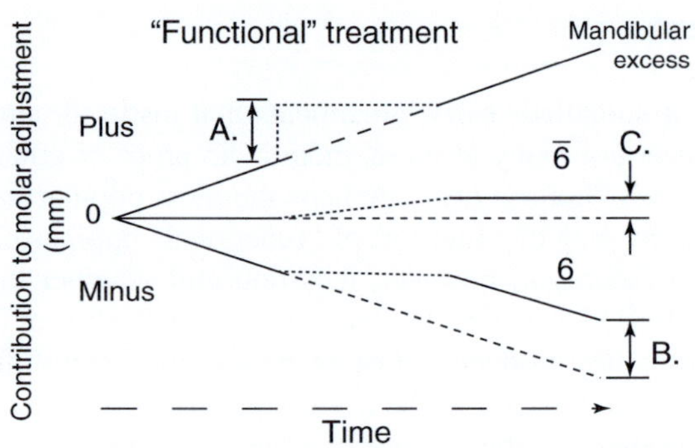

Fig. 3.8 Early treatment with functional appliances. *A*. Mandible advancement by the functional appliance (which advancement is assumed to have no impact on the normal, favorable pattern of growth). *B*. For a time, the usual excess condylar growth would produce no maxillary dentoalveolar compensation, thereby allowing the normal pattern of mandibular excess to produce a change in the occlusion. *C*. Lower anchorage loss, 1 mm or perhaps a bit more with Herbst treatment. The sum, $B + C$, more or less equals the changes required to convert a distal step/Class II to a Class I/normal occlusion. Both contemporary approaches to Class II treatment—two-stage and one—make use of the usual pattern of growth (mandible advancing relative to maxilla) by controlling maxillary dentoalveolar compensation. The choice between the two is a practice management decision, although the functional appliance probably would produce a slightly more protrusive dentition (Reproduced from Tsourakis et al. [13])

Fixed-Appliance Class II Treatment

By way of regional superimposition guided by Björk's implant studies, it is possible to estimate the various components of an extraction or nonextraction treatment. Serial superimposition in a wide variety of treatments shows that, in growing children, 50–75 % of the Class II correction is due to mandibular advancement relative to the midface. In the absence of treatment, the upper dentition will advance almost in lock step with this differential [14]. Fixed-appliance treatment interrupts this interaction, thus allowing the two dentitions to be moved independently of each other. Again, all roads lead to the maxilla.

In passing, it should be noted that the idea that bicuspids are extracted to achieve a molar correction is short-sighted and beside the point. Extraction and subsequent space closure—2 mm in the maxilla and 3 mm—produces only about 1 mm of net molar correction [14]; its real purpose is to alleviate crowding and reduce profile protrusion. A long-term comparison between first-bicuspid extraction and nonextraction in samples matched by discriminant analysis ("borderline"—discriminant scores near zero—by the standards of Saint Louis University in the 1960s and 1970s) showed that the average impact of extraction is a 2-mm "flatter" profile [23]. More pertinent to the present topic, fixed-appliance treatment uncouples the two dentitions so that maxillary anchorage loss is, on average, less than the usual excess mandibular displacement, thereby allowing "growth" to assist in correcting the molar relationship and in reducing the overjet. Nonextraction and bicuspid-extraction treatments, however, differ in terms of maxillary anchorage loss.

In the non-extraction treatments that I have studied [14], the mandibular excess is about 2 mm. Instead of going forward 2 mm, the uppers tend to be driven *distally* a millimeter or so by Cl II elastics and extra-oral traction; however, when bicuspids are extracted, maxillary space closure plus dentoalveolar compensation for the sum of mandibular excess and lower space closure (~3 mm) combines to overpower conventional Class II mechanics. As with nonextraction treatment, the upper dentition is, to a degree, shielded from the displacement of the lower. As a result, the 2 mm or so of upper-molar anchorage loss is less than might be expected, although this reduced loss is still highly correlated with growth intensity as inferred from the integration of growth curves [2] or actual mandibular excess measured from serial cephalograms [14]. Indeed, it is not until growth has more or less stopped that conventional mechanics can hold the upper molars in place. This observation is consistent with Prof. Xu's group's report that upper anchorage loss is a function of age and sex [9, 10]. Clearly, the use of TADs in growing children would ameliorate this anchorage problem and increase the probable speed of treatment. Finally, it must be noted that, in the absence of growth, the total molar correction tends to be diminished, presumably because it would be due entirely to tooth movement [14]. Therefore, the normal pattern of facial growth is a silent, important aid to the achievement of a Normal occlusion but only if its importance is recognized and its effects are used properly.

Conclusion

The purpose of this chapter was to discuss the importance of controlling maxillary anchorage in the development and management of Class II malocclusions. Indeed, I would argue that if one were to examine well-treated or managed Class II malocclusions, no matter what the treatment—fixed or functional; early or late—much of the success will have been achieved by controlling the position of the *upper* buccal segments, either by holding them against mesial dentoalveolar compensation or by actual distal movement. All roads lead to Rome; all roads to Class II prevention and correction lead through the upper dentition. *QED.*

References

1. Lande MJ (1952) Growth behavior of the human bony facial profile as revealed by serial cephalometric roentgenology. Angle Orthod 22:78–90
2. Johnston LE Jr (1998) Growth and the Class II patient: rendering unto Caesar. Semin Orthod 4:59–62
3. Bishara SE, Hoppens BJ, Jakobsen JR, Kohout FJ (1988) Changes in the molar relationship between the deciduous and permanent dentitions: a longitudinal study. Am J Orthod Dentofacial Orthop 93:19–28
4. Solow B (1980) The dentoalveolar compensatory mechanism. Br J Orthod 7:141–161
5. Steiner CC (1960) The use of cephalometrics as an aid to planning and assessing orthodontic treatment. Am J Orthod 46:721–735
6. Lundström A, McWilliam JS (1984) Dentoalveolar compensation for antero-posterior variations between the upper and lower apical bases. Eur J Orthod 6:116–122
7. Southard TE, Behrents RG, Tolley EA (1989) The anterior component of occlusal force, Part 1. Measurement and distribution. Am J Orthod Dentofacial Orthop 96:493–500
8. Southard TE, Behrents RG, Tolley EA (1990) The anterior component of occlusal force, Part 2. Relationship with dental alignment. Am J Orthod Dentofacial Orthop 97:41–49
9. Su H, Bing H, Li S, Na B, Ma W, Xu TM (2014) Factors predisposing to maxillary anchorage loss: A retrospective study of 1403 cases. PLoS One 9:e109561
10. Xu T-M, Zhang X, OH HS, Boyd RL, Korn EL, Baumrind S (2010) Randomized clinical trial comparing control of maxillary anchorage with 2 retraction techniques. Am J Orthod Dentofacial Orthop 138:544e1–544e9
11. McNamara JA Jr (1981) Components of a Class II malocclusion in children 8–10 years of age. Angle Orthod 51:177–202
12. Moorrees CFA, Grøn AM, Lebret LML, Yen PKJ, Fohlich FJ (1969) Growth studies of the dentition: A review. Am J Orthod 55:600–616
13. Tsourakis AK, Johnston LE Jr (2014) Class II malocclusion: the aftermath of a "perfect storm". Semin Orthod 20:59–73
14. Johnston LE Jr (1986) A comparative analysis of Class II treatments. In: Vig PS, Ribbens KA (eds) Science and clinical judgment in orthodontics, 19. Center for Human Growth and Development, Ann Arbor, pp Ć103–Ć148
15. Johnston LE Jr (1996) Balancing the books on orthodontic treatment: an integrated analysis of change. Br J Orthod 23:93–102
16. Johnston LE Jr (1996) Functional appliances: a mortgage on mandibular position. Aust Orthod J 14:154–156

17. Jakobsson SO (1967) Cephalometric evaluation of treatment effect on Class II, Division 1 malocclusions. Am J Orthod 53:446–457
18. Wieslander L (1993) Long-term effect of treatment with the headgear-Herbst appliance in the early mixed dentition. Stability or relapse? Am J Orthod Dentofacial Orthop 104:319–329
19. Gianelly AA (1995) Leeway space and the resolution of crowding in the mixed dentition. Semin Orthod 1:188–194
20. Gianelly AA (1998) A strategy for nonextraction Class II treatment. Semin Orthod 4:26–32
21. Dugoni SA, Lee JS, Varela J, Dugoni AA (1995) Early mixed dentition treatment: Postretention evaluation of stability and relapse. Angle Orthod 65:311–320
22. Dugoni SA (1998) Comprehensive mixed dentition treatment. Am J Orthod Dentofacial Orthop 113:75–84
23. Paquette DE, Beattie JR, Johnston LE Jr (1992) A long-term comparison of non-extraction and bicuspid-extraction edgewise therapy in "borderline" Class II patients. Am J Orthod Dentofacial Orthop 102:1–14

Concept of Physiologic Anchorage Loss

4

Tian Min Xu

Abstract

Anchorage loss is believed to be caused by reaction of orthodontic force in correcting malocclusion teeth. Traditional anchorage control is therefore applied when anchor molar is receiving such reaction. The measures to tip molar back before using them as anchorage is then called anchorage preparation in classical Tweed technique. However, more and more studies show anchorage loss relates to age, sex, treatment time, skeletal pattern, etc. in addition to orthodontic mechanics. Orthodontists should therefore look back at fundamental field in dentistry—Craniofacial Growth and Occlusion Development—rather than always pursue fancy brackets. This chapter collects all available information to us about physiologic characteristics of anchor molar during craniofacial growth, occlusal development, oral function, extraction orthodontic treatment, etc. The behavior of buccal teeth, the rhythm of physiologic anchorage loss during growth, and orthodontic treatment will be revealed by recent studies. The strategy of taking advantage of these physiologic characteristics for orthodontic anchorage control will be discussed.

Anchorage loss is represented typically by molar forward displacement during orthodontic extraction treatment. Orthodontists believe that's because of reaction force of retraction of anterior teeth. So the strategy of preventing molar anchorage loss is to resist the reaction force exerted on molar. And orthodontists believe if we can prevent molar forward movement less than 1/4 of premolar extraction space, we achieve maximum anchorage control. However, our prospective randomized

T.M. Xu
Department of Orthodontics, Peking University School and Hospital of Stomatology, Beijing, China
e-mail: tmxuortho@163.com

T.M. Xu (ed.), *Physiologic Anchorage Control*,
DOI 10.1007/978-3-319-48333-7_4

clinical trial showed upper molar moved forward 4.3 ± 2.1 mm on average with straight wire appliance even with headgear during 2.5 years' orthodontic treatment [1], much larger than the definition of maximum anchorage control in orthodontics. And Prof. Johnston's recent study [2] showed upper first molar moved forward about 2 mm during 12–14 years of age without orthodontic treatment (Figs. 3.1, 3.2, 3.3, and 3.4). We therefore infer that the molar forward displacement of 4.3 mm in our treatment sample may actually include two parts, one from reaction force of orthodontic appliance (mechanical anchorage loss) and the other from natural growth (a part of physiologic anchorage loss).

Why should we differentiate physiological anchorage loss and mechanical anchorage loss from the whole anchorage loss as we described in the traditional way?

Let's look at the features of these two kinds of anchorage loss, respectively. Firstly, we look at mechanical anchorage loss. It is believed to be caused by reaction force. As in four premolars extraction cases, when we use elastic force to retract anterior teeth, the reaction pulls posterior teeth forward, causing molar anchorage loss. To prevent this kind of anchorage loss, orthodontists use TPA or Nance bar to disperse the reaction on molars, use conventional headgear to resist the reaction on molars, or use TAD to detour the reaction to mini-screw implants. Now, we look at physiological anchorage loss. It's not so apparent to orthodontists as mechanical anchorage loss, because the force is not from appliance but from biological body.

Basically, there are probably three sources of biological force that may cause molar anchorage loss during extraction orthodontic treatment. The first is from craniofacial growth, the second is from occlusal force, and the third is from periodontal ligament.

Craniofacial Growth

From Chap. 3 by Prof. Johnston, we have realized upper molars go along with mandible forward growth. The amount of upper molar mesial movement approximates to mandible outgrowing maxilla in the most cases. That explains why Class II cannot correct itself to Class I. The most conceivable force for the above upper molar mesial movement is intercuspated force after establishment of occlusal contact. The other possible force also includes the eruption of second or third molars. Therefore the physiologic anchorage loss of upper molar during orthodontic treatment will mostly depend upon growth pattern of individuals and eruption time of posterior molars. Solow's metallic implant study [3] on upper molar growth demonstrated that individual's mandible rotation pattern counts for much. In Solow's study on a sample of 14 females by implant superimposition, upper molar moved about 8 mm downward and 3 mm forward on average from 9 to 25 years old. But one forward grower in his sample, upper molar grew forward more than 7 mm! What if in orthodontic case? Figure 4.1a shows 12-year-old girl with Class II facial profile before treatment in our prospective randomized clinical trial sample. She was extracted four first premolars and treated with MBT straight wire using headgear as anchorage. After 3 years of treatment, her face changed dramatically to a

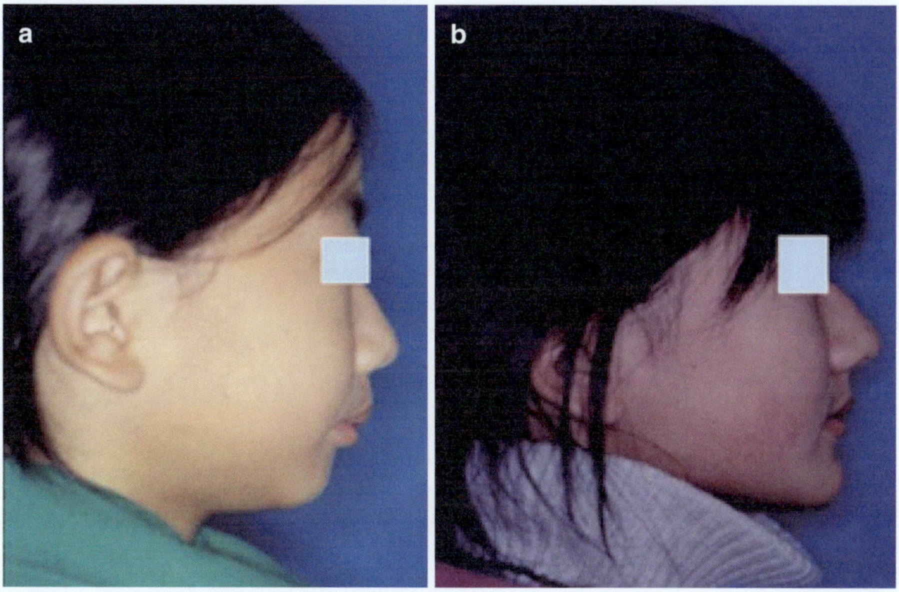

Fig. 4.1 (**a**, **b**) A 12-year-old girl treated with SWA

nice Class I (Fig. 4.1b). Our first impression is we have achieved very good anchorage control for her. But by best fit superimposition on maxilla, we measured her upper molar displaced 6 mm mesially (Fig. 4.2a), much larger than the maximum anchorage definition of 1/4 of premolar extraction space. Then why did her face improve so much in spite of the poor anchorage control? Superimposition on her anterior cranial base shows her mandible grew forward apparently (Fig. 4.2b) during orthodontic treatment. She is certainly a forward grower. If we suppose headgear can refrain molar from mesial movement less than 2 mm according to maximum anchorage control definition of less than 1/4 of a premolar extraction space, which, I believe, was based on the observation of adult orthodontic extraction cases, then her physiological anchorage loss is about 4 mm. Even in Johnston's normal growth pattern sample, the mesial movement of upper molar can reach 2 mm during 12–14 years of age. Since it amounts to the same order of magnitude of the traditional anchorage loss classification, we believe it's appropriate to differentiate it from the whole anchorage loss and define it as physiologic anchorage loss (PAL) and the rest mechanical anchorage loss (MAL).

Occlusal Force

The second biological force that might cause physiologic anchorage loss is the anterior component of occlusal force that is believed to be one of the major forces to keep tight interproximal contact between teeth in dentistry. The anatomical basis for this anterior component is probably due to the relationship among the orientation of masticatory muscle, the direction of functional occlusal plane and teeth

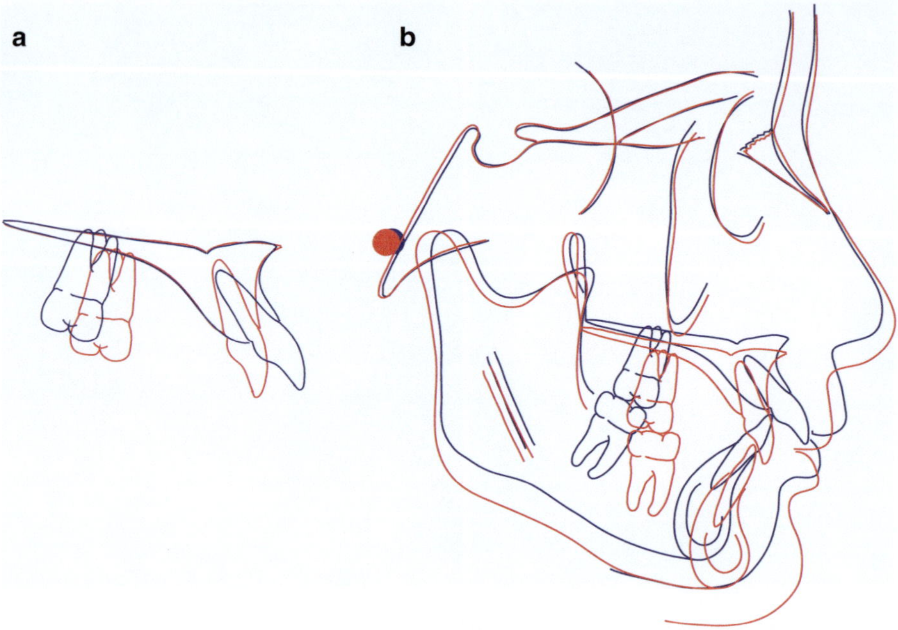

Fig. 4.2 (**a**, **b**) Superimposition shows upper molar lost 6 mm anchorage while mandible grew forward apparently

Fig. 4.3 Occlusal force coming from masticatory muscles

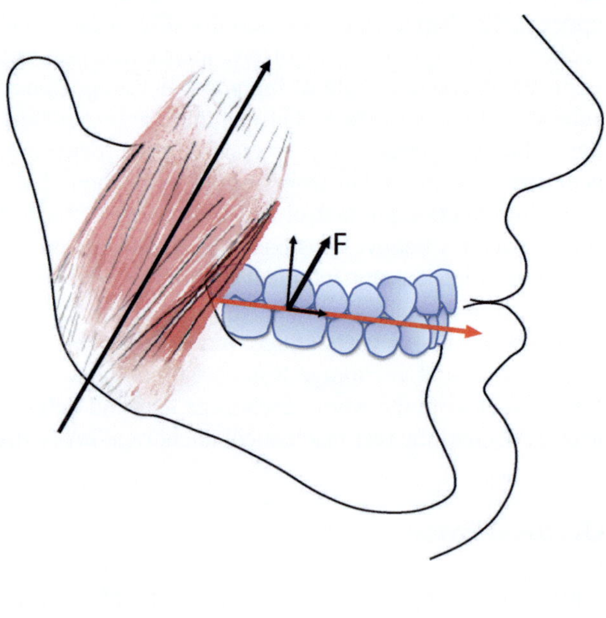

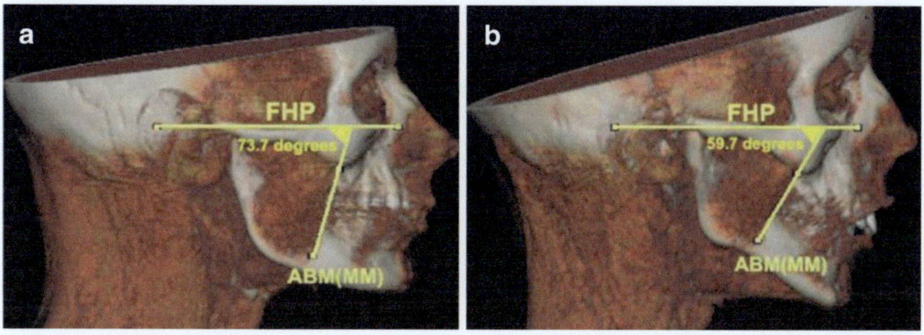

Fig. 4.4 Different orientation of superficial masseter muscle with different craniofacial morphology (Reprinted from Chan et al. [9] with permission from AJODO)

angulation (Fig. 4.3). When biting food, the occlusal force can be decomposed into a vertical force along the teeth axis and a horizontal force along the occlusal plane. By quantitative measurements on 15 subjects, Southard [4, 5] found an occlusal load of 20 pounds on the second molar could create 5 pounds of anterior component against the premolars and 1 pound against the canines, and this force crossed the dental midline and continued around the arch to the canine of the contralateral side in some subjects. Their experiments showed the distribution and dissipation of the anterior component of the occlusal force anteriorly approximated an exponential decay function. And some orthodontists [4–6] believe this anterior component can cause teeth forward tipping and therefore relates to anterior crowding or protrusion. If this is true, one can easily deduce that molars will lose anchorage by this physiologic force after extraction of premolar even without reaction of mechanical force from anterior teeth retraction. This can be easily approved by the observation of tilting toward extraction site of the neighboring teeth in patients of prosthodontic clinic. Weber's investigation on a sample of 54 cases aged 9.6 years on average showed that after first premolar enucleation for 2.5 years, upper first molar tipped forward 3° on average and mesially moved about one-half of the total space closure comparable to canine distal movement [7]. Robertson et al. even found that 91 % of the first premolar extraction space was taken up by the mesial movement of the molars without orthodontic appliance [8]. From the perspective of anchorage control, we may interpret it as molar tends to lose anchorage apparently after extraction of premolars even without receiving reaction force from orthodontic appliance. And the source of the occlusal force is from masticatory muscle. The orientation, strength, and location of these muscles are various. Figure 4.4 shows the different orientation of superficial masseter muscle [9], which is believed to associate with different craniofacial morphology. It's reasonably believed that the strength of the masticatory muscle determines the magnitude of occlusal force, and the orientation of the muscle affects the distribution ratio of its components on posterior teeth in axial and horizontal direction and therefore the inclination of posterior occlusal plane. Less anterior component and more axial component of occlusal force may save more anchorage in orthodontic extraction case.

Periodontal Ligament

In the aforementioned situation, although the anterior component of occlusal force can explain molar forward tipping and displacement into extraction space, it cannot explain why the teeth anterior to extraction site are drifting backward into the extraction space. Picton and Moss's studies [10–13] show transseptal fiber is another important source of teeth drifting. We will talk about teeth drifting more in Chap. 7.

The Strategy of Physiologic Anchorage Control

The common character of physiologic anchorage loss is that it is caused by continuous biologic force, in contrast to mechanical anchorage loss caused by orthodontic appliance. Because of that, headgear can't resist it enough time because it is only worn at night; TAD doesn't control it if it is only used to retract anterior teeth. The way that orthodontists perceive the pattern of anchorage loss dictates the strategy of our anchorage control.

If we perceive anchorage loss is solely caused by reaction of orthodontic force, we deal with retraction force only. For example, we use TPA or Nance bar to disperse the reaction on molars; we use headgear to resist the reaction on molars; or we use TAD to avoid loading molars with the reaction. So the strategy of preventing mechanical anchorage loss is as long as there is a reaction force on anchor molar, we apply a measure to resist it. If we perceive molar anchorage loss is in bodily movement pattern, we apply force to CRE of molar, for example, bending outer bow of cervical headgear upward 20° to let action line go through CRE of upper molar [14]. To deal with physiological anchorage loss, we need to know the pattern of physiological anchorage loss of upper molar at first. The metallic implant marked growth study by Bjork [15] showed upper molar tipped forward during growth. American implant study [16] showed the same pattern, implying a tip back moment may help.

If we perceive the anchorage loss is related to differential growth of maxilla and mandible, we will pay more attention to growth rhythm of craniofacial complex. To investigate how molar grows with jaws, we turned to a longitudinal craniofacial growth sample with metallic implants in AAOF craniofacial images legacy collection website curated by Sheldom Baumrind. Permitted by Prof. Baumrind, we measured 11 untreated individuals (seven males and four females) with more than six time points on the series of oblique films by implant superimposition, using functional occlusal plane (FOP) of 14 years old as reference plane. The reason we chose this age is that it is the age when all cases enter permanent dentition with premolars in occlusion in the sample. The results show upper molar tipped forward 6.7 ± 6.9°

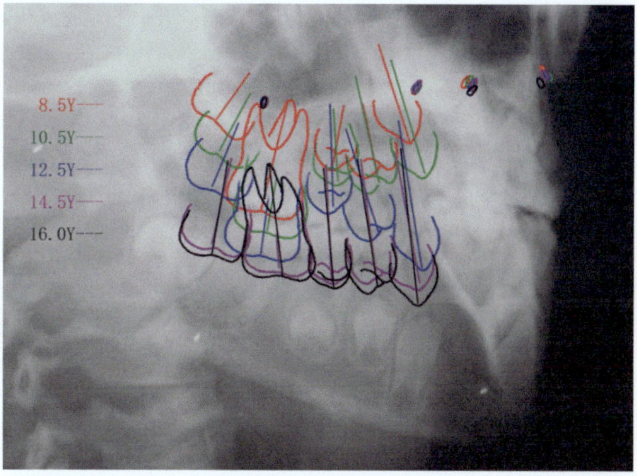

Fig. 4.5 Implant superimposition on oblique film

and the crown displaced forward 3.7 ± 1.1 mm along functional occlusal plane from 10–16 years of age. The peak velocity is 1.4 ± 0.7 mm/year during 12–14 years of age, implying that the most efficient period to prevent physiologic anchorage loss in this sample should be during 12–14 years of age, coinciding to the growth peak of mandible for male adolescence. The FOP/PP decreased 1.3 ± 4.4°. Figure 4.5 is maxillary implant's superimposition on oblique films showing growth pattern of buccal teeth of Case No. 1 in that sample.

When the rhythm is important in physiologic anchorage control, we investigated a longitudinal craniofacial growth sample collected in the Peking University School of Stomatology by Prof. Jiu-Xiang Lin. In this sample, 30 adolescents (ten males and 20 females) with individual normal occlusion were followed by taking cephalometric films from 10–14 years of age. These films were traced and superimposed using the method introduced by Johnston [17]. When the maxilla were superimposed, the U6 displacement and inclination relative to the functional occlusal plane (FOP) were measured. The results show that the mean forward tipping of U6 was 9.6 ± 3.5° and the mean mesial displacement of U6 was 5.1 ± 1.6 mm from 10 to 14 years old. Total FOP/PP decreased 1.3 ± 1.2° from 11 to 14 years old (missing FOP data at 10 years of age because most of premolars have not erupted yet). During the 4 years we observed, the peak growth period happened during 10–12 years of age. U6 tipped forward 6.1 ± 3.0° and displaced mesially 3.0 ± 1.2 mm in these 2 years. The peak velocity for U6 mesial displacement is 1.6 ± 0.7 mm/year during 10–12 years of age, implying that the most efficient period to prevent physiologic anchorage loss in this sample should be during 10–12 years of age, coinciding to the growth peak of mandible for female adolescents. The differences between the Chinese sample and American sample may come from sample sizes, male and female ratio, projection angles (oblique vs. lateral), and races. The further study on larger samples will certainly provide more useful information on physiologic anchorage loss rhythm. In this sense, the craniofacial image legacy collection project supported by AAOF (www.AAOFLegacyCollection.org) may play an important role for future anchorage control method.

If we perceive the anchorage loss is from anterior component of occlusal force, we may turn our attention to bite force. Although we are not sure if we can utilize the force of masticatory muscles to enhance anchorage control right now, there are some indirect evidence to support this possibility. The most obvious one is the common sense that molar anchorage is stronger in low angle case than high angle case. Alexander's study shows either intra-arch or inter-arch obstacle affects teeth movement [18]. From this perspective, occlusal force may enhance molar anchorage by increasing the inter-arch obstruction. Antonarakis et al. studied the relationship between maximum bite force/masseter muscle thickness and the functional appliance treatment outcomes in Class II[1] malocclusion children and found children with lower pretreatment maximum molar bite force showed more mesial movement of mandibular first molars, distal movement of maxillary first molars, and larger change in molar relationship during treatment. They conclude children with thinner pretreatment masseter muscles or weaker bite force show greater dentoalveolar changes [19]. Although it's not practical to strengthen whole masticatory muscle force to enhance molar anchorage in extraction treatment, it is possible to decrease the anterior component of occlusal force and increase axial component to increase inter-arch obstruction by tipping molar back to the angle approximate to the direction of resultant of masticatory muscle force. From this point of view, tipping posterior teeth back in Tweed and Begg techniques may save more anchorage than leveling upper arch in straight wire appliance.

If we perceive the physiologic anchorage loss is caused by continuous biological force, we may use a continuous gentle force or moment to stop it. The most possible material to provide such a force or moment is NiTi wire. We will introduce how to take advantage of this special material to prevent physiologic anchorage loss in next chapters. If we perceive this continuous gentle force is from periodontal ligament, we may provide molar a light continuous moment to prevent it from forward tipping and lower the friction on canine so it may drift back along the archwire without anchorage loading on molar. The mechanics of achieving this controlled drifting will be discussed in the Chaps. 6 and 7.

When we recognize the dentition is a dynamic and functional biologic body, not just a static object, and its surrounding tissues also provide biologic force on it, anchorage control may shift its paradigm again from relying on mechanical force only to partly relying on mechanical force and partly on physiological force. Controlling physiologic anchorage loss by preventing molar from forward tipping during growth and function may keep molar in relative backward tipping position in aligning stage of orthodontic extraction treatment. And when we progress to the space closing stage and use molars to retract anterior teeth, they may work like anchorage prepared as in Tweed technique (refer to classical anchorage control in the first chapter).

Acknowledgment The work was supported, in part, by International Science & Technology Cooperation Program of China No. 2014DFA31800.

References

1. Xu TM, Zhang X, Oh HS et al (2010) Randomized clinical trial comparing control of maxillary anchorage with 2 retraction techniques. Am J Orthod Dentofacial Orthop 138(5):544 e1–9
2. Tsourakis AK, Johnston LE Jr (2014) Class II malocclusion: The aftermath of a "perfect storm". Semin Orthod 20(1):59–57
3. Iseri H, Solow B (1996) Continued eruption of maxillary incisors and first molars in girls from 9 to 25 years, studied by the implant method. Eur J Orthod 18:245–256
4. Southard TE, Behrents RG, Tolley EA (1989) The anterior component of occlusal force, part 1: Measurement and distribution. Am J Orthod Dentofacial Orthop 96:493–500
5. Southard TE, Behrents RG, Tolley EA (1990) The anterior component of occlusal force, part 2: Relationship with dental alignment. Am J Orthod Dentofacial Orthop 97:41–49
6. Dewel BF (1949) Clinical observations on the axial inclination of teeth. Am J Orthod 35:98–115
7. Weber AO (1969) A longitudinal analysis of premolar enucleation. Am J Orthod 56:394–402
8. Robertson NAE, Cavina R, Moss JP (1979) The effect of the extraction of lower first premolars on the migration of teeth in the human dental arch. J Dent Res 58:1252–1256
9. Chan HJ, Woods MG, Stella DL (2008) Mandibular muscle morphology in children with different vertical facial patterns: A 3-dimensional computed tomography study. Am J Orthod Dentofacial Orthop 133(1):10 e1–13
10. Picton DCA, Moss JP (1973) The part played by the transseptal fiber system in experimental approximal drift of the cheek teeth in monkeys (Macaca irus). Arch Oral Biol 18:669–680
11. Moss JP, Picton DCA (1974) The effect on approximal drift of cheek teeth of dividing mandibular molars of adult monkeys (Macaca irus). Arch Oral Biol 19:1211–1214
12. Picton DCA, Moss JP (1978) The effect of reducing cusp height on the rate of approximal drift of cheek teeth in adult monkeys (Macaca irus). Arch Oral Biol 23:219–223
13. Picton DCA, Moss JP (1980) The effect on approximal drift of altering the horizontal component of biting force in adult monkeys (macaca irus). Arch Oral Biol 25:45–48
14. Melsen B, Dalstra M (2003) Distal molar movement with Kloehn headgear: Is it stable? Am J Orthod Dentofacial Orthop 123:374–378
15. Bjork A, Skieller V (1972) Facial development and tooth eruption. An implant study at the age of puberty. Am J Orthod 62(4):339–383
16. Baumrind S, Ben-Bassat Y, Bravo LA et al (1996) Partitioning the components of maxillary tooth displacement by the comparison of data from three cephalometric superimpositions. Angle Orthod 66:111–124
17. Johnston LE, Xu TM, Teng QM (2011) Johnston's cephalometrics handbook, Peking University Medical Press
18. Alexander D, Catherine G, Stavros KG (2013) Factors related to the rate of orthodontically induced tooth movement. Am J Orthod Dentofacial Orthop 143:616–621
19. Antonarakis GS, Kiliaridis S (2015) Predictive value of masseter muscle thickness and bite force on Class II functional appliance treatment: a prospective controlled study. Eur J Orthod 37(6):570–557

Mechanical Properties of Various Archwires and Their Clinical Application in the PASS System

5

Ching-Chang Ko, Si Chen, and Haiping Zhang

Abstract

Clinical studies have revealed that maxillary molar mesialization could occur in physiological drifting and during orthodontic treatment. The straight wire appliance (SWA) using a continuous wire made of shape memory alloy (SMA) might result in an undesired maxillary molar mesialization or an anchorage loss in the initial aligning stage. Recent findings suggest that a maxillary molar tube including a –25° auxiliary tube might minimize this anchorage loss. It was theorized that this auxiliary tube serving as a reserved v bend could preclude the possibility of molar mesialization in SWA. This chapter introduces the clinical implications of this new appliance, called the PASS system. The archwire sequence for the PASS is similar to that of SWA, except that the –25° auxiliary tube is only used for SMA at the initial stage. The mechanical properties of various material types of archwires associated with the PASS system are reviewed. Analysis was completed on the interactions between the archwire and the PASS system, such as the stress-strain relationship and frictional forces. Both low-friction and distalization forces are revealed from our data.

C.-C. Ko (✉)
Department of Orthodontics, University of North Carolina, Chapel Hill, NC 27599-7450, USA
e-mail: Ching-Chang_Ko@unc.edu

S. Chen
Department of Orthodontics, Peking University School and Hospital of Stomatology, Beijing, China
e-mail: elisa02chen@gmail.com

H. Zhang
Beijing Stomatological Hospital, Capital Medical University, Beijing, China
e-mail: haiping@email.unc.edu

T.M. Xu (ed.), *Physiologic Anchorage Control*,
DOI 10.1007/978-3-319-48333-7_5

Anterior-posterior control of the inter-arch relationship is one of the essential procedures in orthodontic treatment. There are numerous means for molar distalization including headgear, Herbst, Xbow, Forsus, elastics, molar tip-back bend, pendulum, temporary skeletal anchorage, etc. Molar anchorage not only represents an important biomechanical modality in Class II treatment but also is a manifest mechanical control in the Class I patient. Unfortunately, during adolescent growth and development, physiological mesial drift of maxillary molars has been demonstrated in non-treated, healthy individuals. It is hypothesized that molar mesial drift may be partially attributed to occlusal force-induced mesialization movement and changes in arch length over time [1, 2]. Arch length (defined as the perpendicular distance from a line joining the mesial of the first permanent molars or distal of the second primary molars and the incisal edge of the central incisors) is influenced by significant events during the transition from the primary to the permanent dentition [3]. Arch length decreases as space is lost due to early mesial shift and closing of posterior Leeway spaces. There is an anchorage loss associated with the change in arch length up to 18 years of age in a normally developing individual.

Historically, Tweed and Begg used a tip-back bend of stainless steel (SS) wires to prevent molar mesialization and to maximize anchorage [4]. The tip-back technique with loops was an important part of the orthodontic technique in the 1960s–1980s. On the contrary, the modern straight wire appliance (SWA) initiates with a continuous wire of shape memory alloys (SMA) that tends to yield mesial tipping of molar crowns due to the positive angulation of the molar tube, curve of Spee, and upper molar backward tipping compensation to distal mandible et al [5]. Thus, SWA can result in an undesired tooth movement in the initial stage (Stage 1). To rescue SWA's disadvantage, many clinicians have applied a tip-back bend in the second stage of the treatment. However, some of anchorage loss in Stage1 is irreversible. Recently, temporary anchorage device (TAD) use has become a popular means for anchorage control [6–9]. Although TAD provides a great anchorage, there are a few drawbacks: (1) the method requires alignment and leveling in the premolar/molar region prior to the TAD placement; there is a potential anchorage loss before TAD installation; and (2) it involves additional costs and surgical procedures. Most recently, Xu added a –25° auxiliary tube into a maxillary molar tube [10]; he theorizes that this auxiliary tube acting as a reserved v bend can preclude the possibility of molar mesialization in SWA. Historically, Level Anchorage bands (Unitek) were designed with the Tweed technique without the need for the second-order bends that were an important part of the original technique used in the mandible [11]. The XBT Buccal Tube (abbreviated XBT) (Fig. 5.1) instead focuses on maxillary anchorage [10]. The clinical implication, wire elasticity, and biomechanics of the XBT system will be discussed and reviewed in the following sections.

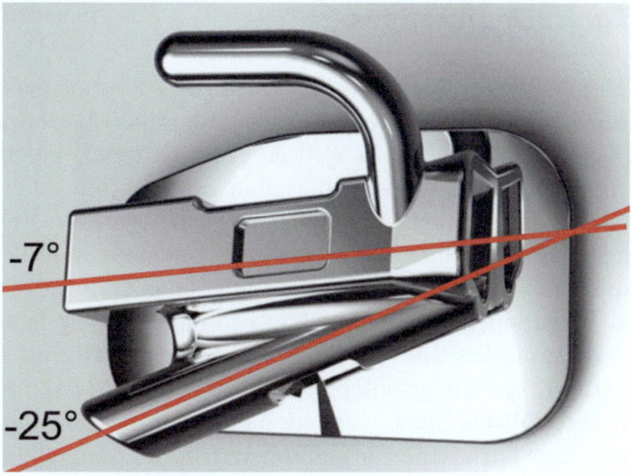

Fig. 5.1 XBT buccal tube (Reproduced from Chen et al. [10])

Clinical Implication of the PASS System

Biomechanical Designs of the PASS System

The PASS system is composed of two parts, the XBT and the multilevel low-friction (MLF) bracket, which emphasize the effectiveness of the interaction between the brackets and archwires [10].

The XBT consists of a –7° main tube and a –25° tip-back auxiliary tube. Two tubes cross at the mesial end, analogous to the letter X, and thus the inventor calls it XBT to differentiate it from the existing parallel buccal tube designs. Unlike the mainstream molar tube which has positive degrees of tipping prescription (e.g., +5° for SWA), negative degrees were designed into XBT to enhance molar anchorage by preventing it from mesial tipping. The initial archwire will be inserted into the tip-back tube, thereby creating a protection moment for molar anchorage from the very beginning of the treatment. With this design, it is therefore expected that crown distal tipping can be reinforced even with the use of very light NiTi wire and without any wire bending.

The MLF bracket has a cervical constriction which can hold the ligature tie and stop it from compressing the archwire; hence reduction of the normal force shall result in low friction in the alignment stage. When the archwire progresses gradually to a larger size, the ligature tie will touch the archwire and generate the proper constrained force for better expression of the prescribed design of the bracket. In addition to this different prescription versus other bracket systems, the slot size is set as 0.020″ for incisors for better torque control and 0.022″ for the rest of the teeth for improved sliding mechanics.

Clinical Implications

The PASS technique can be used for any kind of malocclusions and is especially suitable for all extraction cases including Class I severe crowding, Class II increased overbite and overjet, as well as Class III cases. For the Class I severe crowding cases, alignment can be achieved in a shorter time due to the low-friction characteristic of the brackets. In low-friction environments, gentle force from lip pressure and tissue regeneration in extraction wounds may be utilized to facilitate tooth movement. Due to the unique design of the XBT, the moment generated on the labially positioned canine (which is a common finding in anterior crowding cases) will result in guided distal drift of the canines without the use of laceback. Simultaneously, posterior anchorage will be preserved while anterior crowding is relieved. For Class II deep OB/OJ cases, prevention of molar mesial tipping indubitably enhances the posterior anchorage for anterior retraction. Meanwhile, engaging the initial NiTi wire used for alignment from the gingival direction into the anterior brackets will be helpful to open the anterior overbite from the very beginning. The double-tube design also facilitates the early use of a piggyback wire during alignment to control the upper incisor vertical position and assist bite opening in deep bite cases. For Class III cases, reinforcement of upper molar anchorage could ensure both the efficient use of the extraction space for anterior alignment and enough anchorage provided for inter-maxillary Class III elastics. For periodontally compromised cases, the light force generated and distributed by the PASS system will be helpful to reposition the teeth without overloaded periodontal burden.

These biomechanical assumptions of PASS remain to be tested. Some of the theoretical predictions will be discussed later in this chapter. The following case (Figs. 5.2, 5.3, and 5.4), perhaps, reveals clinical effects of the device.

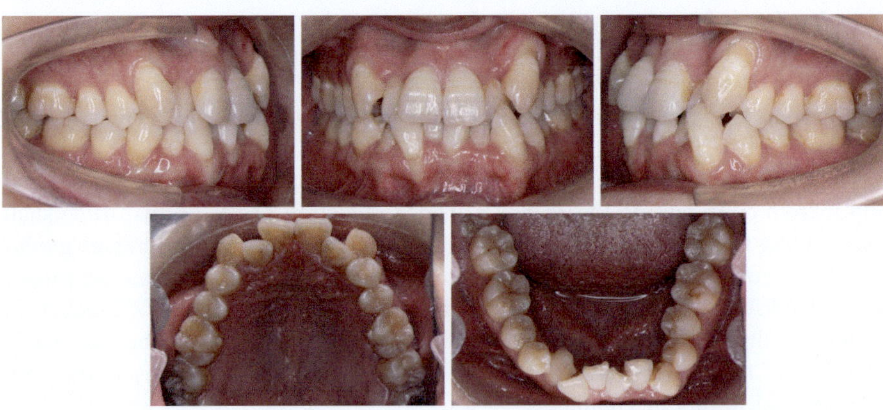

Fig. 5.2 A PASS case illustration. Case description: a 33yearold female presented with the chief complaint of crooked teeth. The patient had a Class I malocclusion with severe anterior crowding of 10 and 8 mm in maxillary and mandibular dentition, respectively. Two maxillary lateral incisors were in crossbite. Chronic periodontitis-related gingival recession was found, with buccal bone loss of the maxillary canines (Reproduced from Chen et al. [10])

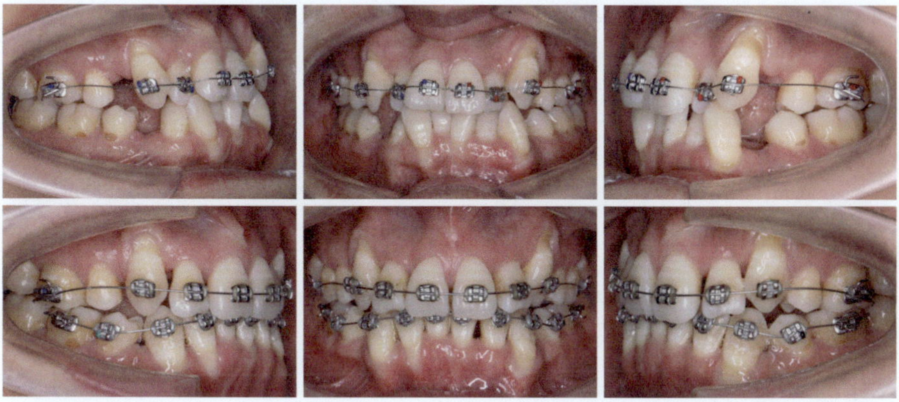

Fig. 5.3 0.014″ NiTi wire was inserted into the tip-back tube of the XBT to facilitate canine distal drift and anterior alignment. Note the XBT technique skipped the premolar, and the wire connected the canine to the molar directly. Six months later, initial upper dentition alignment was achieved using 0.016″ NiTi wire, without periodontal deterioration. Mild upper molar tip-back could be noticed (Reproduced from Chen et al. [10])

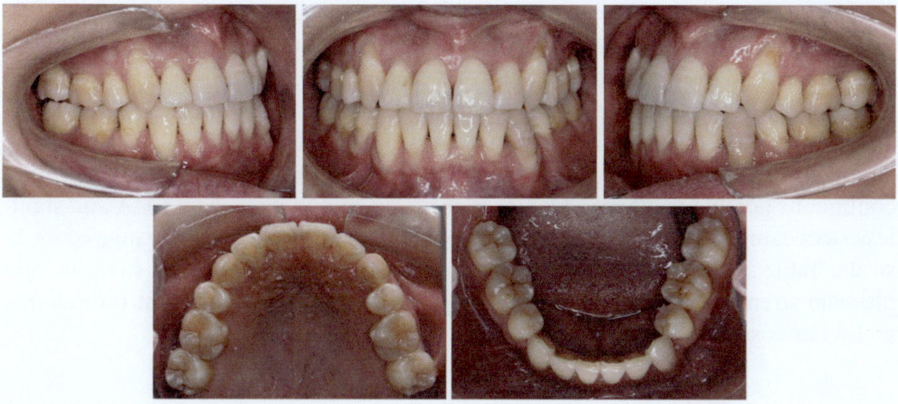

Fig. 5.4 Posttreatment results showed the upper molar position was well maintained, and the extraction space was efficiently used without any other anchorage reinforcement device (Reproduced from Chen et al. [10])

Progress of Biomechanical Effects

After routine periodontal treatment and inflammation control, four first premolars were extracted to provide space for orthodontic movement. The light force NiTi wires with the XBT and MLF were initially used to align the periodontal compromised teeth. Distal drift of the canine, molar anchorage, and incisal upright were observed by the use of PASS techniques (Figs. 5.3 and 5.4). If using conventional SWA brackets and tubes a canine laceback or tieback is needed to pull canine back to relieve anterior crowding, which might accompany a loss of molar anchorage

Table 5.1 Mechanical properties of various archwire materials

	E (GPa)	WR (%)	σ_{yl} (MPa)	σ_{ult} (MPa)
Stainless steel (SS)	191	0.9	1760	1351
Elgiloy (Co-Cr)	205	0.7	1558	1795
TMA (β-titanium)	69	1.3	885	1250
Au	70	<1	209	334
Classic SMA	37	6	455	754
Austenite active SMA	50	10	690	895
Martensitic active SMA	50	10	140	895

SMA Shape memory alloy, *E* Young's modulus, *WR* working range in strain unit, σyl yield strength, σult ultimate tensile strength [13–18]

[12]. Another approach was to segment the wire at the incisor section; this method may require a longer treatment time and still requires some sort of anchorage accessories.

Mechanical Properties of Archwires

An advantage of the PASS system as demonstrated in the above case is the distalization force and moment at the XBT-bonded molar. Within the elastic range, the molar and canine hold the archwire and act in a manner of an inverted v bend. The elastic rebound of the archwire results in distal molar crown tipping. The –25° tube is designed to work with the NiTi archwire that has a great elastic range of 6–10 % strain. The system suits the contemporary orthodontic technique of applying initial continuous flexible archwires. However, the rigid archwires such as TMA and stainless steel cannot be used for the –25° tube due to their limited elastic range of <1 % strain. Table 5.1 shows the Young's modulus, elongation range, yield strength, and ultimate strength of various alloys. Comparative analysis of different orthodontic archwires is summarized below.

Linear Elastic Material [19]

The conventional, non-shape memory alloys (CA) possess a linear elastic behavior followed by plastic deformation as depicted in Fig. 5.5. The typical orthodontic CAs are stainless steel (SS), TMA (β-titanium), Elgiloy (Co-Cr), and gold alloys. The basic characteristics of the CA are low elastic range, high stiffness, high yield strength, and high formability, with few exceptions (e.g., Au). The elastic range of the CAs is typically less than 1 % strain, which allows the small working range for initial alignment. Unfortunately, the orthodontic patient usually presents a high irregular tooth position yielding a high strain (deformation >1 %) in a straight wire once engaged. In the past, the orthodontist would form

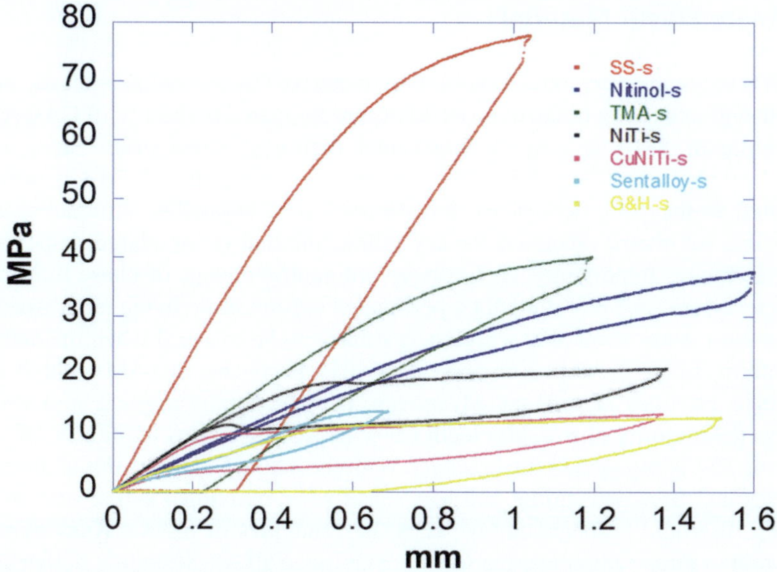

Fig. 5.5 The stress-deflection plots of three-point bending and unbending data for various metallic orthodontic archwires. The stainless steel (*SS*) and TMA show a typical linear elastic behavior followed by plasticity with unrecoverable deformation. All shape memory alloys (*Nitinol*, *NiTi*, *CuNiTi*, *Sentalloy*, and *G&H NiTi*) show nonlinear elastic behavior with full recovery of deformation

loops for CAs to increase elastic range, which is technically challenging and time consuming. The modern orthodontic approaches tend to avoid loops and instead use flexible NiTi of high work range for aligning and leveling. Another feature of the CA is its high stiffness that possesses the property of a high Young's modulus. The higher the archwire stiffness is, the greater the generated force and stress is by the same amount of deformation. SS and Co-Cr provide greater force values than TMA. The gold alloy yields the lowest force level. As such, SS, Elgiloy, and TMA with high stiffness are used in sliding mechanics for space closure. Recently, 0.018″ SS, 0.016 × 0.022″ SS, 0.017 × 0.025″ SS, and TMA have been frequently utilized in space closure. The highly stiff archwire with the greater dimensions and greater Young's modulus could minimize the adverse dumping effect of the teeth adjacent to the extracted tooth space. In the PASS, the CAs can only insert to the –7° tube for the Stage 2 mechanics; it will cause permanent deformation of the archwire or bracket debonding if the wire was enforced to the –25° tube in the initial stage (this will be illustrated later in our simulation data). Finally, the CA has high ductility. Once yielding, the material will undergo plastic deformation with a high percentage of elongation (~50 %) before breakage. Because of high formability, the CAs have been used to form closing loops and finishing bends.

Nonlinear Elastic Materials

The NiTi shape memory alloy (SMA) is characterized by its nonlinear elastic behavior with a greater work range of 6–10 % strains compared to the 1 % of CAs. A typical feature of SMA is a nearly horizontal region of stress-strain curve, called superelastic behavior (Fig. 5.5) [20]. The nonlinear elasticity of SMA is primarily attributed to the congruent phase transformation of crystalline structures, which results in a volumetric change in the crystalline unit that yields a large shape change of the archwire. Importantly, such a large volumetric change of phase transformation is reversible and therefore not a permanent deformation. In the other word, this deformation stores reversible work energy that will be released when the deformation returns. In 1973, Andreasen and Barret [21] discovered that SMA's high working range provides significant advantages in orthodontic aligning and leveling because the majority of irregular teeth cause exceeding strains in the AW, of >1 %, when the AW is engaged to the brackets. With the use of SMA, the initial alignment becomes less time consuming and less sensitive to individual skills, such as wire bending. It would be beneficial to learn the principles of SMAs. Kusy classified SMA into to three categories: martensitic-stabilized alloys, austenitic-active alloys, and martensitic-active alloys [22, 23].

Martensitic-Stabilized Alloys This material is a nonsuperelastic NiTi alloy containing substantial quantities of heavily cold-worked and stable martensite. The alloy has a high austenitic transformation temperature, much greater than the temperature of the oral environment. The stress-strain curve of this material is nearly linear without exhibiting a flat region because of the lack of a phase transformation. Nevertheless, the material possesses a lower modulus and a greater working range (~6 % strain) than that of CAs. The first NiTi wire, Nitinol, was introduced by Andreasen and belongs to this category, which has become one important landmark in the contemporary SWA [24]. In most irregularly positioned teeth, Nitinol can easily engage to the brackets. However, in severe malposition (e.g., rotation), special tools are required to tie the Nitinol due to its relatively stiffer stress-strain behavior versus the other two SMAs.

Austenitic-Active Alloys The alloy starts with austenitic NiTi phase and undergoes a stress-induced martensitic (SIM) transformation [14]. The constitutive law of the stress-strain relationship reveals a superelastic behavior – a flat region with a nearly zero slope. The superelastic wire displays a large deformation (up to 10 % strain) at a constant stress with a return to 0 % deformation (austenitic phase) upon fully unloading. The adaptation of wire to the malpositioned teeth is easier than that of Nitinol. Examples are Nitinol SE and Sentalloy wires.

Martensitic-Active Alloys The alloy's shape memory is subject to the thermoelastic effect [25, 26]. The archwire is initially in the martensitic phase at room temperature. In the oral environment, the temperature raises and deforms the wire

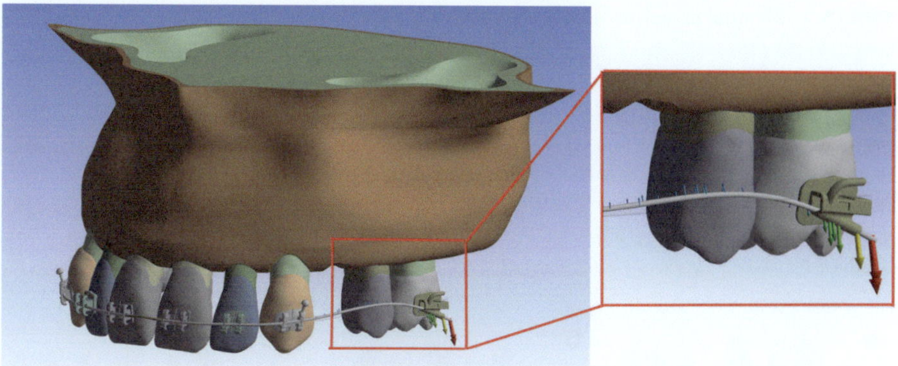

Fig. 5.6 CAD model showing XBT molar tube and a round archwire going into the –25° tube. The model is adapted from FJORD model created by the author [14]

through the austenitic phase transformation. Similar to the Sentalloy, this type of wire exhibits a flat region in stress-strain behavior. The wire is extremely flexible (dead soft) in cool conditions, which allows engagement to severely rotated or displaced teeth, and becomes rigid (modulus ~50–70 GPa) in the mouth. The rigid phase wire can generate enough forces and moments for aligning and leveling, although the force magnitude generated usually is the lowest among the three types of SMA. The high working range can go up to 10 % strain. Examples are CuNiTi and Neo Sentalloy.

Biomechanics of AWs in the XBT Tube

A half maxillary finite element model (Fig. 5.6) was constructed to simulate biomechanics of the PASS system for initial aligning and leveling. The model consists of ten teeth with enamel, dentin and pulp, PDL, trabecular and cortical bone, 0.022″ brackets, and archwires. The CAD program SolidWorks was used to construct parts from geometry files (e.g., .iges, .step) of the solid model obtained by CT or μCT [27]. The .iges model was then imported to Ansys for element automeshing. Forces applied to the dentition and surrounding structures were simulated utilizing the birth-death technique as described in our previous publication [28]. Briefly, to simulate the insertion of an active archwire to the –25° XBT tube, a two-step computer technique was utilized. First, displacement of the wire into the tube removes/deactivates the overlap with the bracket and loads stored energy in the wire and adjacent teeth. Second, the deactivated elements of the contact area were reactivated and the elastic rebound of the deformed wire was acting on the molar. The convergence was confirmed for computation. The three archwires investigated were the 0.014″ CuNiTi, 0.016″ CuNiTi, and 0.016″ SS. The virtual XBT was used. The interfaces between the wire and the brackets and tooth-tooth interfaces were simulated as contact interface. Table 5.2 shows the material

Table 5.2 Material properties used in the FEM

	Young's modulus (GPa)	Poisson's ratio
Enamel	84.1	0.33
Dentin	18.3	0.31
Pulp	0.002	0.45
Periodontal ligament	Mooney-Rivlin constitutive constants [26]	
Lamella dura	15.0	0.33
Cortical Bone	15.0	0.30
Cancellous Bone	0.25	0.30

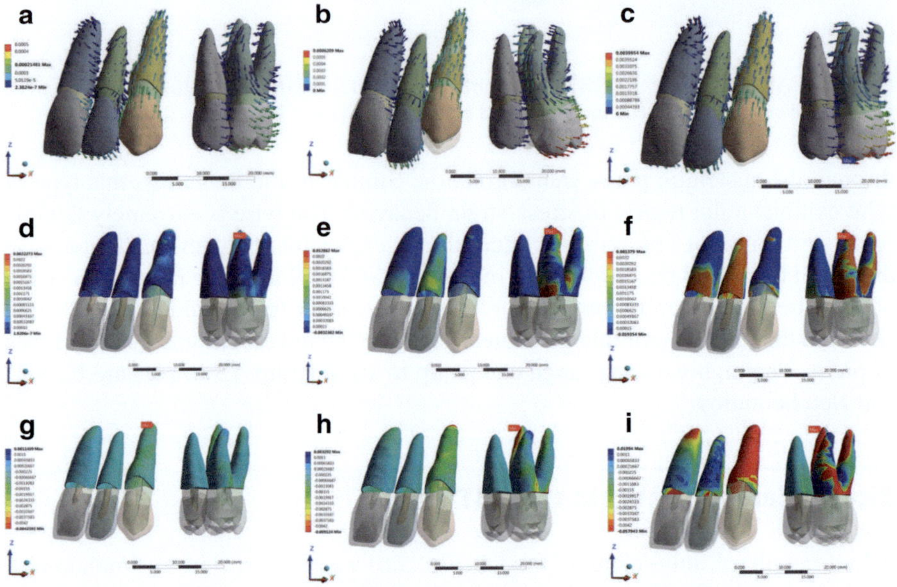

Fig. 5.7 Results of the FEA. Top row shows displacement vectors with deformation of the teeth. (**a**) 0.014″ CuNiTi; (**b**) 0.016″ CuNiTi; (**c**) 0.016″ SS. Middle row shows maximum principal stress distribution of (**d**) 0.014″ CuNiTi; (**e**) 0.016″ CuNiTi; and (**f**) 0.016″ SS. Bottom row shows minimum principal stress distribution of (**g**) 0.014″ CuNiTi; (**h**) 0.016″ CuNiTi; and (**i**) 0.016″ SS

properties used for the present FEM. The Mooney-Rivlin hyperelastic property was assigned to the periodontal ligament as described in the literature [29–31]. Stress distribution and deformation vectors through the dentition and surrounding tissue were calculated and compared.

The results showed that the XBT design yielded a distal molar crown rotation, a canine intrusion, and an incisor retraction and extrusion (Fig. 5.7). Some, but not all, of the predictions agreed with the tooth movement of the clinical case. The predictions of molar anchorage and incisor retraction and extrusion could be supported by the clinical data. The canine distal drifting, however, could not be proven. It is possible that the vertical position and angulation of the malpositioned canine

Table 5.3 Reaction force and displacement on the maxillary molar (UL6) and the maxillary canine (UL3) and maximum equivalent stress on wire

	0.014″ NiTi	0.016″ NiTi	0.016″ SS
Reaction force on UL6 bracket	0.060933 N	0.11848 N	0.79004 N
Max deformation UL6	0.1517×10^{-8} m	6.209×10^{-8} m	39.95×10^{-8} m
Max deformation UL3	1.374×10^{-8} m	2.716×10^{-8} m	171.7×10^{-8} m
Equivalent stress on wire	247.4 MPa	312.2 MPa	2077.3 MPa

in the clinical case may affect the predictions and transseptal fiber force was not simulated in this model. The magnitude of the displacement was proportional to Young's modulus and wire size: 0.016″ SS > 0.016″ CuNiTi > 0.014″ CuNiTi. Similar to the displacement, stress values were also proportional to the modulus and the wire size. The general pattern showed that the compressive stresses were concentrated at the mesial root tip and distal alveolar crest of the molar, which would induce bone resorption. On the contrary, the high tensile stresses were located on the distal root tip and mesial alveolar crest leading bone formation. The prediction of the –25° auxiliary tube for initial aligning and leveling showed preliminary promise of molar anchorage (distal rotation). However, our prediction implied an intrusive movement of the canine with minimum rotation. Note that our simulation bracket used zero prescription, which might not be appropriately representing the actual tipping effect that required a future investigation. Other effects as observed in the clinical case, including lingual and extrusive movement of the incisors, were also supported by the FEA. The FEM provides indeterminate biomechanical analysis for assessment of the XBT design beyond the simplified v bend theory [32].

One important outcome via our FEA indicated that the 0.016″ SS was not suitable material to be used for the –25° tube. The peak von Mises stress on the wire was 2077 MPa (Table 5.3) and exceeded the yield strength of the steel [33–35]. It is reasonable to believe the tube will debond before the wire gets deformed. The net force acting on the XBT molar by the 0.016″ SS again showed an extraordinary high value of 800 g. The SS may be used after initial alignment but not at the beginning.

Frictional Effect Between the AW and the MLF Bracket

The design of the PASS multilevel low-friction (MLF) brackets is expected to prevent ligatures from pressing the archwire (Fig. 5.8). It was assumed that a small-size archwire in the MLF bracket would experience low frictional force in the leveling and aligning stage [11]. We therefore designed a study to compare the frictional force (FF) of the PASS bracket with the traditional twin bracket (Ormco, OptiMesh™) for simulated rotation correction. Both brackets were made of stainless steel with a 0.022″ slot characterized in Table 5.4. Two archwires, 0.014″ and 0.016″ CuNiTi, and a ligature of elastic module (Power "O," Ormco) were used for testing.

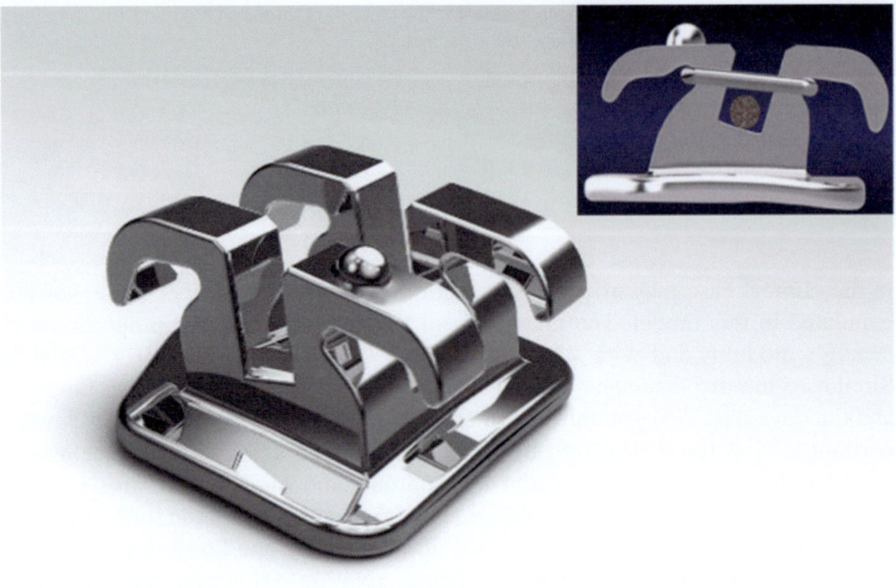

Fig. 5.8 PASS multilevel low-friction (MLF) brackets (Reproduced from Chen et al. [10])

Table 5.4 Prescription of the two bracket types

	Ormco bracket	PASS bracket
Position	Maxillary bicuspid	Maxillary first bicuspid
Slot size	0.022″	0.022″
Angulation	0°	−1°
Torque	0°	−4°

A rotary stage was used to attach a bracket to simulate the rotational status of the crooked tooth, with rotations of 0°, 10°, 20°, and 30°. The bracket on the rotary table was aligned between two Teflon blocks serving as the adjacent brackets, with a fixture where the rotation angle was defined as a relative angle to the neighboring tooth (Teflon blocks) (Fig. 5.9) [36]. The setup is designed to simulate three adjacent posterior brackets that are approximately one premolar width apart from each other (7.5 mm from bracket center to adjacent bracket center). The fixture and the rotary table were mounted to an Instron machine (Model 4411, Instron Corp., Canton, Massachusetts). The pulling test with a static load cell of ±500 N was performed at a crosshead speed of 10 mm/min over 10 mm lengths of archwire. The drawing forces versus the drawing distance were recorded, and the friction force (FF) was calculated as the force averaged from 1 to 10 mm drawing distance. Each combination of the bracket, archwire, and rotation prescription was tested five times.

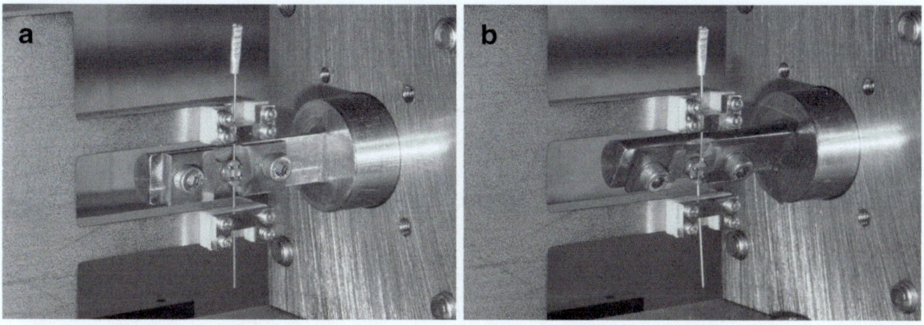

Fig. 5.9 Frictional test with Instron by simulating the rotation with a three-bracket scenario where the Teflon blocks are located at both sides of the testing bracket. (**a**) 0° rotation; (**b**) 30° rotation. Prior to rotating the bracket to the predetermined angle, three "brackets" and the load cell were aligned using a 0.021 × 0.025″ AW. After alignment, the 0.016″ round AW was tested at 0° for 1 mm to get a baseline friction and then tested at the predetermined rotation angle for the test 9 mm

Table 5.5 Statistical summary of the friction force (FF) of Ormco and PASS brackets

		Ormco (Mean ± SD gF)		PASS (Mean ± SD gF)	
Archwire	Rotation	Baseline (0° rotation)	Desired rotation	Baseline (0° rotation)	Desired rotation
0.014″	0°	147.4 ± 23.6	147.4 ± 23.6	122.7 ± 4.1	122.7 ± 4.1
	10°	143.2 ± 31.9	189.8 ± 34.8	126.6 ± 18.8	143.2 ± 16.21
	20°	133.9 ± 41.2	248.2 ± 63.0	125.1 ± 38.8	201.9 ± 40.1
	30°	172.7 ± 35.0	396.2 ± 81.3	127.5 ± 29.6	267.7 ± 28.2
0.016″	0°	151.7 ± 20.8	151.7 ± 20.8	116.4 ± 12.5	116.4 ± 12.5
	10°	164.0 ± 23.1	190.1 ± 20.9	120.7 ± 6.3	155.5 ± 17.5
	20°	154.8 ± 10.7	263.8 ± 24.1	115.0 ± 7.5	191.0 ± 24.7
	30°	171.0 ± 10.8	372.7 ± 44.8	110.0 ± 7.8	263.9 ± 38.9

The mean FF of both brackets was compared using ANOVA, and the data is presented in Table 5.5 and Fig. 5.10. The effects of bracket type ($F = 12.298$, $P = 0.001$) and rotation angle ($F = 151.310$, $P = 0.000$) on FF were significant, while the archwire size ($F = 0.102$, $P = 0.750$) did not have a significant effect on the FF. The interaction of the bracket type and the rotation angle was also significant ($F = 5.114$, $P = 0.003$). As expected, the MLF bracket did result in a lower FF than the Ormco twin bracket; the percent decrease ranged from 16 to 32 %. The 0.016″ archwire would slide more easily in the PASS MLF bracket than the conventional twin bracket in the simulated angulations of 0°, 10°, 20° and 30°. The FF at 0° was consistent with those reported in the literature [37].

Acknowledgment The work was supported, in part, by NIH/NIDCR R01DE022816-01.

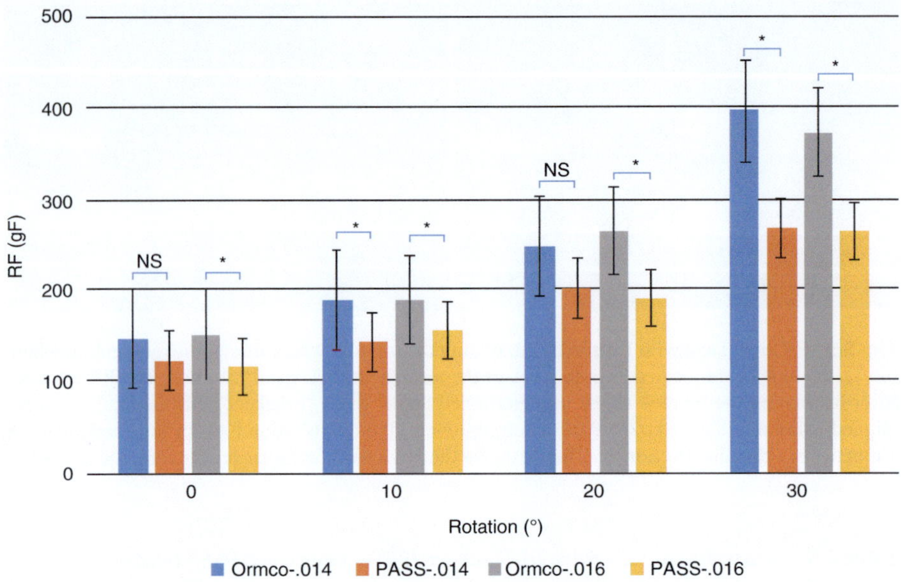

Fig. 5.10 Comparison of the FF between the PASS bracket and Ormco bracket under different rotation corrections. The PASS MLF bracket generated less frictional force than the Ormco brackets at 0°, 10°, 20°, and 30° rotation. * indicates statistical significance

References

1. Kim YE, Nanda RS, Sinha PK (2002) Transition of molar relationships in different skeletal growth patterns. Am J Orthod Dentofacial Orthop 121(3):280–290
2. Su H, Han B, Li S et al (2014) Compensation trends of the angulation of first molars: retrospective study of 1403 malocclusion cases. Int J Oral Sci 6:175–181
3. Sillman JH (1947) Changes in the dental arches as a factor in orthodontic diagnosis. Am J Orthod 33(9):565–581
4. Zhang Y, Xia X, Deng F et al (2012) Analysis of tip back bend on initial displacement of the maxillary first molar in Tip-Edge force system by three-dimensional finite element method. Hua Xi Kou Qiang Yi Xue Za Zhi 30(3):329–332
5. Su H, Han B, Li S (2014) Factors predisposing to maxillary anchorage loss: a retrospective study of 1403 cases. PLoS One 9(10):e109561
6. Tseng YC, Hsieh CH, Chen CH et al (2006) The application of mini-implants for orthodontic anchorage. Int J Oral Maxillofac Surg 35:704–707
7. Sawa Y, Goto K, Suzuki N et al (2001) The new method for the maxillary retraction of the anterior teeth using a titanium microscrew as anchorage. Orthodontic Waves 60:328–331
8. Creekmore TD, Eklund MK (1983) The possibility of skeletal anchorage. J Clin Orthod 17:266–269
9. Melsen B (2005) Mini-implants: where are we? J Clin Orthod 39:539–547
10. Chen S, Chen G, Xu T (2015) Clinical application of the PASS technique. J Clin Orthod 49(8):508–515
11. Proffit WR (2000) Contemporary orthodontics, 3rd edn. Mosby, St. Louis
12. McLaughlin RP, Bennett JC, Trevisi HJ (2002) Systemized orthodontic treatment mechanics. Elsevier Science, Los Angeles

13. Goldberg AJ, Morton J, Burstone CJ (1983) The flexure modulus of elasticity of orthodontic wires. J Dent Res 62:856–858
14. Burstone CJ, Qin B, Morton JY (1985) Chinese NiTiwire-A new orthodontic alloy. Am J Orthod 87:445–452
15. Burstone CJ, Goldberg AJ (1980) Beta-titanium: a new orthodontic alloy. Am J Orthod 77:121–132
16. Literature P (1977) Elgiloy and Truchrome Stainless Steel Orthodontic treatment wires. Rocky Mountain/Associates International, Denver
17. Kusy RP, Greenberg AR (1982) Comparison of the elastic properries of nickel-titanium and beta-titanium arch wires. Am J Orthod 82:199–205
18. Kusy RP, Mims L, Whitley JQ (2001) Mechanical characteristics of various tempers of as-received cobalt-chromium archwires. Am J Orthod Dentofacial Orthop 119:274–291
19. Kusy RP (1997) A review of contemporary archwires: their properties and characteristics. Angle Orthod 67:197–208
20. Brantley WA (2001) Theodore eliades. In: Orthodontic materials- scientific and clinical aspects. George Thieme Verlag, Stuttgart
21. Andreasen GF, Barrett RD (1973) An evaluation of cobalt-substituted nitinol wire in orthodontics. Am J Orthod 63(5):462–470
22. Kusy RP (2000) Ongoing innovations in biomechanics and materials for the new millenium. Angle Orthod 70:366–376
23. Kusy RP (2002) Orthodontic biomaterials: from the past to the present. Angle Orthod 72(6):501–512
24. Andreasen GF, Brady PR (1972) A use hypothesis for 55 nitinol wire for orthodontics. Angle Orthod 42:172–177
25. Santoro M, Nicolay OF, Cangialosi TJ (2001) Pseudoelasticity and thermoelasticity of nickel-titanium alloys: a clinically oriented review. Part I: temperature transitional ranges. Am J Orthod Dentofacial Orthop 119:587–593
26. Santoro M, Nicolay OF, Cangialosi TJ (2001) Pseudoelasticity and thermoelasticity of nickel-titanium alloys: a clinically oriented review. Part II: deactivation forces. Am J Orthod Dentofacial Orthop 119:594–603
27. Ko CC, Rocha E, Larson M (2012) Past, present, and future of finite element analysis in dentistry. In: Moratal D (ed) Finite element analysis – from biomedical applications to industrial developments. InTech-Open Access: http://www.intechopen.com, Croatia, pp 3–24
28. Canales C, Larson M, Grauer D (2013) A novel biomechanical model assessing orthodontic, continuous archwire activation. Am J Orthod Dentofacial Orthop 143(2):281–290
29. Natali AN, Pavan PG, Scarpa C (2004) Numerical analysis of tooth mobility: Formulation of a non-linear constitutive law for the periodontal ligament. Dent Mater 20(7):623–629
30. Qian L, Todo M, Morita Y et al (2009) Deformation analysis of the periodontium considering the viscoelasticity of the periodontal ligament. Dent Mater 25(10):1285–1292
31. Uhlir R, Mayo V, Lin PH (2016) Biomechanical characterization of the periodontal ligament: orthodontic tooth movement. Angle Orthodontist (in press). DOI: 10.2319/092615-651.1
32. Burstone CJ, Koenig HA (1988) Creative wire bending – the force system from step and V bend. Am J Orthod Dentofacial Orthop 93:59–67
33. Shackelford JF (1988) Introduction to materials science for engineers, 2nd edn. Macmillan, New York, pp. 70–88
34. Callister WD Jr (2013) Materials science and engineering: an introduction. Wiley
35. Courtiney TH (1990) Mechanical Behavior of Materials. McGraw-Hill Inc., New York, pp. 1–45
36. Gibson C (2016) Limiting factors affecting stage I treatment: a biomechanical perspective. MS Thesis, University of North Carolina, Chapel Hill
37. Articolo LC, Kusy RP (1999) Influence of angulation on the resistance to sliding in fixed appliances. Am J Orthod Dentofacial Orthop 115:39–51

6 Biomechanics of Physiologic Anchorage Control

Tian Min Xu

Abstract

In Edgewise time, doctors control force system by making a certain bending angle and locating it in a certain position, both the angle and the position count. In straight wire time, although wire-bending angle can be substituted by pre-adjusted angle in bracket or tube, we don't control position of bends any more, which affects not only the magnitude but also the direction of moments on neighboring teeth. According to Burstone's geometry classes of force system from an idea arch, we can deduce the most malpositioned tooth with the largest wire-slot angulation will dominate the direction of net moment and therefore the equilibrium forces. Orthodontists then lose the control power of force system with contemporary straight wire technique. From the anchorage perspective, molars should avoid receiving forward tipping moment from the very first arch wire. The new solution is trying to put the largest wire-slot angle (or dominant moment) on anchor molar instead of any malpositioned teeth in front of it. To make molar dominate the system moment, an additional tip back tube is added to anchor molar. Mechanism of differential moments to protect molar anchorage and correct malocclusion will be discussed. Vertical control with tongue anchorage pad will also be introduced.

Treatment mechanics should reflect orthodontists' recognitions of malocclusion occurrence and tooth movement efficiency. There are two basic treatment mechanics, one emphasizes controlled tooth movement represented by Edgewise technique and the other emphasizes free tipping represented by Begg technique. While

T.M. Xu
Department of Orthodontics, Peking University School and Hospital of Stomatology, Beijing, China
e-mail: tmxuortho@163.com

T.M. Xu (ed.), *Physiologic Anchorage Control*,
DOI 10.1007/978-3-319-48333-7_6

controlled tooth movement has demonstrated excellent anchorage control ability on posterior teeth, free tipping exhibited advantage in relieving anterior irregularity or proclination. Modern fixed appliances try to take advantages of both at different stages. For example, when using thin NiTi wire in self-ligating appliance, teeth can be moved freely at aligning stage; when progressing to space closing stage, thick stainless steel rectangular wire is used, and it can enhance molar anchorage to retract anterior teeth. The problem is when physiologic anchorage loss is concerned, anchorage control is no more the matter of retraction stage. It should start at the very beginning and last throughout the whole treatment. In that case, the conventional thin NiTi archwire, although may facilitate anterior teeth correction in aligning stage, it also accelerates physiologic anchorage loss especially when a straight archwire is engaged in the 0° buccal tube. Why is that?

Let's analyze the growth of dentition first. From Chaps. 3 and 4, we realize that molars change their positions and directions during growth and stomatognathic function. Upper molars are used to tipping forward and lower molars tend to be uprighted. What about other teeth during the growth? Since it's difficult to discern bilateral teeth images in cephalogram considering the projection of the curved arch form on sagittal plane, we turned to a unique sample. In AAO Legacy Collection, there is a longitudinal growth sample with metallic implants collected by Prof. Mathews, now curated by Prof. Sheldon Baumrind [1]. Thirty-six cases were included; some of them got minor orthodontic treatment. The most striking thing is all cases have 45° oblique films with metallic implants in each time point. Since the oblique film is almost parallel to buccal segment, we believe that is the best film to show the growth of all buccal teeth. From the 36 cases, we selected 11 of them without any orthodontic treatment and evaluated yearly changes of buccal teeth angulation by superimposition on metallic implants of each year's tracing from the age of 8.5 to 15.5. The results show upper molars tipped forward and canines and premolars tipped backward in general during eruption. The interesting finding is the apex of upper first molar is relatively stable while the apices of premolar and canine displaced mesially and second molar apex displaced distally (Fig. 6.1). After all teeth coming into occlusion, buccal teeth tend to tip forward in general, which are probably due to anterior components of occlusal force transferred through interproximal contacts. And teeth angulation changes also demonstrate pubertal growth stage. Figure 6.1 illustrates buccal teeth angulation change of the Case No. 12 among these samples. The rapid PAL happened during 12–14 years of age. The upper molar tipped forward 6.6° and moved 4.3 mm mesially. If we treated this patient at 12, bonding a 0° buccal tube on upper first molar and engaging a straight wire would give molar a forward tipping moment that would accelerate upper molar's PAL (Fig. 6.2a–c) and change the occlusal plane that will make Class II protrusion correction even more difficult. Braun and Legan [2] studied the geometric and mathematical relationship between dental occlusion and rotation of the occlusal plane. They found that upward and forward rotation of occlusal plane tends to develop Class II relationship, and each degree of rotation of the occlusal plane would result in a 0.5 mm change in molar relationship. Figure 6.3 shows even all teeth align on a straight wire with the six keys' normal angles, different occlusal plane may affect the dental protrusion.

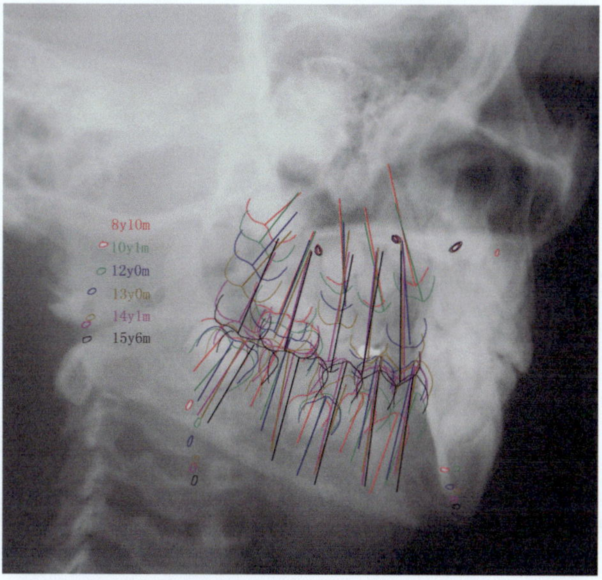

Fig. 6.1 Superimposition on maxilla implants of oblique films showing the growth of buccal segment teeth of Case 12

In contemporary straight wire system, all standard normal angulations of teeth are relative to Andrews plane or a straight rectangular archwire, not necessarily normal relative to craniofacial physiologic structure. In another word, modern straight wire prescriptions don't define what is normal functional occlusal plane first, which should be determined by the function of posterior teeth. Among those posterior teeth that composed functional occlusal plane, upper first molar is believed to be the key of the occlusion since Dr. Angle. Studies on craniofacial growth show upper molar tips forward to compensate mandible excess during growth [3, 4], so it has its own physiologic norms relative to jaws in different growth stages. If we tip it forward as in Fig. 6.2, we change its angulation relative to the resultant force direction of masticatory muscles at that stage, which may induce more anterior component of occlusal force and lose more anchorage. From mechanical point of view, with straight wire mechanics, not just the first molar being tipped forward, second premolar will also be tipped forward and be intruded as canine is extruded, which will make functional occlusal plane decreased prematurely than the individual's nature growth stage (Fig. 6.4). Although we don't know what's its influence on the posttreatment function and stability of the dentition, it's safer to let nature find its physiologic angulation for posterior teeth function. Since we know there is no nature force to tip molar back, I believe preventing molar forward tipping from the first stage of orthodontic treatment is a more logical strategy than allowing it free forward tipping on NiTi wires then uprighting it on stainless steel wires with headgear or TAD.

To prevent molar forward tipping on initial NiTi alignment wires, we designed a cross buccal tube (Fig. 6.5) that consists of two tubes, one −25° round tube with the diameter of 0.018 inch for thin NiTi wires in early stage of treatment and

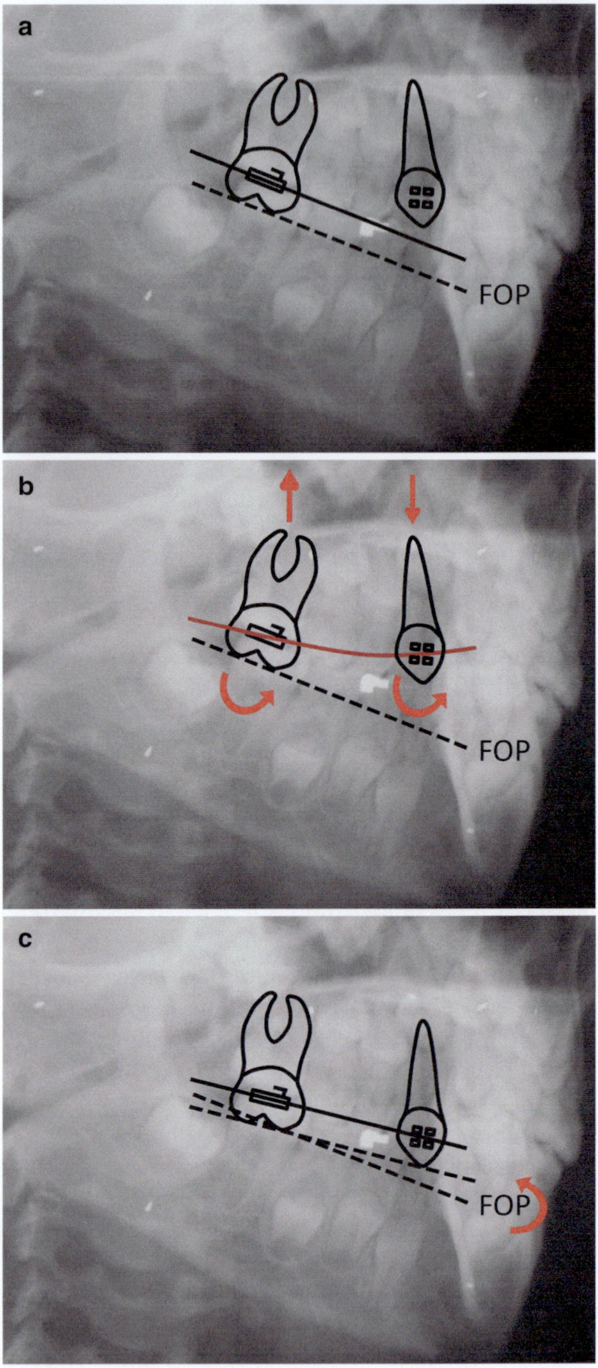

Fig. 6.2 (**a**) The development stage of dentition in 12 years of age of the Case 12 when canine has not erupted into occlusion. (**b**) Engaging a straight wire will give molar a tip forward moment to accelerate molar forward tipping growth. (**c**) To align the molar and canine on a straight archwire, functional occlusal plane may rotate more than normal growth tendency in counterclockwise direction

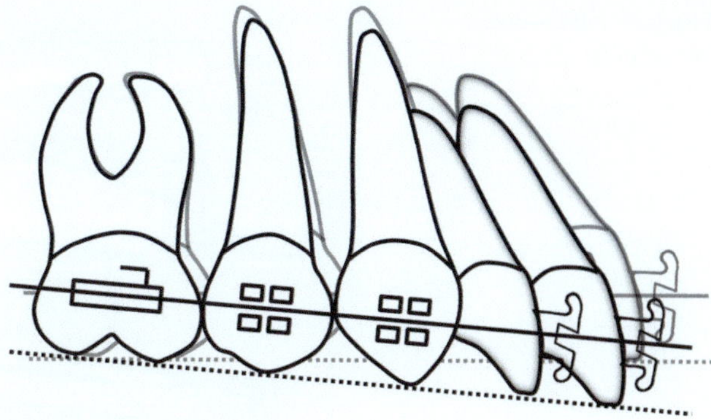

Fig. 6.3 The same bracket description on the straight archwire, forward tipped upper first molar will flatten posterior occlusal plane to increase upper arch protrusion

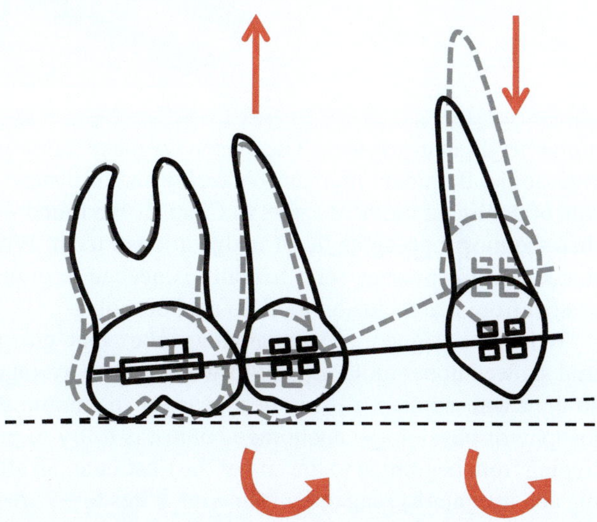

Fig. 6.4 In the first premolar extraction case, initial NiTi archwire will tip posterior teeth forward and change the FOP when aligning the high canine

another −7° rectangular tube sized 0.022 × 0.027 inch for thick round wires and rectangular wires in the following stages of treatment. Two tubes cross at mesial entrance, so we call it cross buccal tube and brief it as XBT.

Why we designed a thin −25° round tube? From the pattern of PAL, we know upper molars tend to tip forward during growth. To prevent this kind of anchorage loss, we need a tip back moment. Contemporary straight wire appliances use thin NiTi archwire to align anterior teeth; the 0.018 round tube can accommodate 0.012–0.016 thin NiTi wires that are usually used in aligning stage. Small diameter of this round tube can not only increase tip back moment by decreasing the clearance between archwire and tube but also save the room in the molar area. We found when putting the tube in the middle of the molar crown height, more than −25° will stick the distal end of the tube below the occlusal plane for a lot of cases. In other words, −25° is the largest angle for a 0.018″ round tube allowed in the occlusal half of upper

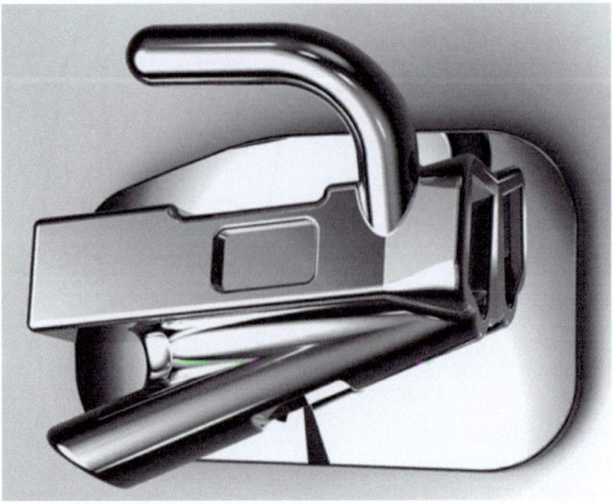

Fig. 6.5 XBT—cross buccal tube

molar height in most cases. The reason we make this angle as large as possible is we want to put dominant moment on anchor molar instead of malocclusion teeth. The role of dominant moment refers to Chap. 1. We found −25° has already been larger than the most tipping angle of malpositioned teeth. When more than 25° malpositioned tooth is present, wire bending is needed to grab the control power of force system from malocclusion tooth to anchor molar.

Why we designed −7° rectangular tube? Our prospective randomized clinical trial showed upper molar tipped forward 7.2° on average in the sample treated with straight wire appliance using headgear for maximum anchorage control. The philosophy of physiologic anchorage control is to try to prevent upper molar forward tipping from beginning to the end of the treatment. So after relieving anterior crowding and irregularity, engaging following wires to −7° rectangular tube can take over the dominant moment to ensure anchor molar receiving 24 hours tip back moment during the whole orthodontic treatment. In this way, PAL can obtain the best control contraposing its feature of occurrence.

Now let's see the mechanics if we change the conventional buccal tube in Fig. 6.2 to XBT tube. Supposing Case No.12 was an extraction case, upper molar would tend to tip forward because of the interruption of balancing force from anterior teeth and the transseptal fiber force after premolars extraction, besides the forward tipping tendency caused by mandible excess growth than maxilla. To prevent this kind of PAL, a tip back moment is needed. By engaging a 0.014″ NiTi archwire in −25° tip back tube and in anterior teeth brackets (Fig. 6.6), we provide upper molar a gentle continuous tip back moment.

Now let's analyze the force system on upper molar. Since −25° tip back on molar is usually larger than the angulation of anterior teeth, we know dominant moment will be on the first molar when the NiTi archwire is used to align abnormally angled

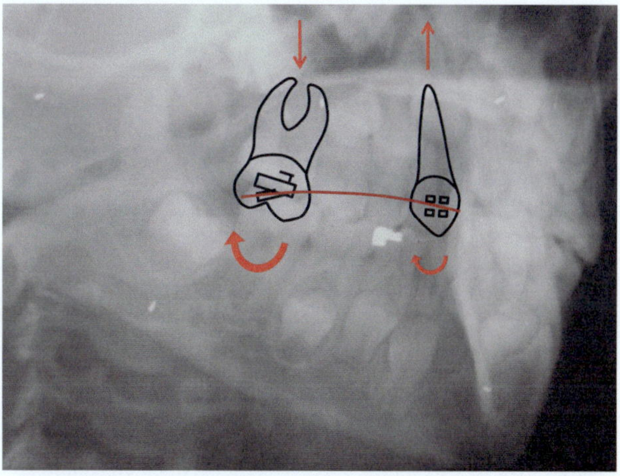

Fig. 6.6 Changing conventional buccal tube in Fig. 6.2 into XBT tube, the force system reversed

teeth in the front. Let's look at the characteristics of anterior teeth in extraction case. The most common indications for typical extraction treatment in orthodontics are apparent crowding or protrusion. In crowding cases, canines were usually in high position due to lack of eruption space because upper canines were the last ones in the eruption sequence before the first molars. In protrusion cases, canines were lucky to squeeze into dentition in time, but the anterior components of occlusal force from the back teeth and also probably the eruption force of the second or third molar, considering the forward tipping growth pattern of these teeth, would tip canines' crown forward that might cause incisors' labial inclination by transferring the force through interproximal contacts. In cases with strong lip muscle, canines might be tipped distally. So upper canines are most susceptible to the influence of environmental factors among the buccal segment. Now let's compare the force systems in the above three situations with conventional 0° buccal tube or −25° tip back tube, respectively.

Figure 6.7 shows canine is in high position. When using 0° buccal tube (Fig. 6.7a), both teeth will get tip forward moment as in Burstone Class I or Class II. Molar tends to lose anchorage. If using −25° tip back tube (Fig. 6.7b), molar gets tip back moment while canine gets tip forward moment as in Burstone Class V or Class VI. Molar tends to gain anchorage.

Figure 6.8 shows canine is in forward tipping angulation. When using 0° buccal tube (Fig. 6.8a), the larger wire-slot angle is on canine. So canine dominates the system moment, 0° wire-slot angle on molar makes this force system just like in Burstone Class III. Molar gets one half of the canine moment with the same direction. If using −25° tip back tube (Fig. 6.8b), both teeth will get tip back moment as in Burstone Class I or Class II. And molar gets larger moment than in Fig. 6.8a.

Figure 6.9 shows canine is in backward tipping angulation. When using 0° buccal tube (Fig. 6.9a), the larger wire-slot angle is on canine. So canine dominates the

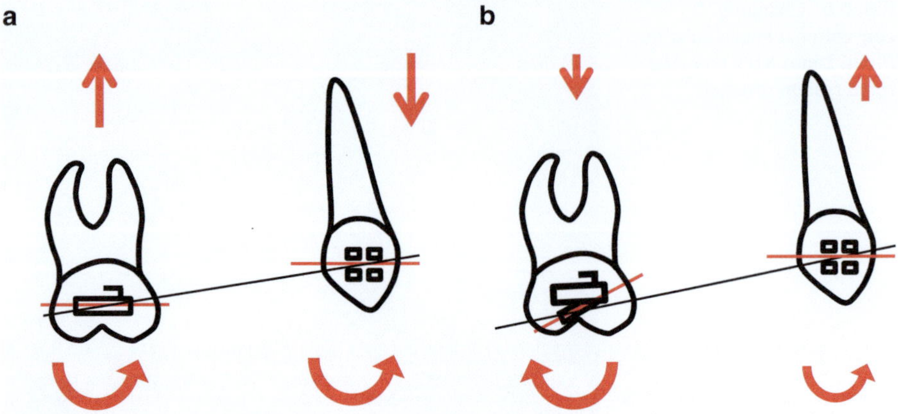

Fig. 6.7 (**a**, **b**) Comparing force system between conventional buccal tube and XBT tube when canine is in high position

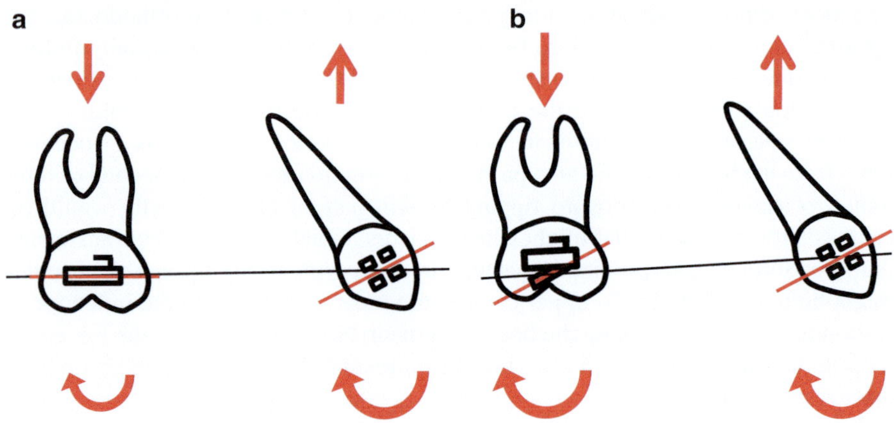

Fig. 6.8 (**a**, **b**) Comparing force system between conventional buccal tube and XBT tube when canine is in forward tipping position

system moment, 0° wire-slot angle on molar makes this force system as Burstone Class III, but the direction of the moment and force are just opposite to those in Fig. 6.8a. Molar tends to lose anchorage in this situation. If using −25° tip back tube (Fig. 6.9b), molar gets tip back moment while canine gets tip forward moment as in Burstone Class V or Class VI. Molar tends to gain anchorage.

From the above three situations, we learn if using conventional 0° buccal tube (Figs. 6.7a, 6.8a, and 6.9a), molar will get either forward or backward tipping moments depending on the position and angulation of anterior malocclusion teeth. Using −25° tip back tube in Figs. 6.7b, 6.8b, and 6.9b gives molar the best chance to get dominant moment. From Burstone six basic geometry classifications, we

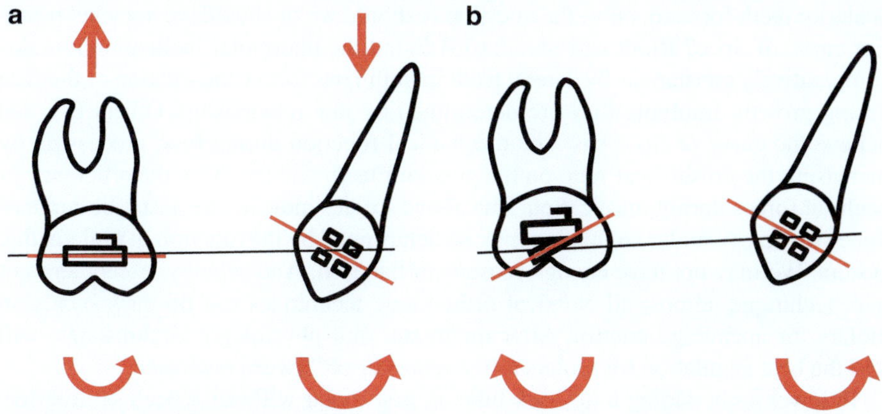

Fig. 6.9 (**a**, **b**) Comparing force system between conventional buccal tube and XBT tube when canine is in backward tipping position

know only the largest dominant moment can keep the consistent direction insusceptible to other teeth angulation.

If we keep upper molar in backward tipping angulation, the dental arch won't be as straight as contemporary straight wire appliance or self-ligating appliance do for the six keys' goal, will that be OK?

More than 120 years ago, Dr. Spee found there is an upward concave occlusal curves exist in human and animals that own tuberculum articulare, which is now called the curve of Spee. Dr. Spee observed "In the beginning, the curve of the masticatory surface of the mandible is sometimes not very clear and is much flatter than in the upper jaw where it is seldom missing. In such cases, the varying pressure exerted on the teeth appears to gradually induce compensation of the curve difference" [5]. It tells us the curve originated from upper arch, and it is becoming flattened gradually during growth but not straight because the mandible could not move straight forward when there is tuberculum articulare in front of condyle according to Dr. Spee. Studies on the size of curve of Spee have shown that different malocclusions have different curve depths, and basically Class II cases have larger curve of Spee than Class I cases, and Class III have the least curve of Spee [6–9]. Orthodontists used to believe the curve of Spee is on lower arch and neglect it originated from upper dentition. Although leveling lower arch is good for both bite opening in anterior teeth and uprighting molars on posterior teeth, leveling upper arch with straight arch wire that is most commonly used in contemporary straight wire technique may extrude both incisors in the front and molars at the back end. The interesting thing is orthodontists are taught leveling 1 mm curve of Spee on lower arch needs around 1 mm space on each side in making extraction decision but forget this is also true for upper arch. Our study shows leveling posterior curve of Spee needs 0.87 ± 0.08 mm on each side [10]. When anchorage control is concerned, leveling posterior curve on upper arch with straight arch wire may lose 1.74 mm extraction space by tipping all posterior teeth forward. Now, the question is should we or should we not level posterior curve of Spee? Bjork and Skieller [3] found the intermolar inclination remains comparatively constant as the lateral teeth in both jaws follow the rotation of the face during growth. Implying they are determined by jaw relationship. Others [11, 12] believe the curve of Spee has a biomechanical function during food processing by increasing the crush/shear ratio on the posterior teeth and therefore the efficiency of occlusal forces during mastication. The above studies indicate the posterior curve of Spee affected by molar angulation may be determined by the function of oral gnathic system. We may not have enough reasons to flatten it. And actually, except straight wire technique, almost all classical orthodontic techniques use tip back bends on molars for anchorage control. After treatment, oral physiologic circumstance will find the best angulation for molars as the recovery of "Tweed occlusion."

In lower arch, adding a tip back tube on first molar will cause occlusal interference. So we just cut a slot on the occlusal wall of the conventional buccal tube (Fig. 6.10a). The slot size allows thin arch wires, usually less than 0.018″ arch wire, to go through. When inserting an arch wire from the mesial entrance and going out of the slot, it will make a −20° tip back angle that makes lower molar dominate the system moment in most cases (Fig. 6.10b). After relieving anterior crowding and irregularity, thicker arch wires are inserted into the conventional rectangular tube that has a −4° prescribed angle in this system, so always keeping the dominant moment on anchor molar.

According to mechanical law, any tip back bend on molar will give molar a tip back moment and an extrusive force while giving anterior teeth an intrusive force to reach static equilibration (Fig. 6.11). The larger the net system moment, the larger the vertical equilibrium forces on molar and anterior teeth. When intrusive force is large enough on incisors, measures must be taken to prevent incisors from flaring out. That's why a J hook in Tweed Edgewise and Class II elastics in Begg technique is a must in the respective technique from the initial archwire. In contemporary

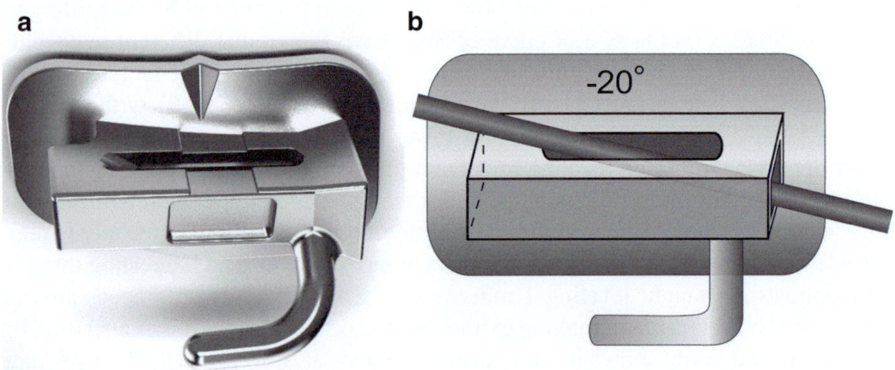

Fig. 6.10 (**a**) Lower XBT tube. (**b**) Inserting an archwire from the mesial entrance and going out from the slot makes a −20° tip back angle

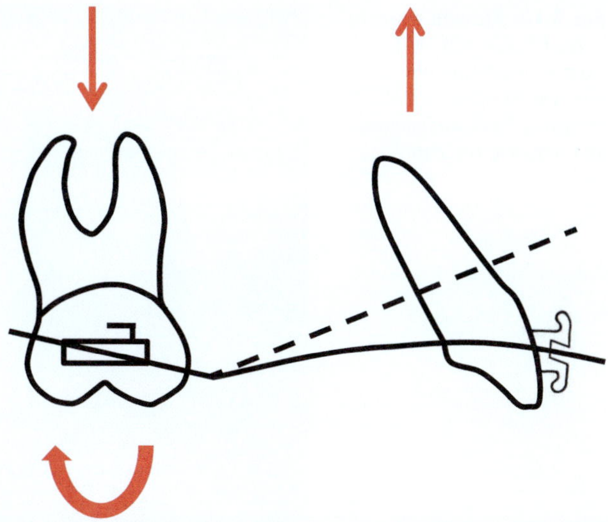

Fig. 6.11 Tip back bend on molar tends to flare incisor out

fixed appliances, the initial archwire is almost always straight NiTi wire. Since there is no tip back moment on molar in this situation, there is certainly no intrusive force on incisors. Instead, for most cases with normal direction curve of Spee on upper arch, a straight NiTi will give upper molar a tip forward moment and anterior teeth an extrusive force (Fig. 6.12). That's why in maximum anchorage cases, headgear goes to molar in modern techniques or other anchorage auxiliaries like Nance, TPA, or TAD are used. Now the question is when engaging a thin NiTi in −25° tip back tube, whether the upper incisors need backward force like in classical Tweed or Begg techniques or molars need anchorage auxiliaries like in contemporary straight wire techniques?

Let's compare the magnitudes of force and moment created by stainless steel wire and NiTi wire first. Burstone's study [13] showed the bending moment of the austenitic NiTi wire is about 1/5 of the same size (0.016 inch) stainless steel wire (Fig. 6.13). So the bending moment created by 0.016 NiTi wire in −25° tip back tube is equivalent to that created by the same size stainless steel wire with −5° tip back bend. When five times difference is concerned, in high canine situation as in Fig. 6.14, molar may get opposite moments when using NiTi archwire in −25° tip back tube (Fig. 6.14a) comparing using the same size stainless steel wire with −5° tip back bend (Fig. 6.14b). When five times' difference is concerned, we can deduce the tip back moment created by 0.012–0.016 inch NiTi wire in −25° XBT tube is much less than 0.016″ Australia wire with 30°–45° tip back bends in Begg technique or thick stainless steel rectangular wire with 10° tip back bend on upper first molar in Tweed technique. The small tip back moment by NiTi wire may not tip molar back; by the same token, it may also not create enough intrusive force to flare incisors out. Prof. Ko's FEM model in Chap. 5 showed upper incisors actually may get lingual and extrusive force when using XBT tube. Then we don't need Cass II

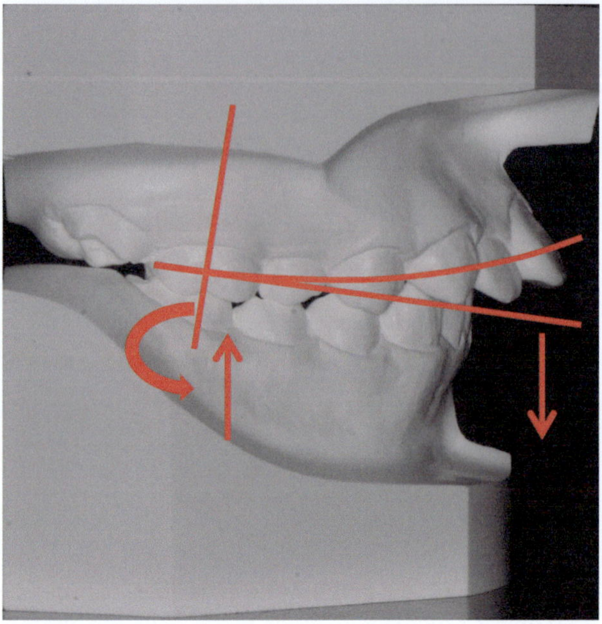

Fig. 6.12 Straight wire on curved dental arch will exert forward tipping moment on upper molars, extrusion force on incisors, and intrusive force on molars

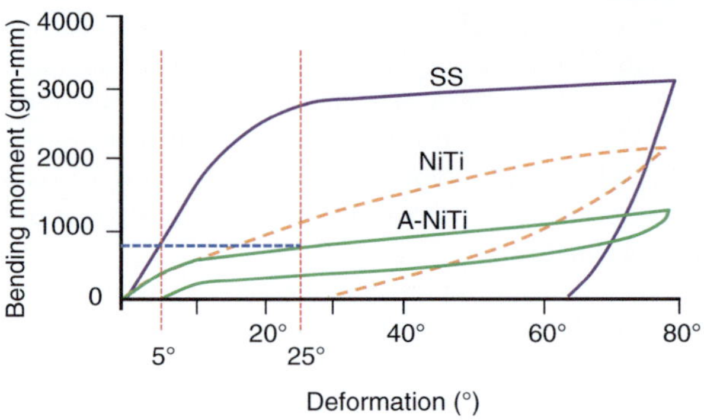

Fig. 6.13 Comparison of the magnitudes of bending moment created by 0.016 inch stainless steel and NiTi wires (Redrawn from Burstone et al. [13])

elastics like in Begg technique or J hook like in Tweed technique for that purpose. Another advantage for tip back tube over tip back bend on wire is we don't need to worry the influence of wire shifting on molar moments. We all know tip back bend position relative to buccal tube affects tip back moment on molar even with the same tip back angle. For example, we dictate 30° tip back bends at 3 mm in front of left and right molar tubes, if archwire shift 2 mm to the left side, the tip back bend will be just 1 mm in front of the left buccal tube but 5 mm in front of the right buccal tube. The tip back moment on the left side will then be larger than the right side. With tip back tube, no matter which side the archwire shifts to, the bending position is always 0 mm in front of buccal tube. And there will never be notching resistance when sliding mechanics is concerned.

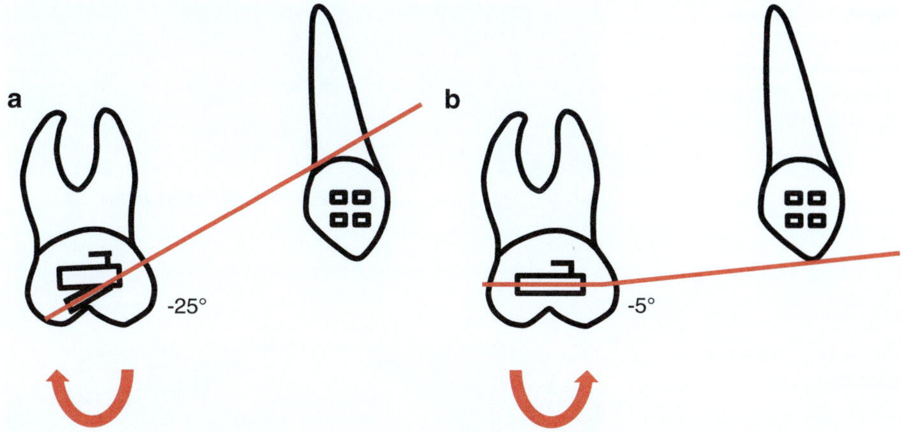

Fig. 6.14 (**a**) –25° tip back tube. (**b**) –5° tip back bend

If the −25° tube design is not aiming to tip molar back, what's its effect? In physiologic anchorage control system, the main purpose of this tip back tube is to prevent molar forward tipping caused by physiologic anchorage loss, or any possible large angles in anterior teeth, or high canine, or just normal curve of Spee when a straight NiTi wire is engaged during aligning stage. The consequence of this kind of early anchorage loss may cause more anterior components of occlusal force when molar tipped forward. Opposite to it, if we keep molar straight up or even tip back a little bit, the axial components of occlusal force is larger, and the muscle anchorage is probably stronger. New studies support intermaxillary occlusal force can inhibit teeth movements [14, 15]. After anterior malpositioned teeth are aligned to near normal position and angulation, or wire-slot angulation less than 7°, thicker wires go through −7° rectangular tube, keeping dominant moment always on anchor molar throughout the whole treatment period. When molars are prevented from forward tipping in aligning and leveling stages, they will be angled relatively backward to the anterior dentition, which is similar to the anchorage prepared in Tweed technique when treatment proceeds to space closure stage. In this way, along with tip back angle in upper premolar and second molar, plus curved main archwires, upper arch will present an upward concave curve after treatment, and lower arch are relatively flattened just like the situation Dr. Spee described at the beginning of occlusal curve formation. According to Dr. Spee, the varying pressure exerted on the teeth will gradually induce compensation of the curve difference.

In high-angle cases, when upper molar extrusion is a real concern, we add a TAP on upper molars. TAP is an acronym of "tongue anchorage pad." It's modified from TPA. The problem with TPA we believe is that the contact area between the U loop and tongue is too small to bear tongue pressure, and its position is arbitrary with no biological base. So it works more like a mechanical device to prevent molar rotation or maintain the arch width. In physiologic anchorage control system, we emphasize

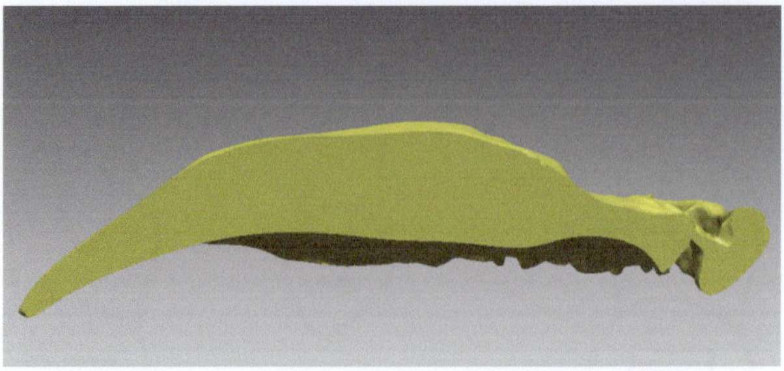

Fig. 6.15 Silicone impression of tongue swallowing height (Reproduced from Xu et al. [19])

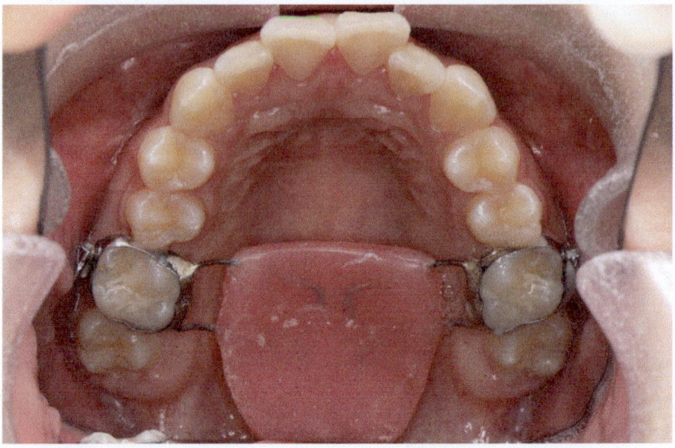

Fig. 6.16 TAP—tongue anchorage pad

to utilize all physiologic force in orthodontic treatment. Tongue is certainly an important source of force. During deglutition, the base of the tongue is moved forcibly upward and backward toward the hard palate, sweeping the fluid backward down the pharynx [16, 17]. This kind of tongue movement creates a considerable force on the hard palate, or any dental appliance positioned in its way during swallowing. A normal person swallows about 2400 times a day [18], and abnormal swallowing habits such as tongue thrust swallowing can also cause malocclusion. If tongue force can create malocclusion, it should also be used to correct teeth if we can transfer it to teeth with appropriate device. We therefore investigated tongue pressure during swallowing and resting on a special location we got by a silicone impression of tongue during swallowing [19, 20]. Figure 6.15 is the sagittal section of the silicone impression. The impression records the distance between the tongue and the hard palate in swallowing and is correlated with tongue strength. And we found different patients have different thickness of the impression, indicating large individual variations. If a conventional TPA locates far away from tongue swallowing height, the tongue pressure is supposed to be less than enough to affect teeth. We therefore made an acrylic pad (TAP) and located it at the tongue swallowing height recorded by impression (Fig. 6.16), and measured the tongue pressure on the pad. The results show the tongue pressure is about 540 g during swallowing and 13 g during resting. Since the swallowing force from tongue is upward and backward on

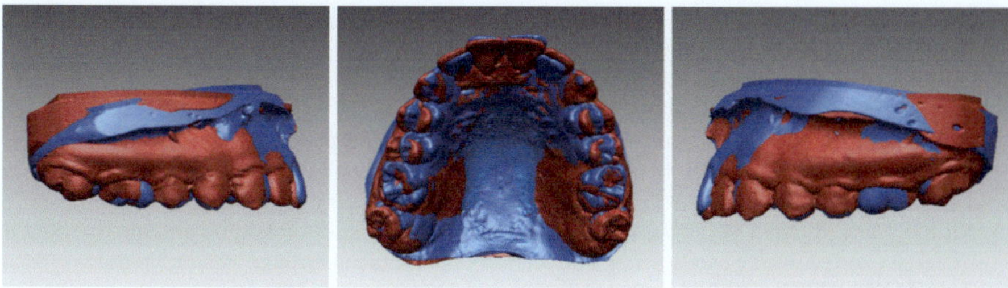

Fig. 6.17 3D digital model superimposition show upper first molar tipped back and intruded

the TAP, it gives upper molar an intrusive and backward tipping force. Figure 6.17 is the superimposition of digital model of the case in Fig. 6.16, which shows upper molar intruded and tipped back. The fabrication of TAP and its clinical application will be introduced in Chap. 9.

References

1. www.AAOFLegacyCollection.org
2. Braun S, Legan HL (1997) Changes in occlusion related to the cant of the occlusal plane. Am J Orthod Dentofacial Orthop 111:184–188
3. Bjork A, Skieller V (1972) Facial development and tooth eruption. An implant study at the age of puberty. Am J Orthod 62(4):339–383
4. Kim YE, Nanda RS, Sinha PK (2002) Transition of molar relationships in different skeletal growth patterns. Am J Orthod Dentofacial Orthop 121(3):280–290
5. Spee FG (1890) The gliding path of the mandible along the skull. Arch Anat Physiol 16:285–294
6. Yu Yue (2014) Spee's curve measurement based on least square curve fitting method. Dissertation, Peking University
7. Farella M, Michelotti A, van Eijden TM et al (2002) The curve of Spee and craniofacial morphology: a multiple regression analysis. Eur J Oral Sci 110(4):277–281
8. Fidler BC, Artun J, Joondeph DR et al (1995) Long-term stability of Angle Class II, division 1 malocclusions with successful occlusal results at end of active treatment. Am J Orthod Dentofacial Orthop 107(3):276–285
9. Shannon KR, Nanda RS (2004) Changes in the curve of Spee with treatment and at 2 years posttreatment. Am J Orthod Dentofacial Orthop 125(5):589–596
10. Yu Y, Xu TM (2015) Spee's curve measurement based on least square curve fitting method. Chin J Orthod 22(2):78–82
11. Monson GS (1932) Applied mechanics to the theory of mandibular movements. Dent Cosmos 74:1039–1053
12. Osborn JW (1993) Orientation of the masseter muscle and the curve of Spee in relation to crushing forces on the molar teeth of primates. Am J Phys Anthropol 92:99–106
13. Burstone CJ, Qin B, Morton JY (1985) Chinese NiTi wire— a new orthodontic alloy. Am J Orthod 87(6):445–452
14. Alexander D, Catherine G, Stavros KG (2013) Factors related to the rate of orthodontically induced tooth movement. Am J Orthod Dentofacial Orthop 143:616–621
15. Antonarakis GS, Kiliaridis S (2015) Predictive value of masseter muscle thickness and bite force on Class II functional appliance treatment: a prospective controlled study. Eur J Orthod 37(6):570–577

16. Sicher H, DuBrul EL (1988) Sicher and DuBrul's oral anatomy, 8th edn. Ishiyaku Euro America, St Louis, pp. 161–199
17. Ovsenik M, Volk J, Marolt MM (2014) A 2D ultrasound evaluation of swallowing in children with unilateral posterior crossbite. Eur J Orthod 36:665–671
18. Staub WJ (1961) Malfunction of the tongue. Part II. The abnormal swallowing habit: its causes, effects, and results in relation to orthodontic treatment and speech therapy. Am J Orthod 47(8):596–617
19. Xu KF, Zeng JJ, Xu TM (2016) Effect of an intraoral appliance on tongue pressure measured by force exerted during swallowing. Am J Orthod Dentofacial Orthop 149(1):55–61
20. Zeng JJ, Xu KF, Gao XM et al (2015) Tongue resting pressure of the tongue anchorage pad in different body positions: a pilot study. J Oral Rehabil 42:414–419

Drift of Dentition and Low-Friction Appliance

7

Ruoping Jiang, Fei Teng, Feiyu Du, Huizhong Chen,
and Tian Min Xu

Abstract

Dentitions drift forward by physiological force from the tongue, bite force, eruption force, etc. until the anterior force from the lips can stop it to reach a balance. Our recent study and others all show after extraction of premolars, anterior teeth drift backward, and posterior teeth drift forward (another source of physiologic anchorage loss). Alexander therefore advocated to delay the bonding of the lower arch to take advantage of natural drifting to relieve anterior crowding, implying teeth will not drift after putting on a fixed appliance. Friction is believed to be a resistance for teeth sliding along the archwire, so theoretically lowering the friction will reduce resistance for canine sliding backward. With XBT buccal tube, molars are prevented from forward drifting from very first thin nickel-titanium (NiTi) archwire. If we can induce canine sliding back along the archwire with low friction, we can relieve anterior crowding without stressing anchor molar with laceback or tieback to save anchorage in initial alignment stage.

Drift of Dentition

In orthodontic extraction treatment, first molars are usually used as anchorage to retract anterior teeth to close the extraction space. Anchorage control strategy therefore normally relates to the methods of reducing stress on anchor molars to leave more space for the relief of anterior crowding or protrusion. Bourdet [1] first described a spontaneous adjustment of dentition after tooth loss and named it as

R. Jiang (✉) • F. Teng • F. Du • H. Chen • T.M. Xu
Department of Orthodontics, Peking University School and Hospital of Stomatology, Beijing, China
e-mail: jiangruoping@126.com; hover_mavis@126.com; feiyudupku@qq.com; poplonglong@163.com; tmxuortho@163.com

T.M. Xu (ed.), *Physiologic Anchorage Control*,
DOI 10.1007/978-3-319-48333-7_7

"physiological drift of teeth" or "physiologic drift," which told us one possibility that anterior teeth may move back after the extraction without stressing anchor molars with orthodontic appliances.

Clinical studies on physiological drift after extraction focused on the mandibular dentition mainly [2–9]. After the lower first premolars were extracted, in Panpadreas' 10-month observation [5], the lower first molars of 20 patients moved mesially about 1.19 mm and tipped forward about 1.90° totally. Jia et al. [7] found first molars moved mesially about 0.7 mm with a 0.7° forward tipping within 7 months. Weber [2] reported that canines moved distally about 4.4 mm during 2.5 years. For the anterior teeth, studies [5, 7] showed the edges of the incisors may move lingually 2.3 mm and 2.53 mm, retroclined 4.5° and 8.8° in 7 and 10 months, respectively. Some researches [2, 10, 11] indicated that only about 1/3–1/4 of the first premolar extraction spaces were taken up by mesial drift of the first molars, whereas most of the space closures were attributed to distal drift of the canines.

Instead of using cephalograms or manual measurement of dental casts, our ongoing study applies 3D digital model superimposition method to investigate drifting phenomena on upper arch after premolars extraction based on the stable area we found from implant-marked study recently [12], that is, the medial 2/3 of the third rugae and the regional palatal vault dorsal to it as shown in Fig. 7.1. The study collected 86 models of 45 patients, which divided into two groups—61 models with

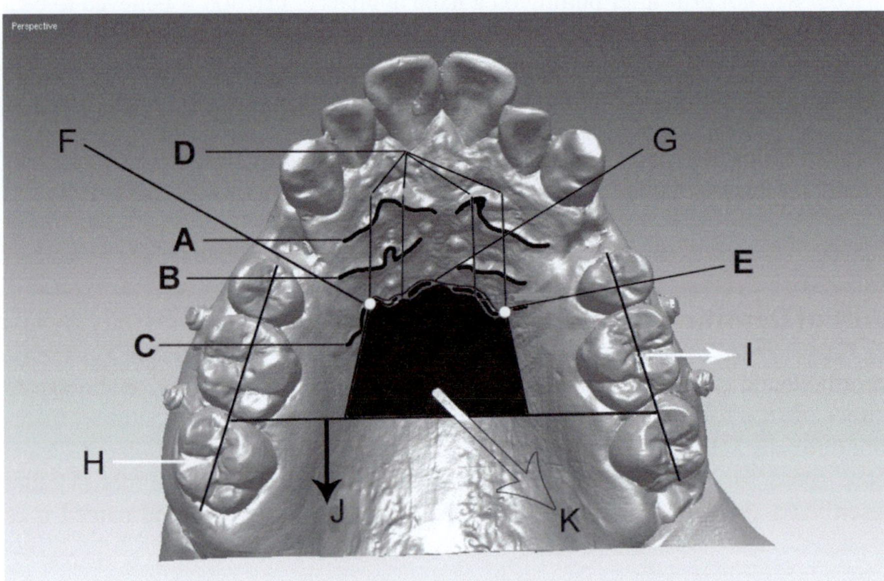

Fig. 7.1 Stable area for 3D superimposition found from our implant marked study. (*A*) Right first ruga, (*B*) right second ruga, (*C*) right third ruga, (*D*) trisection lines of the rugae, (*E*) and (*F*) lateral trisection points of the left third ruga and right third ruga, (*G*) anterior border line of the stable palatal region, (*H*) and (*I*) right and left occlusal line through the central groove of the posterior teeth, (*J*) line in contact with the distal surface of the left and right maxillary first molars, (*K*) stable region (Reproduced from Chen et al. [12])

first premolars extraction as group one and 25 models with second premolars extraction as group two. The sample was observed from 10 to 240 days, the digital models at different time points of each model were registered by the method mentioned above, and then 3D changes of teeth position were measured and compared [13].

We found the individual tooth drift could start as early as 10 days after extraction, and the amount of teeth drift continuously increased, and the phenomena has been observed even until 240 days after extraction. In both groups, the first molars displaced and tipped mesially with a mesial-palatal rotation, while the canines displaced and tipped distally with a distal-palatal rotation after premolars extraction. Since the interval time between every impression taken for each patient was different, linear interpolation method was used to reckon teeth movement at certain time node like the 10th day, 20th day, 30th day, and so on. Only subjects that have the closest time of impression taken to the fixed time node were enrolled. The amount of tooth displacement, inclination, and rotation are shown in Tables 7.1 and 7.2.

The results showed there were no statistical significant differences ($p > 0.05$) in canine drifting between the two groups. However, the differences in displacement and inclination of the first molars were statistically significant ($p < 0.05$). As we can see in Fig. 7.2, the amount of the first molars mesial inclination of group two was greater than that of group one at each time point and so was the amount of the mesial displacement in Fig. 7.3. No difference was found in rotation of the first molars between groups ($p > 0.05$).

Linear interpolation method was also used to reckon the average teeth movement of every 30 days. But we recruited all the samples to make the most usage of the data. Results were showed in Table 7.3 and 7.4. Table 7.3 showed the amount of the mesial displacement of the first molars in every 30 days after the premolars extraction. We found that with the premolars extraction, first molars drifted mesially about 0.5–0.6 mm in the first month then slowed down rapidly during the following 60 days, then kept drifting at a gradually decreased rate and then a relatively stable rate till 240 days. When comparing with the two groups, the amount of every month molar drifting was significantly higher in group two than that of group one,

Table 7.1 Teeth displacement, inclination, and rotation after extraction of upper first premolars

Periods after extraction	Displacement (mm)		Inclination (°)		Rotation (°)	
	First molar	Canine	First molar	Canine	First molar	Canine
10 days	0.18 ± 0.22	−0.17 ± 0.18	0.46 ± 0.64	−0.54 ± 1.12	0.03 ± 0.38	−0.64 ± 0.97
20 days	0.23 ± 0.18	−0.35 ± 0.36	0.94 ± 0.90	−0.94 ± 1.31	0.07 ± 0.41	−1.03 ± 1.85
30 days	0.34 ± 0.28	−0.38 ± 0.27	1.78 ± 0.89	−1.42 ± 2.35	0.40 ± 0.57	−0.90 ± 0.86
60 days	0.77 ± 0.53	−0.83 ± 0.60	2.51 ± 2.13	−1.99 ± 2.60	0.41 ± 1.02	−1.92 ± 1.47
90 days	1.00 ± 0.66	−1.09 ± 0.80	3.08 ± 2.65	−2.78 ± 2.95	0.48 ± 1.33	−2.54 ± 1.92
120 days	1.37 ± 0.69	−1.35 ± 0.97	4.28 ± 3.02	−3.29 ± 3.41	0.80 ± 1.39	−3.05 ± 2.39
150 days	1.62 ± 0.73	−1.51 ± 1.11	4.98 ± 3.41	−3.41 ± 3.73	0.78 ± 1.55	−3.56 ± 2.57
180 days	1.76 ± 0.79	−1.57 ± 1.19	5.41 ± 3.67	−3.28 ± 3.93	0.70 ± 1.68	−3.72 ± 2.69
210 days	1.74 ± 0.76	−2.17 ± 1.09	5.31 ± 3.55	−5.00 ± 4.04	0.32 ± 1.72	−5.06 ± 1.96
240 days	1.96 ± 0.95	−2.58 ± 0.93	6.21 ± 4.52	−5.71 ± 4.06	0.09 ± 2.09	−5.65 ± 2.05

Displacement and inclination: (+) mesial, (−) distal
Rotation: (+) palatal-mesial, (−) palatal-distal

Table 7.2 Teeth displacement, inclination, and rotation after extraction of upper second premolars

Periods after extraction	Displacement (mm)		Inclination(°)		Rotation(°)	
	First molar	Canine	First molar	Canine	First molar	Canine
10 days	0.34 ± 0.19	–0.20 ± 0.12	1.92 ± 1.39	–0.15 ± 0.16	0.67 ± 0.41	–0.24 ± 0.96
20 days	0.46 ± 0.33	–0.27 ± 0.20	1.99 ± 1.87	–0.17 ± 0.63	0.64 ± 0.73	–0.39 ± 1.12
30 days	0.59 ± 0.50	–0.32 ± 0.26	2.62 ± 2.19	–0.50 ± 1.07	0.7 ± 0.83	–0.36 ± 1.80
60 days	1.25 ± 0.50	–0.86 ± 0.42	4.58 ± 2.04	–1.86 ± 1.82	1.46 ± 0.96	–1.20 ± 1.35
90 days	1.59 ± 0.69	–1.15 ± 0.57	5.72 ± 2.25	–2.72 ± 2.27	2.00 ± 1.53	–1.68 ± 1.44
120 days	2.28 ± 0.48	–1.34 ± 0.76	7.56 ± 2.66	–3.67 ± 3.14	2.38 ± 2.01	–2.31 ± 1.62
150 days	2.49 ± 0.47	–1.56 ± 0.72	8.18 ± 2.96	–4.19 ± 3.24	2.07 ± 2.04	–2.88 ± 1.52
180 days	2.77 ± 0.55	–1.86 ± 0.61	8.52 ± 2.25	–4.80 ± 3.26	1.71 ± 2.07	–3.53 ± 1.65
210 days	3.14 ± 0.57	–2.11 ± 0.73	10.19 ± 2.12	–5.75 ± 3.99	1.74 ± 2.64	–4.50 ± 0.88
240 days	3.08 ± 0.29	–2.14 ± 0.87	9.92 ± 2.05	–7.05 ± 4.05	0.91 ± 2.30	–4.28 ± 1.21

Displacement and inclination: (+) mesial, (−) distal
Rotation: (+) palatal-mesial, (−) palatal-distal

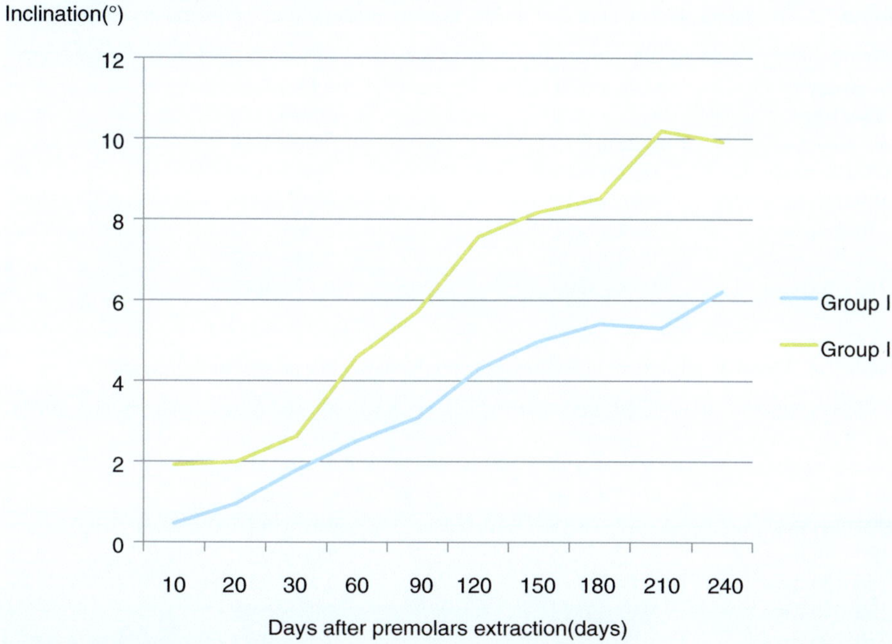

Fig. 7.2 Mesial inclination of first molars after premolars extraction

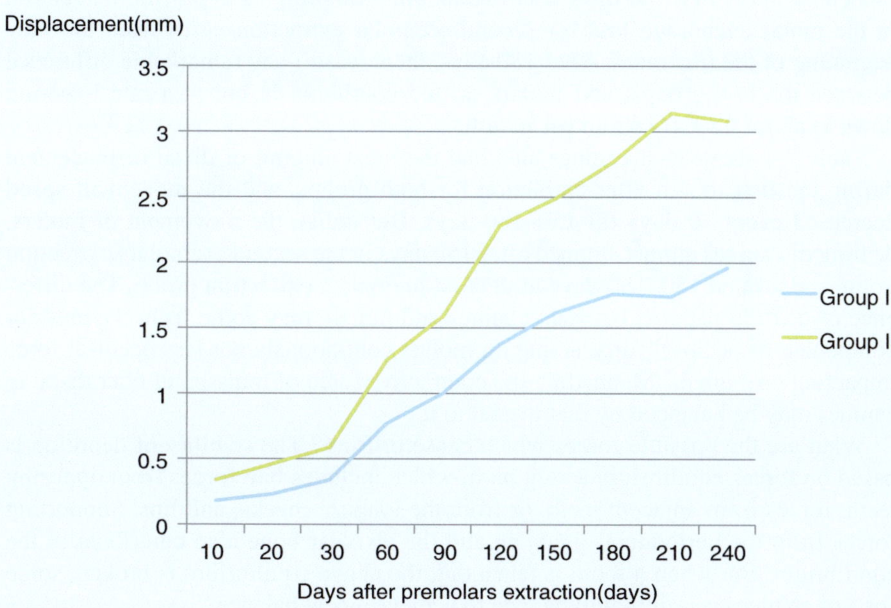

Fig. 7.3 Mesial displacement of first molars after premolars extraction

Table 7.3 Mesial displacement of first molars in every 30 days after the premolars extraction

Periods after extraction	First premolars extraction (mm)s	Second premolars extraction (mm)
0–30 days	0.46 ± 0.51	0.61 ± 0.36
30–60 days	0.32 ± 0.26	0.59 ± 0.26
60–90 days	0.22 ± 0.16	0.39 ± 0.19
90–120 days	0.22 ± 0.11	0.34 ± 0.08
120–150 days	0.16 ± 0.14	0.29 ± 0.08
150–180 days	0.14 ± 0.11	0.28 ± 0.09
180–210 days	0.14 ± 0.08	0.18 ± 0.00
210–240 days	0.14 ± 0.09	0.17 ± 0.17

Table 7.4 Distal displacement of canines in every 30 days after premolars extraction

Periods after extraction	First premolars extraction (mm)	Second premolars extraction (mm)
0–30 days	0.56 ± 0.50	0.37 ± 0.24
30–60 days	0.36 ± 0.28	0.39 ± 0.21
60–90 days	0.27 ± 0.20	0.27 ± 0.24
90–120 days	0.18 ± 0.15	0.16 ± 0.14
120–150 days	0.12 ± 0.14	0.06 ± 0.11
150–180 days	0.06 ± 0.11	0.12 ± 0.11
180–210 days	0.02 ± 0.13	0.03 ± 0.00
210–240 days	0.00 ± 0.04	0.07 ± 0.03

especially in the first 180 days after extraction, prompting us to pay more attention to the molar anchorage loss for second premolar extraction cases from the very beginning of the treatment. After 180 days, there wasn't any remarkable difference between the two groups, and molars drifted continuously but at a rate lowering down to about 0.14–0.18 mm per month.

Table 7.4 shows that canines also had the most amount of distal displacement during the first month after extraction for both groups, and the movement speed decreased every 30 days till 150–180 days. But unlike the movement of molars, drifting of canines almost stopped after 150 days in the second premolars extraction group and around 150–180 days in the first premolars extraction group. The difference of drifting patterns between canines and molars may come from the anterior component of occlusal force acting on molars continuously but less occlusal force impacting on canines. Meanwhile the contractive force of transseptal fiber distal to canines may be balanced by that mesial to it.

What are the possible forces which cause drifting? The stability of dentition is based on forces equilibrium acting on it, which includes bite forces from opposing teeth, forces from adjacent teeth, or from the tongue, cheeks, and lips. Supporting forces from the periodontal ligament and the alveolar bone also contribute to the equilibrium. But when a tooth is taken out, the above equilibrium is broken, some sorts of changes certainly will happen to achieve a new balance.

The anterior component of the occlusal force is speculated to be one of the reasons that drift the teeth when the adjacent teeth are missing [14]. But animal studies [15] have found that the occlusal force would not always accelerate the physiological drift of teeth after extraction, sometimes it may hamper the drift, and there were also studies [15, 16] shown that reduced occlusal force facilitated tooth movement. The controversial outcomes may be resulted from the various directions of the occlusal force, depending on the malocclusion, the contact areas, the cusps abrasion, and so on.

Since the 1960s, animal tests conducted by Murphey, Bulter, Picton, Moss, Xu, and Liu et al. [17–20] have confirmed the physiological drift and concluded that the contractive force came from the healing transseptal fiber after tooth extraction may be one of the possible causes. Murphey studied [17] on *Macaca irus* reported that after the lower right first molar was extracted, the second premolar, which had an original mesial space, moved mesially in the first 2 weeks and then turned back and moved toward the distal. This finding was nearly the same as one of the animal samples in Bulter's study [18]. The reversal of mesial migration of this particular specimen of No. 6 was found coincided with the transseptal fiber reorganizing across the distal alveolar crest. Meanwhile there were two other specimens observed as no reversal of the mesial drifting, of which the transseptal fibers revealed incomplete reorganization. Bulter explained that when the distal transseptal fiber were destructed immediately after the extraction, the second premolar was pulled by fibers in the mesial, but after about 2 weeks when the transseptal fiber reorganized and extended across the interseptal bone crest into the extraction site, the contractive force from the new healing transseptal fibers was higher than the traction force from the mesial, so the premolar started to move distally.

Picton and Moss conducted a series of studies [15, 16, 19, 21] on *Macaca irus*. They [21] found that after the removal of tooth contacts, the distance between pairs of adjacent teeth reduced in only 2 h. It was proposed that the transseptal fiber system produced approximation of the adjacent teeth. By observing the drift of teeth with or without contact with the opposing cusps [15], they also found the small and continuous force from the transseptal fiber system was sufficient to outweigh the intermittent wedging effect when the teeth were brought into occlusion or food was crushed. Moreover, in another study [19], when the transseptal fibers were cut or scraped on one side, the rate of teeth drift on this side was significantly lower than the control side. All these results indicated that the transseptal fiber system played an important part in the physiological drift of teeth.

Southard et al. [22] named the force which could keep teeth contact as "interproximal force (IPF)." He designed a method to measure and calculate the magnitude of IPF of ten volunteers. The bites were disoccluded first in order to exclude the influences from the occlusal forces. He found that IPF was changing according to contacts or circumstances, but the highest force value usually was the one between the lower first molar and the second premolar, which was about 36.7 ± 6.6 g, and could increase to about 57.2 ± 9.1 g after chewing for 5 min. Southard concluded that the source of IPF was the periodontium, and the contractive force of the transseptal fiber might play an important role. From this point of view, we could speculate that the magnitude of the contractive force from the new healing transseptal fibers of an extraction socket might be around the force level of IPF—which was less than 40–60 g roughly.

Fixed Appliance, Friction, and Tooth Movement

For a typical four first bicuspids extraction case, molars are usually used as anchorage to relieve crowding and reduce protrusion. From anchorage protection perspective, reducing the resistance of sliding (RS) on archwire to zero by not bonding the mandibular fixed appliance, in order to allow the lower anterior teeth drift back to take the advantage of the physiological drift, is probably a good strategy [2, 5, 7–9], which was also called as "driftodontics" by Alexander [23]. Usually the lower anterior crowding will be alleviated on some level after a few months indeed (Fig. 7.4). But "driftodontics" is not always wanted because molars could drift forward and lose anchorage too, especially in upper dentition [2, 13]. Under this situation, it is better to put on a fixed appliance to hold up the molars as soon as we can. And the molars should be given a force or moment that can resist this kind of forward drifting tendency. In Tweed technique, orthodontists use headgear for molar anchorage protection or preparation routinely. And tip back bends on Australian wire are used in Begg technique for similar purposes. While in the contemporary straight wire appliance system, a thin round NiTi archwire is usually applied as the initial archwire, it's efficient to align the malpositioned teeth, but the molars won't be hold up when the archwire is in a passive configuration in conventional buccal tube. In high canine or exaggerate curve of Spee upper arch, it may even give upper molars a forward tipping moment to accelerate the anchorage loss. Therefore the XBT tube introduced in Chap. 5 is believed to be a good solution. When the initial light NiTi archwire inserts into the −25° tip back tubes, molars get backward tipping moments to prevent them from drifting forward. While canines may receive the same direction moments in most of the cases, according to Burstone's six classes of geometries introduced in Chap. 2, these moments may actually facilitate canines backward drifting. Under this circumstance, lowering RS on canine brackets will certainly help. Any low-friction brackets may serve this purpose well.

In 1997, Kusy and Whitley [24] described the three components of RS according to the wire-bracket configuration. When the wire-slot angulation (θ) is less than the critical contact angle for binding (θc, the level where the wire contacts both ends of the bracket slot), classic friction (FR) will be the only source of RS. FR=N (normal pressure) $\times\mu$ (friction coefficient). The value of N is the amount of force acting perpendicular to the surface of the object, such as the ligating force.

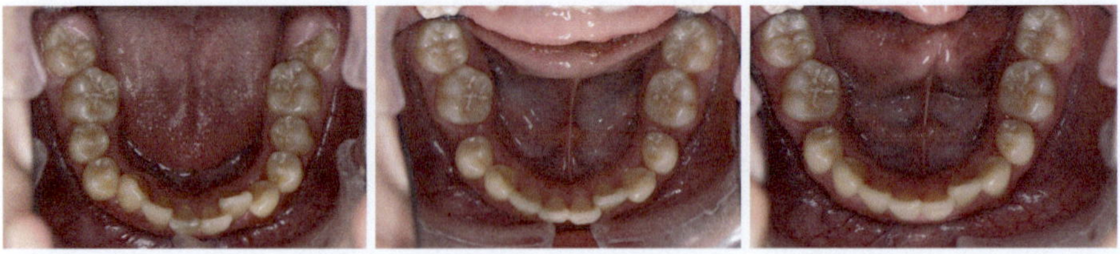

Fig. 7.4 Occlusal views before treatment, and 3 and 6 months after extraction of the lower second premolars

When wire-slot angulation is larger than θc in second-order direction, archwire starts elastic deformation and enters binding (BI) stage. Under this circumstance, there are two normal pressures: the N from ligating in the first order and the force exerted normal to the edges of the bracket slot by the archwire (N_{BI}). The amount of N_{BI} is proportional to correction force, so the thicker, stiffer archwires create more normal force. Hence the RS increases rapidly.

When the wire-slot angulation increases sufficiently to make the wire a plastic deformation, this critical angle is called θz by Kusy, BI becomes notching (No), and the RS increases dramatically that stops tooth sliding.

Theoretically, θc could be affected by two main factors, (1) the clearance between archwire and slot and (2) the width of bracket or buccal tube. In first-order direction, the deeper slot has larger θc. A passive self-ligating bracket has constant θc on a same size archwire, but the θc of an active self-ligating bracket will change depending on the archwire configuration and malocclusion degree. A wider bracket has smaller θc hence increases RS. Self-ligating brackets delay the same size archwire entering binding stage by increasing the first-order θc (Fig. 7.5) or decreasing the bracket's width to increase both the first-order and the second-order θc (Fig. 7.6) comparing with conventional brackets. It decreases the chance of binding and notching in severe crowding dentition with big irregularity. Through these strategies, self-ligating brackets might have some advantages to reduce friction.

However, large wire-slot clearance also decreases teeth control, making mild irregularity correction difficult. As the scene in Fig. 7.7, with one thin archwire, the

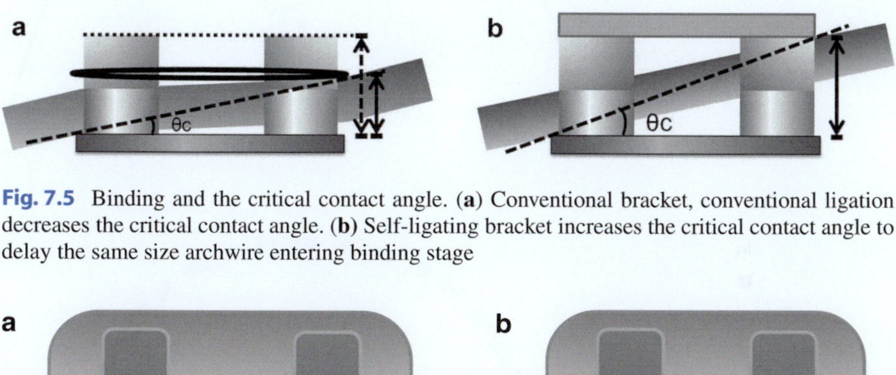

Fig. 7.5 Binding and the critical contact angle. (**a**) Conventional bracket, conventional ligation decreases the critical contact angle. (**b**) Self-ligating bracket increases the critical contact angle to delay the same size archwire entering binding stage

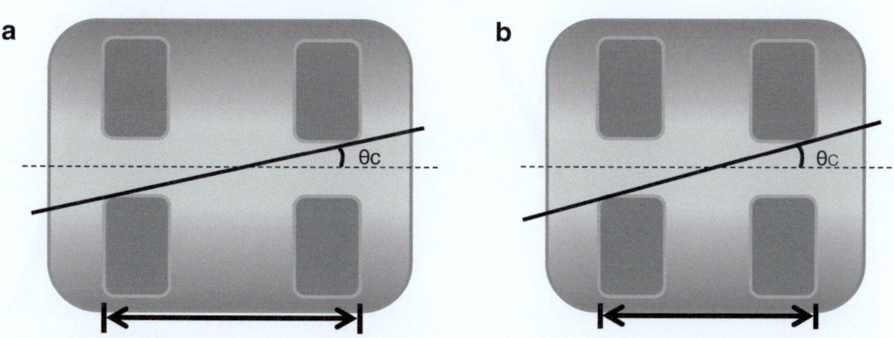

Fig. 7.6 Bracket width and the critical contact angle (*θc*). Narrower bracket has bigger θc when the slot height of brackets are the same (**a**) Wider bracket. (**b**) Narrower bracket

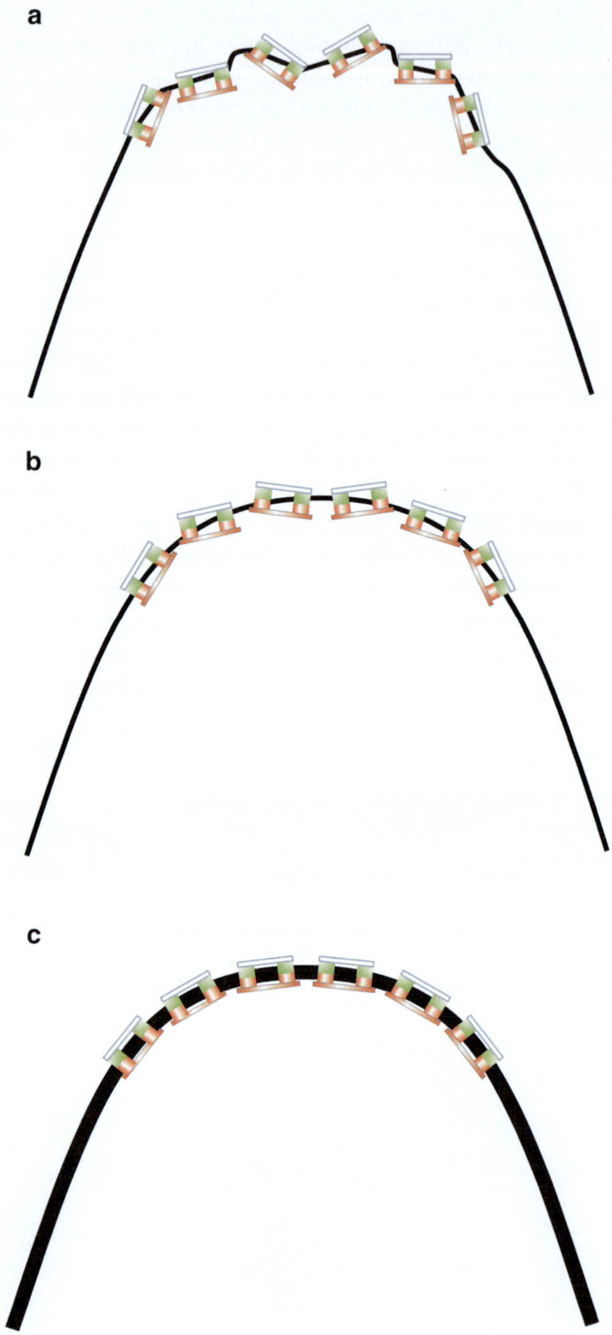

Fig. 7.7 Crowding reliefs by self-ligating brackets with different size of archwires. (**a**) Thin archwire in a crowing arch start to relief the crowding. (**b**) Mild rotations cannot be corrected because the thin archwire have large first-order clearances. (**c**) Rotations corrected by rectangular archwire because of small first-order clearances

most severe rotations are partly corrected, but the mild irregularity is left uncorrected (Fig. 7.7a, b). That's the reason why passive self-ligating bracket system requires changing the second archwire into .014 × .025″ rectangular NiTi wire (Fig. 7.7c) or uses two round archwires to reduce the clearance, instead of the thicker round NiTi archwire which is commonly used in the conventional bracket system.

Kusy [25] pointed out the most efficient tooth movement happened when wire-slot angle θ is approximate to θc, because at this point archwire will just contact to the slot walls hence could exert the correction force on it while RS is lower. But it is not easy to create the situation that θ≈θc for every tooth in one arch with the same type of bracket and one single archwire. Because in most of malocclusion cases, teeth irregularity is various in three dimensions and involves more than one tooth. It is very possible that a wire-slot angle θ is good for the sliding of one tooth but not so good for another one just nearby in the same arch. Hence if a bracket design could give orthodontists the ability to control the balance between low friction and tooth control on one arch, it will be certainly beneficial.

Multilevel Low-Friction (MLF) Brackets

Multilevel low-friction (MLF) bracket (Fig. 7.8) is originally designed to reduce the friction by cutting the outer walls of the slot into slopes to shift up the ligature wire off the archwire to increase the first-order clearance. The unique slope design makes the wire-slot clearance adjustable and so the θc (Fig. 7.9), when coupling various sizes of archwires (.012″, .014″, .016″, .018″) with ligature wires (0.20 mm, 0.25 mm, 0.30 mm) or elastomeric rings to get more than 16 sizes of clearances.

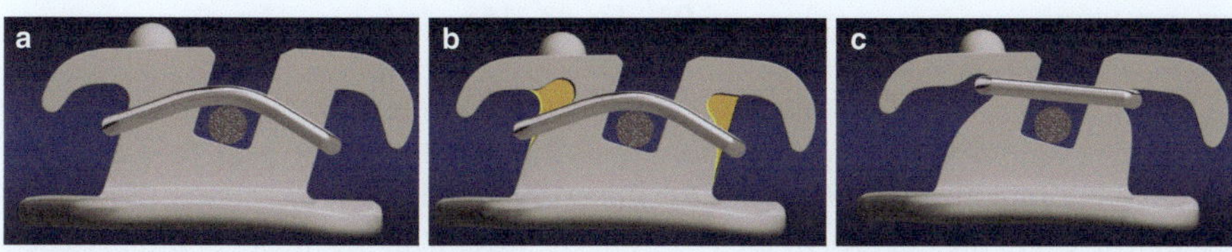

Fig. 7.8 (**a**) Conventional twin bracket. (**b**) Cutting the outer walls of the slot into slopes. (**c**) MLF bracket: the ligature wire is shifted up to increase the wire-slot clearance

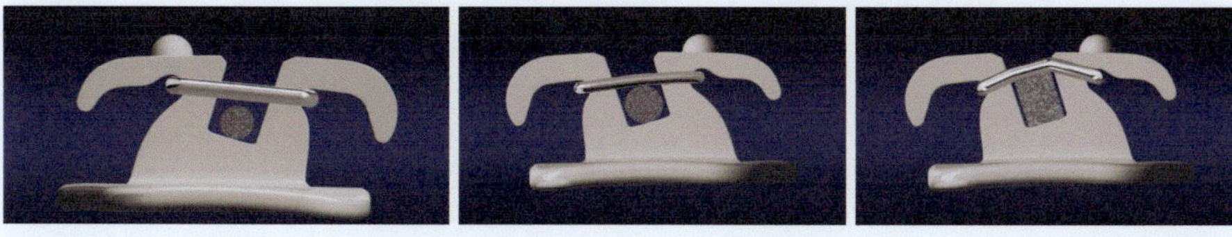

Fig. 7.9 Gradually increasing tooth control when archwire and/or ligature wire getting thicker. Full control of tooth when using rectangular wire

Table 7.5 shows clearance or non-clearance status with different combinations of archwires and ligature wires. When using 0.20 mm ligature wire, all round archwires have clearance. When using 0.25 mm ligature wire, archwire size up to .018″ will just eliminate the clearance. When using 0.30 mm ligature wire, archwire size equal to or thicker than .016″ will leave no clearance. In addition to it, orthodontists can also change a wide twin bracket into a narrow single bracket to increase θc by selecting single wing ligation. In this way, orthodontists can adjust the friction force and correction force on one archwire so that it may have the best chance to realize what Kusy and Whitley [24] suggested the most efficient tooth movement condition—θ≈θc. Since the friction is adjustable, it's called multilevel low-friction (MLF) bracket.

Figure 7.10 illustrates the clinical application of this feature. After extraction of premolars, the lowest RS would be certainly desired to allow the canine drift back, so we can choose 0.20 mm ligature wire on a .012″ or .014″ NiTi archwire. For large deviation tooth as the right lateral incisor, we want large clearance to decrease archwire deformation, so we also choose 0.20 mm ligature wire, and a single wing ligating can also increase θc to reduce binding and meanwhile increase inter-bracket distance to increase elastic range of the archwire. For medium rotated teeth, we can use 0.25 mm ligature, and for mild rotation like right central incisor, we can choose 0.30 mm ligature to increase correction force. So with MLF bracket, orthodontists can adjust the first-order clearance and θc for each tooth on one archwire. This gives orthodontists more control power on teeth correction.

Our ongoing in vitro experiment tests the influence of first-order angulations, thickness of archwires and ligature wires on RS of MLF brackets and conventional brackets. Two nickel-titanium archwires (.014″ round, .018″ round) and two stainless steel ligatures (0.20 mm, 0.25 mm) were coupled with these brackets. The first-order rotation was set at values of 0°, 4°, 8°, 15°, and 20°. The dimensions of brackets were shown in Table 7.6.

The results (Table 7.7) demonstrated the various levels of frictions with different archwire/ligature/rotation combinations in MLF bracket group and revealed that 0.25 mm ligature always had higher RS than 0.20 mm ligature no matter the size of the archwire and the degrees of the rotation. Besides, with the most commonly used

Table 7.5 Clearance with different archwires and ligature wires combination

	Size of ligature wire		
Size of archwire	0.20 mm	0.25 mm	0.30 mm
0.012″	C	C	C
0.014″	C	C	C
0.016″	C	C	NC
0.018″	C	NC	NC
0.016 × 0.022″	NC	NC	NC
0.017 × 0.025″	NC	NC	NC
0.018 × 0.025″	NC	NC	NC
0.019 × 0.025″	NC	NC	NC

C with clearance, *NC* non-clearance

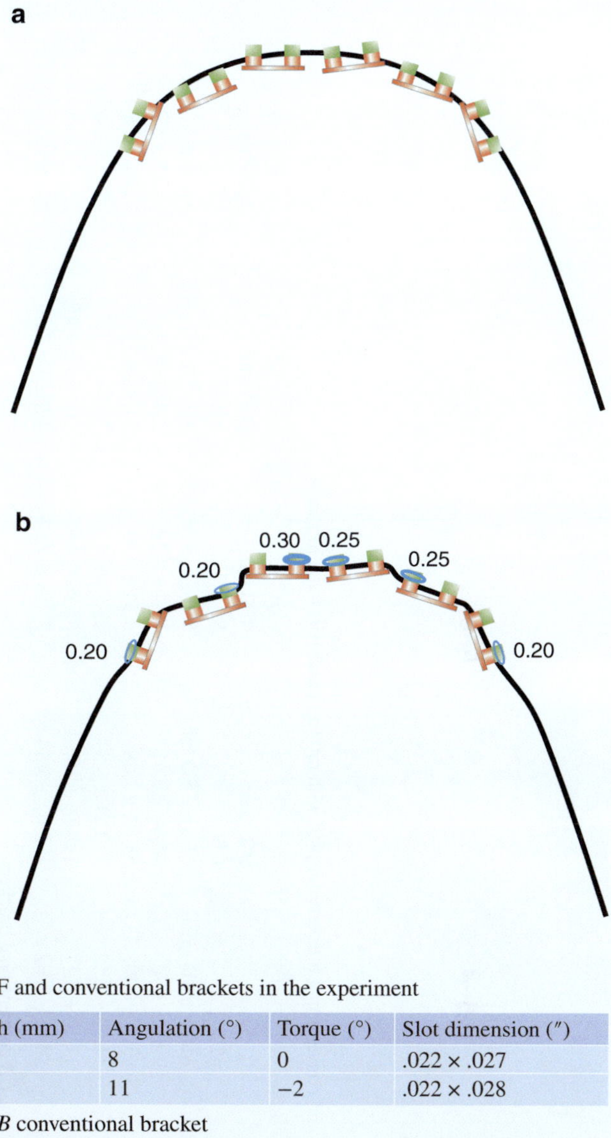

Fig. 7.10 The clinical application of adjusting level of friction for each tooth by choosing size and position of ligature wires. (**a**) The relationships between teeth and the archwire before ligating. (**b**) Choosing different size and position of ligature to adjust the level of friction for each tooth

Table 7.6 Dimensions of MLF and conventional brackets in the experiment

	Bracket width (mm)	Angulation (°)	Torque (°)	Slot dimension (″)
MLF (UR3)	2.78 ± 0.02	8	0	.022 × .027
CB (UR3)	3.35 ± 0.00	11	−2	.022 × .028

MLF multilevel low friction, *CB* conventional bracket

initial wire—.014″ NiTi archwire, coupling with 0.20 mm or 0.25 mm ligature in 20° rotations, the highest values of RS are just about 36 g and 51 g, both of which are within the range of light force. While in conventional bracket group with exactly the same setting, the RS is 176 g with 0.25 mm ligature. The results also revealed that the levels of RS of the conventional brackets were significantly higher than that of MLF brackets, which was unfavorable for teeth sliding at the initial treatment stage. If using elastic module, the first-order clearance will be much less than using ligature wire. North Carolina study showed when ligating a .014″ CuNiTi with

Table 7.7 RS of MLF brackets and conventional brackets coupled with different archwires and ligatures

Archwire	0.014″			0.018″		
Ligature	0.20 mm	0.25 mm	0.25 mm	0.20 mm	0.25 mm	0.25 mm
Bracket type	MLF	MLF	CB	MLF	MLF	CB
Degree	Mean ± SD (gF)	Mean ± SD (gF)	Mean ± SD (gF)	Mean ± SD (gF)	Mean ± SD (gF)	Mean ± SD (gF)
0°	1.12 ± 1.18	2.52 ± 1.70	40.06 ± 6.61	1.64 ± 3.10	2.46 ± 4.70	51.45 ± 6.27
4°	2.98 ± 1.11	6.47 ± 1.40	55.62 ± 7.68	4.50 ± 2.53	31.38 ± 3.20	125.55 ± 6.44
8°	8.32 ± 2.23	11.09 ± 2.52	112.21 ± 6.84	23.96 ± 4.02	70.04 ± 3.37	190.54 ± 4.96
15°	15.76 ± 5.16	17.10 ± 3.17	139.16 ± 15.01	62.90 ± 4.88	108.56 ± 5.45	227.13 ± 5.97
20°	36.09 ± 5.48	50.61 ± 6.62	176.01 ± 5.54	71.54 ± 7.60	126.96 ± 8.50	232.95 ± 8.47

MLF multilevel low-friction bracket, *CB* conventional bracket

elastic module on MLF, the friction force can reach to 201.9 g at 20° rotation (Table 5.5 in Chap. 5). Although the two experimental data can't be compared directly because of different NiTi material and testing machine, larger clearance with thin ligature wire is certainly beneficial to sliding mechanics than smaller clearance with thick elastic module.

Kusy [26] has evaluated the influence on binding of third-order torque to second-order angulation based on an experiment of ten wire dimensions, four bracket widths, and four bracket slots (.018″, .020″, .022″, and .024″). The results found thinner or tender wire (e.g., NiTi wire) provided lighter torque moment comparing with a thicker or stiffer (e.g., stainless steel wire) one. He proposed that using a .020″ slot can accrue practical advantages, on the basis of the contemporary orthodontic treatment philosophy which prefers light and continuous force and torque. But for an extraction case with a .022″ slot system, normally we have to sacrifice the light torque requirement and use a .019 × .025″ archwire to maintain the teeth angulation and torque. If the .020″ slot system can be introduced into the clinic, smaller wires can be applied to gain both light torque moment and good tooth control, because of the reduction of the wire-slot clearance.

Theoretically, for a .019 × .025″ archwire in a .022″ slot, the value of torque play can be calculated from trigonometric functions as 7.3° [27]. But as Brauchli et al. had mentioned, in reality the third-order clearance should be larger because neither the dimensions of the slot nor the dimensions of the archwire are 100 % precise. Therefore they believed that the measured torque play in vitro can be expected to be about 15° for the abovementioned combination [28, 29]. So every .001″ clearance will cause 5° torque loss for a combination of .019 × .025″ archwire in a .022 × .028″ slot. This was similar with the experimental results from Xing and Feng [30] and Meling et al. [31].

MLF bracket has dual slot size: .020 × .027″ slot for incisors and .022 × .027″ for other teeth. Table 7.8 shows prescriptions of MLF brackets and XBT tubes in PASS. The purpose of setting the .020″ slot is to decrease the third-order slot-wire clearance to get better torque control with lighter force. And compared with a .018″ slot, it fits most of the frequently used rectangular archwires and gives orthodontists more clinical flexibility.

Wainwright et al. [32–37] believed the moment of 15–20 Nmm is clinically optimal or effective for torque application. The torsional stiffness of archwire is essential for torque moment delivering. Meling et al. [31] tested the torsional properties of rectangular stainless steel and NiTi wires. They found the torsional stiffness of stainless steel wires was obviously higher than that of NiTi wires. Huang et al. [38] confirmed that for a .019 × .025″ stainless steel wire, just 3° torsion can yield 20 Nmm torque moment, and for a .018 × .025″ stainless steel wire, the 4° torsion will do the same. Such a narrow range of torque twist needed to apply on the wire is hard to deliver precisely by hands. Therefore they both suggested better to gain the torque control through the bracket rather than the wire, and a rectangular NiTi archwire or thinner stainless steel rectangular archwire was recommended as well.

Considering the wire stiffness requirement for space closing or arch form maintaining and the light force demanding for patient's comfort and teeth health, the

Table 7.8 Prescriptions and dimensions of MLF brackets and XBT tubes

Tooth	Torq. (°)	Ang. (°)	Distal offset (°)	M/D width or length (mm)	Slot dimension (″)
U1	16	4	0	3.0	0.020 × 0.027
U2	14	6	0	2.8	0.020 × 0.027
U3	0	8	0	2.8	0.022 × 0.027
U4	−4	−1	0	2.8	0.022 × 0.027
U5	−4	−3	0	2.8	0.022 × 0.027
U6 (auxiliary tube)	−10 (0)	−7/(−25)	10 (15)	4.5	0.022 × 0.027/(0.018)
U7	−20	−9	5	3.2	0.022 × 0.027
L1	−3	0	0	2.2	0.020 × 0.027
L2	−3	0	0	2.2	0.020 × 0.027
L3	0	3	0	2.8	0.022 × 0.027
L4	−10	0	0	2.8	0.022 × 0.027
L5	−15	−2	0	2.8	0.022 × 0.027
L6	−15	−4/(−20)	0	4.2	0.022 × 0.027/(0.018)
L7	−10	−6	0	3.0	0.022 × 0.027

.018 × .025″ and .019 × .025″ stainless steel archwires are the most common used archwires by the majority of orthodontists. Among them, .018 × .025″ stainless steel is considered as the best choice in PASS' dual slot size system. For the anterior teeth which need more labial-palatal inclination control, there is about 5° third-order clearance less with this wire in the .020″ slot than the conventional combination of .019 × .025″ stainless steel wire in a .022″ slot. Thus, a better incisor torque expression can be expected with MLF brackets. On the other hand, Oliver's study [39] showed third-order torque in posterior dental segments can generate frictional resistance during anterior retraction using sliding mechanics. A substantial increase in frictional resistance occurs if the torque in a bracket slot exceeds the third-order clearance angle of the wire-slot combination. So for the posterior segments in which low frictions are desired to facilitate the wire-slot sliding, the configuration of .018 × .025″ stainless steel archwire in a .022″ slot in PASS system will have about 20° third-order clearance, which means having 5° more clearance than a .019 × .025″ stainless steel wire does. Therefore the larger torque clearance of the .018″–.022″ wire-slot configuration could reduce the friction force obviously.

According to Kusy's study [26], the torque effect of the .019 × .025″ archwire in a .020″ slot is similar to a .021 × .025″ archwire in the .022″ slot; they have the same amount of small torque clearance, only about 5°. Thus we should be careful of applying this kind of wire-slot combination, for the high torsional stiffness of a .019 × .025″ stainless steel archwire makes it difficult to keep the torque moment within the physiological limit precisely. So if .019 × .025″ stainless steel archwire is needed for strong torque control, using .019 × .025″ NiTi archwire beforehand is suggested. For cases that have less torque control demanding, a .017 × .025″ stainless steel or other less size archwire could be chosen alternatively.

The main worry of using undersized archwire in retraction stage is tipping control on posterior teeth when anchorage control is critical. Unlike most of the straight wire system, PASS designed a gradually increasing distal tipping angle from the first bicuspids to the second molars for both arches (Table 7.8). This embodies part of the curve of Spee in upper arch and simulates the anchorage preparing in lower arch as Tweed anchorage preparation. Individualized curve of Spee can be made up on archwire according to the compensation needs of specific malocclusion.

Acknowledgment The work was supported, in part, by Beijing Municipal Science & Technology Commission No. Z141107002514054.

References

1. Bourdet M (1957) Researches et Observations Sur toutes les parties de'l art du Dentiste, Paris
2. Weber AD (1969) A longitudinal analysis of premolar enucleation. Am J Orthod 56(4):394–402
3. Campbell-Wilson M (1975) Preliminary investigation into the movement of the lower labial segment following loss of first premolars. Br J Orthod 2(1):25–28
4. Robertson NAE, Cavina R, Moss JP (1979) The effect of the extraction of lower first premolars on the migration of teeth in the human dental arch. J Dent Res 58:1252
5. Papandreas SG, Buschang PH, Alexander RG et al (1993) Physiologic drift of the mandibular dentition following first premolar extractions. Angle Orthod 63(2):127–134
6. Swessi DM, Stephens CD (1993) The spontaneous effects of lower first premolar extraction on the mesio-distal angulation of adjacent teeth and the relationship of this to extraction space closure in the long term. Eur J Orthod 15(6):503–511
7. Jia QL, Gao XM, Fu MK (1995) Physiological drift of the mandibular dentition after first premolar extractions. Chin J Stomatol 30(1):23–25
8. Jia QL, Gao XM, Fu MK (1995) Physiological drift of the mandibular dentition after second premolar extractions. Chin J Orthod 2(2):58–60
9. Wei S, Jing LI, Zhou YH (2013) Three-dimension model analysis for physiological drift of the mandibular dentition after extraction of mandibular second premolars of Angle class II patients. J Peking Univ Health Sci 45(1):81–86
10. Glauser R (1973) An evaluation of serial extraction among Navajo Indian Children. Am J Orthod 63(6):622–632
11. Kinne JH (1975) Untreated first premolar serial extraction: long term observation. Dissertation, University of Washington, Seattle
12. Chen G, Chen S, Zhang XY et al (2011) Stable region for maxillary dental cast superimposition in adults, studied with the aid of stable miniscrews. Orthod Craniofac Res 14(2):70–79
13. Du FY, Xu TM (2014) An exploratory study of physiologic drift of the dentition following the extraction of maxillary premolar. Dissertation, Peking University School and Hospital of Stomatology, Beijing
14. Beek HV, Fidler VJ (1977) An experimental study of the effect of functional occlusion on mesial tooth migration in macaque monkeys. Arch Oral Biol 22(4):269–271
15. Picton DC, Moss JP (1978) The effect of reducing cusp height on the rate of approximal drift of cheek teeth in adult monkeys (Macaca irus). Arch Oral Biol 23(3):219–223
16. Picton DC, Moss JP (1980) The effect on approximal drift of altering the horizontal component of biting force in adult monkeys. Arch Oral Biol 25(1):45–48
17. Murphey WH (1970) Oxytetracycline microfluorescent comparison of orthodontic retraction into recent and healed extraction sites. Am J Orthod 58(3):215–239
18. Bulter T (1969) Comparative histologic study of heavy intermittent and light continuous forces. Am J Orthod 55(3):304–305
19. Picton DC, Moss JP (1973) The part played by the trans-septal fibre system in experimental approximal drift of the cheek teeth of monkeys (Macaca irus). Arch Oral Biol 18(6):669–680

20. Liu XL, Chen X, Lin H et al (2004) An experimental study of tooth movement. J Xi Jiao Tong Uni Med Sci 24(5):510–513
21. Picton DC, Moss JP (1982) Short-term changes in the mesiodistal position of teeth following removal of approximal contacts in the monkey (Macaca fascicularis). Arch Oral Biol 27(3):273–278
22. Southard TE, Southard KA, Tolley EA (1992) Periodontal force: a potential cause of relapse. Am J Otrhod Dentofac Orthop 101(3):221–227
23. Alexander RG (1983) The Vari-simplex discipline. Part 3: extraction treatment. J Clin Orthod 17(8):537–547
24. Kusy RP, Whitley JQ (1997) Friction between different wire-bracket configurations and materials. Semin Orthod 3(3):166–177
25. Kusy RP (2000) Ongoing Innovations in Biomechanics and Materials for the New Millennium. Angle Orthod 70(5):366–376
26. Kusy RP (2004) Influence on binding of third-order torque to second-order angulation. Am J Orthod Dentofacial Orthop 125(6):726–732
27. Joch A, Pichelmayer M, Weiland F (2010) Bracket slot and archwire dimensions: manufacturing precision and third order clearance. J Orthod 37(4):421–429
28. Brauchli LM, Senn C, Wichelhaus A (2011) Active and passive self-ligation — a myth? Angle Orthod 81(2):312–318
29. Brauchli LM, Steineck M, Wichelhaus A (2012) Active and passive self-ligation: a myth? Part 1: torque control. Angle Orthod 82(4):663–669
30. Xing LT, Feng YX (2013) Torque performance of the different bracket systems and how torque angle affects on frictional resistance. Dissertation, Shanxi medical university, Shanxi
31. Meling TR, Odegaard J, Meling EO (1997) On mechanical Properties of square and rectangular stainless steel wires tested in torsion. Am J Orthod Dentofacial Orthop 111(3):310–320
32. Wainwright WM (1973) Faciolingual tooth movements: its influence on the root and cortical plate. Am J Orthod 64(3):278–302
33. Burstone CJ (1966) The mechanics of the segmented arch techniques. Am J Orthod 36(2):99–120
34. Feldner JC, Sarkar NK, Sherican JJ et al (1994) In vitro torque deformation characteristics of orthodontic polycarbonate brackets. Am J Orthod Dentofacial Orthop 106(2):265–272
35. Jarabak JR, Fizzel JA (1973) Technique and treatment with light-wire edgewise appliances. Am J Orthod Dentofacial Orthop 64(3):317–318
36. Reitan K (1957) Some factors determining the evaluation of forces in orthodontics. Am J Orthod 43(1):32–45
37. Reitan K (1964) Effects of force magnitude and direction of tooth movement on different alveolar bone types. Angle Orthod 34:244–253
38. Huang N, Gu M, Han XL et al (2008) The properties of different orthodontic rectangular arch wires in torsion. W China J Stomatol 26(2):152–155
39. Chung M, Nikolai RJ, Kim KB et al (2009) Third-order torque and self-ligating orthodontic bracket–type effects on sliding friction. Angle Orthod 79(3):551–557

Physiologic Anchorage Control System

8

Tian Min Xu

Abstract

Based on the physiologic characteristics of craniofacial growth, dentoalveolar compensation, and the function of posterior curve of Spee, combining with mechanism of differential moments and advantages of NiTi wire, a corresponding appliance has been developed to simplify the treatment mechanics with the very basic bracket structure. It composes of XBT buccal tube and MLF bracket. Combined with archwires with the curve of Spee, we try to follow physiologic features of dentition as much as possible and take advantage of it while doing orthodontic treatment. We call this new appliance Physiologic Anchorage Spee-wire System or PASS. The main difference between PASS and contemporary straight wire appliance (SWA) is that SWA's prescription is based on optimal occlusion when occlusion development is completely finished, while PASS pays more attention to the dynamic process of occlusal development and dental compensation characteristics when jaw relationship is not optimal. The knowledge of how dentoalveolar compensation occurs will give orthodontists clues on how to retard it or even reverse it. A striking feature of this technique is that we try to keep the physiologic or compensated curve of Spee in posterior segment for function while straightening anterior teeth for esthetics.

In above seven chapters, we have introduced the fundamental theory of physiologic anchorage control system. The treatment philosophy of PASS is based on best available knowledge of malocclusion occurrence and research progress on craniofacial growth and biomechanics at the present time.

T.M. Xu
Department of Orthodontics, Peking University School and Hospital of Stomatology, Beijing, China
e-mail: tmxuortho@163.com

T.M. Xu (ed.), *Physiologic Anchorage Control*,
DOI 10.1007/978-3-319-48333-7_8

Dynamic Process of Occlusal Development

Björk's metallic implant studies told us that the forward rotation is a general feature of the facial development, and the rotation of the mandible is more than twice as great as that of the maxilla. From biomechanical point of view, if mandible outgrows maxilla in sagittal plane and rotates more than twice as maxilla counterclockwise, the occlusal contact relation will tip the upper molar forward. Figure 8.1a–d illustrates the dental compensation during facial growth based on Björk implant study data [1]. Growth studies [2, 3] on upper molars seem to support this deduction.

If the upper molar is tipped forward, it will push teeth before it to shift forward (Fig. 8.1d). This anterior force may also transit through interproximal contact of teeth to reach incisors or even cross the dental midline in the way Southard [4, 5] found for the dissipation of the anterior component of the occlusal force until the resistance from the opposite direction to reach an equilibrium state (Fig. 8.2). During this process, if premolars or canines erupt into dentition in time, incisors may be pushed forward to create protrusion, while if premolars or canines erupt late or outside the normal dental arch, the upper molar might tip forward more to shorten the dental arch length and cause crowding. Figure 8.3 shows a situation when the second premolar erupts later than mandible growth spurt, the upper molar may tip much more than it should be, which may later on change functional occlusal plane when aligning buccal segment teeth on a straight line with the first molar. When protrusion or crowding reaches to a certain limit, extraction orthodontic treatment is inevitable.

Dental Compensation of Abnormal Skeletal Relationship

If mandible growth is the cause of the compensatory change of molar angulation, abnormal skeletal relationship should result in different molar angulation. To test this hypothesis, we investigated a large sample of 1403 subjects seeking orthodontic treatment at the orthodontic clinic of Peking University School of Stomatology [6]. Pretreatment cephalometric films were measured. According to the cephalometric data of Chinese normal occlusion (ANB $2.7 \pm 2.0°$; MP/SN $32.5 \pm 5.2°$) [7], we classified the skeletal sagittal and vertical jaw relationships into skeletal Class I to Class III and low- to high-angle groups. The upper molar to palatal plane and lower molar to mandibular plane angulations were measured and comparisons were made among the six groups. The results are summarized in Table 8.1.

From Table 8.1, we can find in skeletal Class II cases where the lower teeth or mandible were in a relatively distal position compared with the opposing counterpart, the maxillary first molar would be more distally inclined, whereas the mandibular first molar would be more mesially inclined. The opposite was true in skeletal Class III cases. This indicates that molar angulation compensates to sagittal jaw relationship. If we check vertical jaw relationship, we can find that in

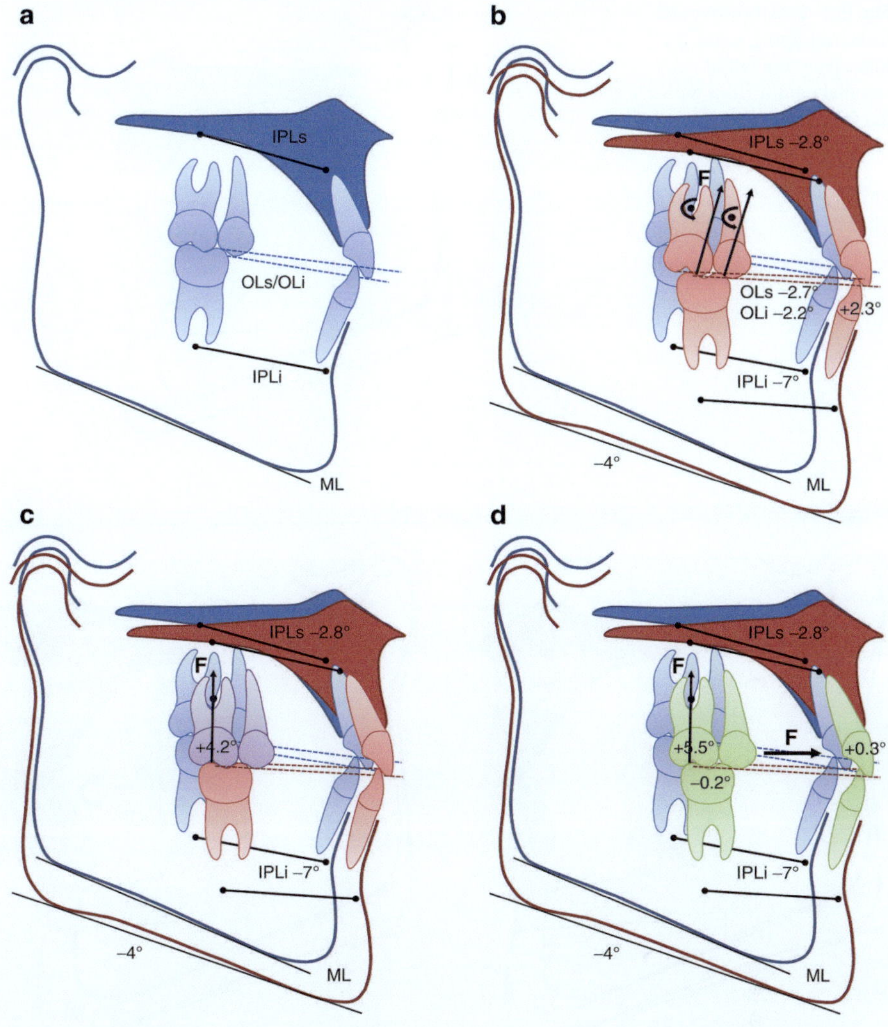

Fig. 8.1 (**a**) IPLs represents implant line in maxilla; IPLi represents implant line in mandible. OLs represents maxillary occlusal line and OLi represents mandible occlusal line following Björk study. (**b**) In Björk sample of 19 cases with metallic implants, mandible rotated −7° on average while maxilla rotated −2.8°, which may change molar occlusal contact and give upper molar and premolar forward tipping moment. Upper and lower occlusal plane also compensated for the difference between maxilla and mandible rotation by more than −2° through posterior teeth eruption. (**c**) Meanwhile, the upper molar may tip forward to compensate the difference between mandible and maxilla rotation (7°–2.8°= 4.2°) too. (**d**) According to Johnston's study, when mandible outgrows maxilla, it brings upper molar forward, which may explain why in Björk sample, the upper molar tipped 5.5°, larger than the difference between mandible and maxilla rotation. And the forward tipping force of posterior teeth may transfer through interproximal contacts to incisors and tip them labial too. The reaction may tip lower molar back a little bit too (Redrawn from Björk and Skieller [1])

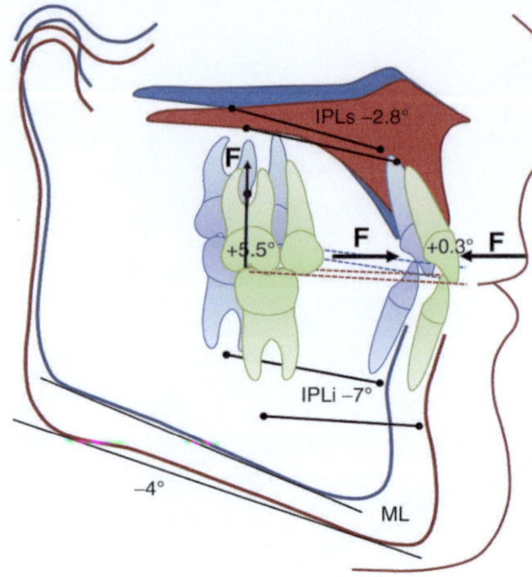

Fig. 8.2 Incisors stopped forward tipping when the force from the labial reached equilibrium with the force from the backward

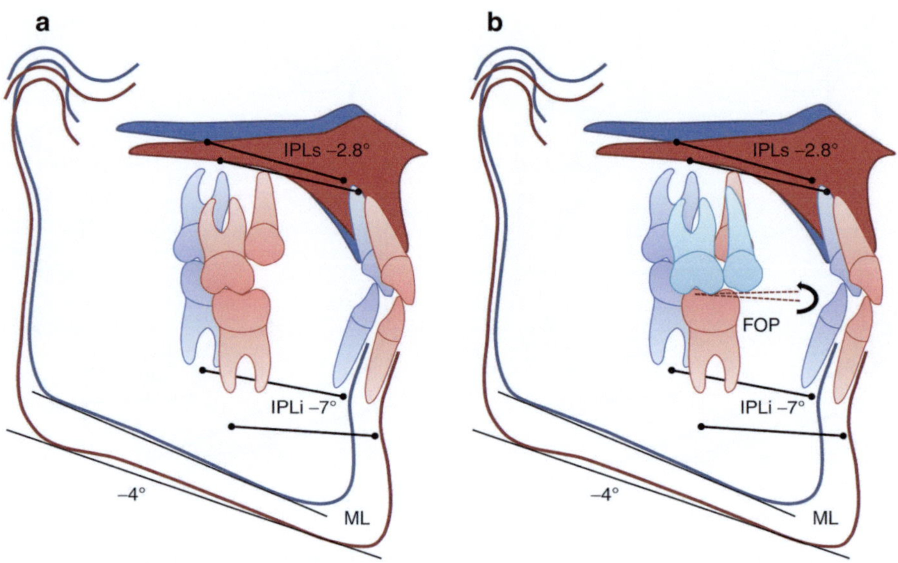

Fig. 8.3 (**a**) When delayed eruption of second premolar happened, upper molar may tip forward more to occupy part of premolar space. (**b**) Forward-tipping upper molar may tip premolars forward than normal and also decrease occlusal plane

high-angle cases, both upper and lower molars were more distally tipped, and in low-angle cases, both molars were mesially tipped. These results agree with Liao's study on normal occlusion with different vertical jaw relationships , and indicate that molar angulation compensates to vertical jaw relationship too. We can therefore imagine the upper molar may tip back most in Class II high-angle case. When engaging a straight NiTi wire in extraction case, upper molars in this kind of skeletal jaw relationship would certainly get more forward tipping moment than other

Table 8.1 The upper molar to palatal plane and lower molar to mandibular plane angulations (°)

		UM/PP		LM/MP	
Classification	*N*	Mean ± SD	*P* value	Mean ± SD	*P* value
Sagittal			0.000		0.000
Class I	588	80.4 ± 5.4		96.9 ± 5.6	
Class II	646	78.2 ± 5.7		95.6 ± 5.6	
Class III	169	82.5 ± 6.2		98.1 ± 5.6	
Vertical					
Low	56	81.6 ± 6.3	0.000	91.5 ± 4.5	0.000
Average	703	80.2 ± 6.0		94.6 ± 5.1	
High	644	78.8 ± 5.5		98.9 ± 5.3	
Total	1403	79.6 ± 5.9		96.5 ± 5.7	

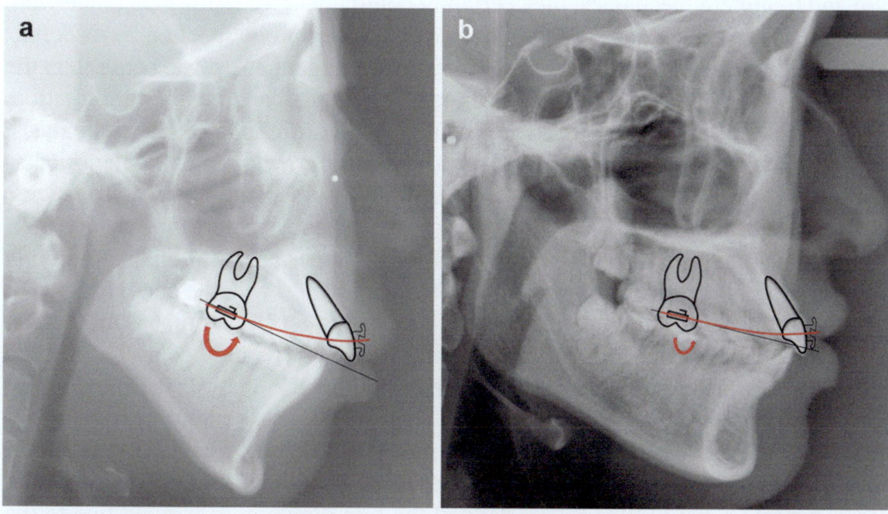

Fig. 8.4 (**a**, **b**) Straight wire gives upper molar more forward tipping moment in high-angle Class II with apparent curve of Spee than in low-angle Class I

skeletal patterns that have relatively uprighted molars (Fig. 8.4a, b). Will that lead to more upper molar forward tipping or anchorage loss? To answer this question, we made a further investigation on posttreatment cephalograms in the above sample of 1403 subjects. The independent sample t-test for the analysis of the change of UM/PP and treatment-related factors showed that the UMs tipped forward more in premolar extraction cases than non-extraction cases with statistical significance. When using the change of UM/PP as dependent variable and possible relative factors as independent variables, the pretreatment UM/PP angle stuck out as the most significant factor contributing to anchorage loss. The more distally tipped the UMs are before treatment, the more they will tip mesially during treatment [9]. That questions our daily practice of putting straight archwire into any malocclusion as a routine technique.

Key Role of Functional Occlusal Plane

Occlusal plane is an important reference for orthodontists to align upper and lower teeth on it. Prof. Johnston [10] called it "bottom line," because treatment must ultimately be felt at the level of the occlusion for it to have an effect on the molar relationship. Basically there are four defined occlusal planes in orthodontics: functional occlusal plane, Down's occlusal plane or anatomic occlusal plane, upper occlusal plane, and lower occlusal plane. Each serves different purpose by their respective definitions. When making treatment plan, which one should we aim at? This question is often asked in full-mouth denture restoration, but has never been asked in orthodontics. Since the last three definitions of the occlusal planes involved upper and lower incisors that predispose to be influenced by different types of malocclusion and treatment mechanics, they certainly could not serve as the goal plane well. Functional occlusal plane (FOP) relates more to posterior bite function by its definition and may serve our purpose of orienting posttreatment bite plane better than the other three although it tends to reduce its cant following mandible forward rotation. Johnston also uses this one as "bottom line" to constitute the pitchfork analysis. From biomechanical point of view, if mandible is outgrowing maxilla, the orientation of masticatory muscles attached to mandible would change with it. To reach a new balance of force and improve posterior bite efficiency, molars may change their angulation along with mandible growth. When all upper posterior teeth are tipping forward and going downward to compensate mandible growth, the curve of Spee of upper arch decreases and that of lower arch increases to form compensation curve as Dr. Spee described. The final result is still a curve. The flat occlusal plane is a simplification of the curved one to facilitate cephalometric analysis in orthodontics. FOP used to represent posterior occlusal plane cant decreases along with the above changes of the curve of Spee. The process should also be regarded as dentoalveolar compensation to mandible growth. Now the question is how to simplify the posterior curve into a flat FOP? Osborn defined the bite direction as vertical line to the tangent of the posterior curve of Spee composed by the last two upper molars [11]. But in orthodontics, since the second molar usually is not fully erupted at the beginning of treatment, orthodontists used to simplify functional occlusal plane as a straight line bisecting the occlusion of the first molar, second premolar, and first premolar instead. We therefore should know, when using a straight line to represent a curved occlusal plane, we could have different directions depending on the definition (Fig. 8.5). And one of the directions might represent the best for bite efficiency determined by physiologic circumstance of individual's oral-gnathic system, although we don't know which one it is.

Now, let's check the effects of our contemporary orthodontic appliance on the functional occlusal plane. Take extraction of four premolars case as an example. After extraction, the original force equilibrium of dentition as showed in Fig. 8.2 is interrupted, the anterior components of occlusal force, eruption force from end molars, and transseptal fiber force will tend to tip upper molar forward, especially when we engage a straight NiTi wire in a curved occlusal plane, which will give upper molar a forward tipping moment as in Fig. 8.6. This situation will be worsened when canines are in high position as in Fig. 6.4, or second premolars are extracted, ectopic eruption or

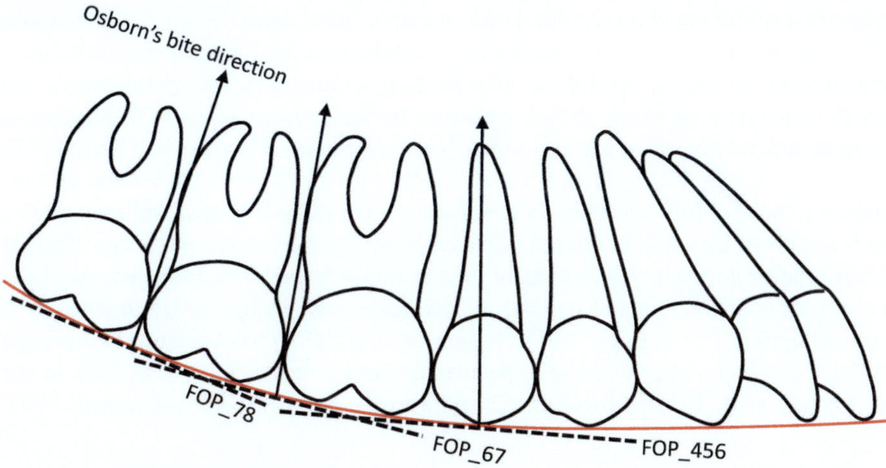

Fig. 8.5 Straighten curve of Spee of upper arch equivalents to make tangents of this curve, which will end up with different FOP directions

Fig. 8.6 Upper M1and PM2 are prone to be tipped forward in aligning stage if no anchorage control measure is applied on posterior teeth especially when they are in backward-tipping position either due to growth stage or compensation of skeletal jaw relation, which may change the FOP

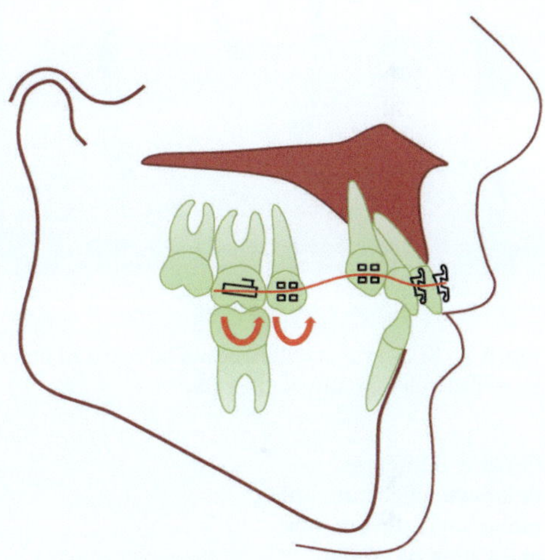

delayed eruption as in Fig. 8.3. When changing to thicker wires, occlusal plane may compromise the vertical difference between anterior teeth and posterior teeth on a curve to a straight line. There will be no problem to align all teeth according to six keys on any straight line as in Fig. 8.7, because six keys' standard does not define normal angle of teeth to jaws or face, but to a straight archwire. And our contemporary orthodontic techniques emphasize aligning teeth on a straight line or a flat occlusal plane for esthetics but neglect which direction of the occlusal plane is appropriate to individual's chewing function and posttreatment stability. I assume that we should treat anterior and posterior teeth for different purposes, straightening anterior teeth for esthetics and keeping posterior curve for function. That comes back to the question of orientation of functional occlusal plane. When posterior segment is a curved one, leveling it with a straight wire will end up with different FOP inclination depending on upper first molar angulation control and treatment mechanics. Mckinney and Harris [12] compared Begg lightwire, standard Tweed edgewise, and straight wire techniques and showed the change of FOP is −0.6° in Begg technique, −1.8° in Edgewise, and −3.2° in SWA. Five times' difference exists between the smallest FOP rotation in Begg technique that always uses tip back bend with Class II elastics and largest FOP rotation in straight wire technique that is usually without tip backs. So we end up with different "bottom line" in different techniques. According to Braun and Legan [13], each degree of forward rotation of occlusal plane tends to increase 0.5 mm Class II molar relationship, which is accordant to our clinical impression on the effects of the three techniques on Class II correction. The respective change in U6 angulation is forward tipping 1.3° in Begg, 2.0° in Edgewise, and 5.6° in SWA relative to averaged FOP [12], in accordance with the respective mechanics we perceived (Fig. 8.8). In our RCT study [14], U6 tips forward 7.2° on average relative to PP plane with MBT

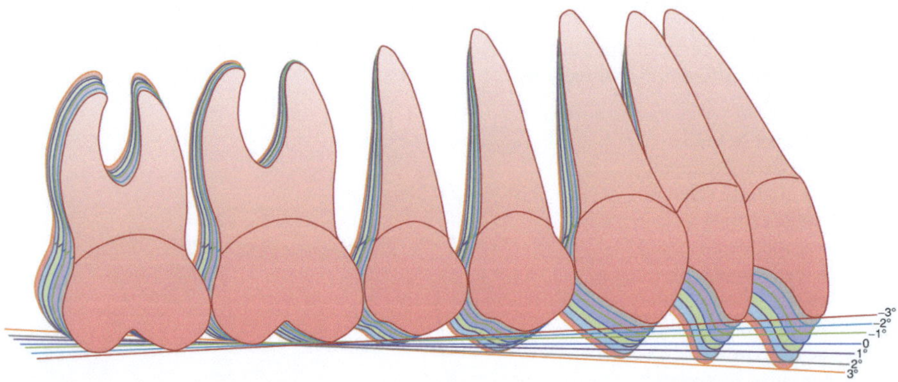

Fig. 8.7 Six keys' standard could be realized on any occlusal planes, orthodontic treatment therefore could change this *bottom line*

Fig. 8.8 Different treatment mechanics affect molar angulation and the inclination of FOP in different ways. *Begg* +molar tip back bend plus +Class II elastics, *Tweed* +molar tip back bends plus −J hook, *SWA* −molar tip forward. *Note* "+" represents FOP increasing direction or clockwise rotation, "−" FOP decreasing direction or counterclockwise rotation that is the tendency of normal growth. Different treatment mechanics may reduce or accelerate it

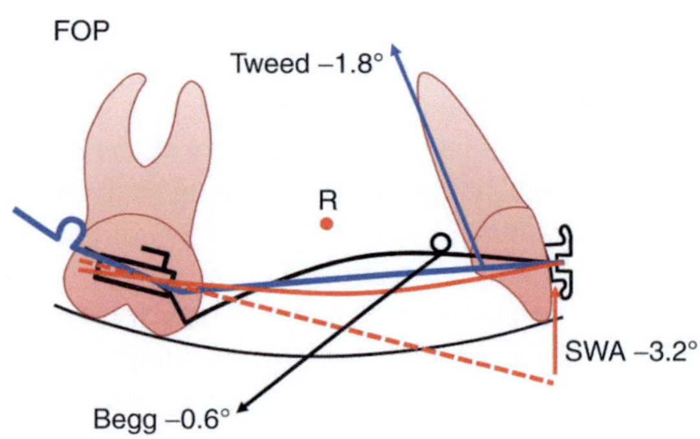

straight wire technique in a maximum anchorage sample. Why orthodontists usually can't discern this kind of change in molar angulation? Probably because when we check the lateral view occlusion or take intraoral lateral view photos, we always align occlusal plane with our camera's horizontal (Fig. 8.9). If U6 angulation plays key role to FOP inclination and teeth can be aligned on any FOP direction with six keys' standard as in Fig. 8.7, then should we follow straight wire mechanics to accelerate FOP forward rotation? Or should we follow Begg mechanics to delay or reduce the FOP forward rotation? Or should we even reverse FOP rotation?

Supposing there is a nature decided ideal occlusal plane at certain age, say 13 years, and we start treatment at 11 years when occlusal plane is on its way toward

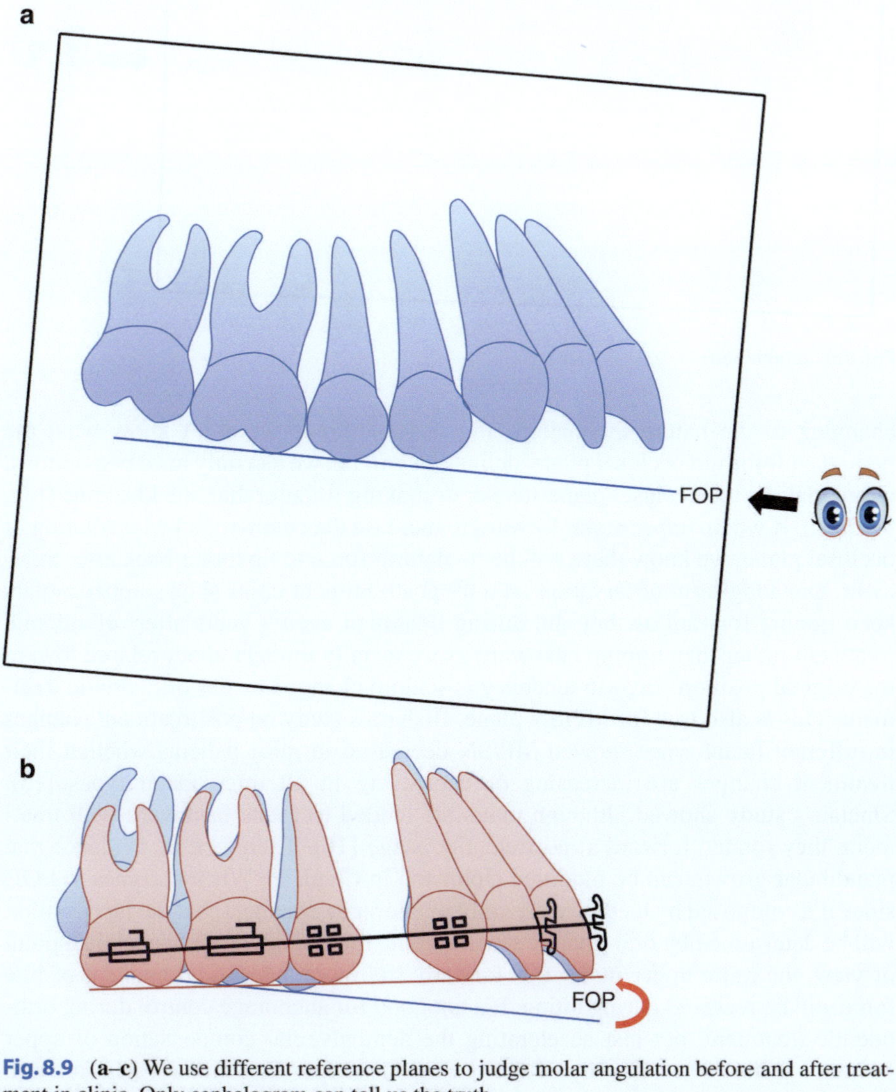

Fig. 8.9 (**a–c**) We use different reference planes to judge molar angulation before and after treatment in clinic. Only cephalogram can tell us the truth

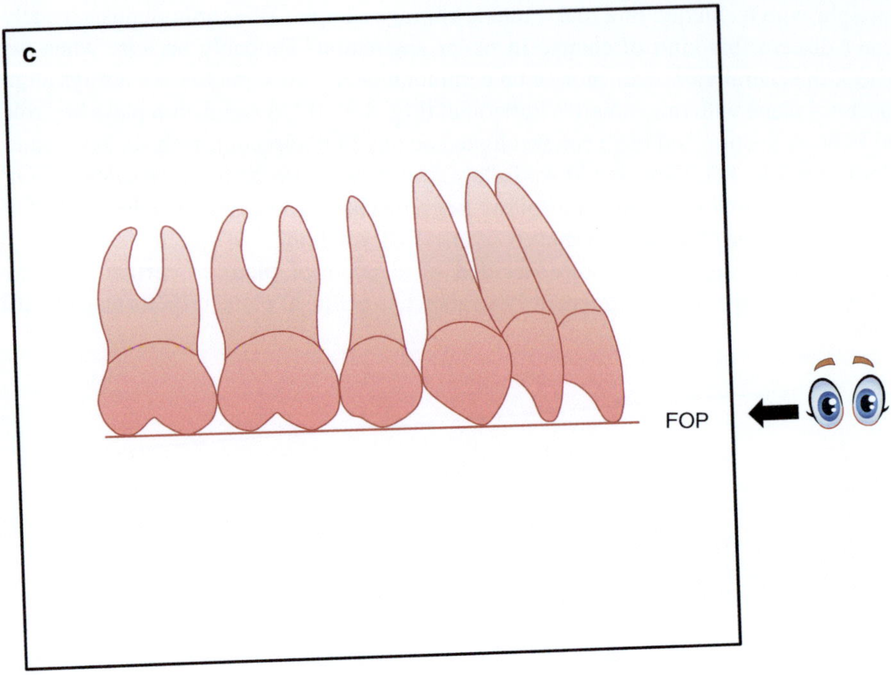

Fig. 8.9 (continued)

changing to the nature inclination (Fig. 8.10a). Since we don't know what the natural equilibrium occlusal plane inclination will be, we can only have two options, either making the occlusal plane steeper or making it flatter than the ideal one (Fig. 8.10b, c). If we tip upper molar forward to increase the counterclockwise rotation of occlusal plane, we know there will be no natural force to tip molar back after treatment. Our long-term observation on a 49 posttreatment cases shows upper molars keep tipping forward as they did during treatment even 3 years after orthodontic treatment rather than tipping backward as we usually thought about relapse toward the original position. Growth tendency is seldom changed by our orthodontic treatment. This is also true for MP/SN plane. Bishara's study on posttreatment changes in different facial types showed MP/SN decreased in most patients whether their treatment changes are increasing or decreasing in all three facial types [15]. Sinclair's study showed although mandible tended to rotate backward with treatment, they rotated forward at postretention stage [16]. There is little evidence that mandibular growth can be modified (Johnston in Chap. 3). When it comes to FOP, since it's composed by teeth, we can only temporarily change it, but the last position will be determined by oral-gnathic system of the individual. From mechanical point of view, the more upper molar tips forward, the more anterior component of bite force will be received during biting. It's not good for anchorage control during orthodontic treatment, not just accelerating the dentoalveolar compensation of upper posterior teeth. When the key of the occlusion—upper first molar—tips forward,

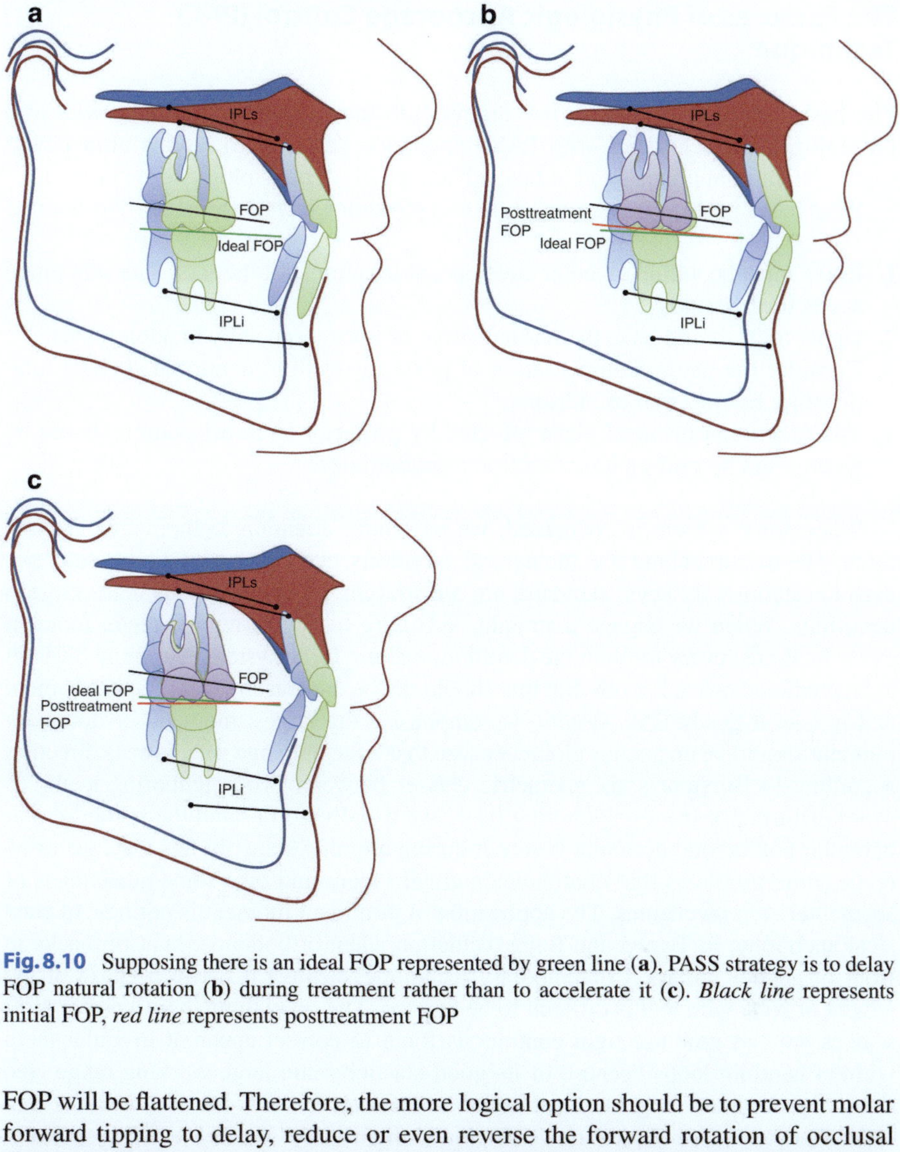

Fig. 8.10 Supposing there is an ideal FOP represented by green line (**a**), PASS strategy is to delay FOP natural rotation (**b**) during treatment rather than to accelerate it (**c**). *Black line* represents initial FOP, *red line* represents posttreatment FOP

FOP will be flattened. Therefore, the more logical option should be to prevent molar forward tipping to delay, reduce or even reverse the forward rotation of occlusal plane, rather than to accelerate it. Just as Prof. Johnston mentioned in Chap. 3, "the final expression at the occlusion is in large measure a prevention, reduction, or reversal of maxillary dentoalveolar compensation" for Class I and Class II subjects. After treatment, with mandible growth, the intercuspation force may tip upper molar forward and flatten the occlusal plane inclination until it reaches a new natural equilibrium position. The role of orthodontic treatment is to give occlusion a second chance to match the mandible growth and function and to give patient straight anterior teeth for esthetics. The physiologic anchorage control technique is based on the above philosophy.

The Features of Physiologic Anchorage Control (PAC) Technique

The basic principle of PAC is moving teeth to the position in harmony with oral physiologic characteristics with PASS appliance designed to reduce unfavorable force system in appliance and to take advantage of all physiologic force in mouth.

What is the position in harmony with oral physiologic characteristics? We assume:

1. Roots must be within alveolar envelope, at least most of the root. The safe range needs further study.
2. Upper arch should have the normal curve of Spee, especially in adolescents.
3. Consider the nature compensation of posterior teeth to abnormal skeletal relationship, not just that of incisors.
4. The functional occlusal plane affected by posterior teeth orientation should be determined by oral-gnathic function of individuals.

When force system is concerned, we pay more attention to moments, not just force. The reason behind it is the natural dentitions, even the optimal ones Andrews used to establish six keys' standard, are not straight, let alone various malocclusion dentitions. When we engage a straight NiTi wire to align irregular teeth, moment exists in almost every tooth in the dentition, making force system extremely difficult to be predicted on each tooth. But that should not be the reason we forget the moment and just let it go. In PAC system, we emphasize the largest moment, or dominant moment should be on anchor molar because that's the only one we know its direction according to Burstone's six geometric classes between two neighboring teeth. To avoid disturbance from neighboring teeth, we usually don't bond the second molar behind it and second premolar before it during aligning stage. In this way, we overcome some problems that continuous archwire faces and take some advantages of segmental arch mechanics. The application of dominant moment is not new to classical anchorage in Tweed and Begg technique when orthodontist bent tip backs in front of anchor molars. Contemporary techniques neglect it partly because of the advent of NiTi wire that is difficult to be bended. The good thing, however, for NiTi wire is we can now use light continuous force to correct apparent irregular teeth without bending loops because of its good elasticity and large working range (see Chap. 5). Another progress in orthodontic appliance is low-friction brackets that reduce the resistance of teeth movement under light force. The above two progress in orthodontic appliance hardware make contemporary orthodontic treatment differ from classical appliances by one possibility, that is, the expression of physiologic force, which is almost impossible on heavy thick wires. What are the physiologic forces in the mouth? The following should be considered in orthodontic treatment:

1. Muscles of lip, bucca, and tongue
2. Tooth eruption force
3. Bite force
4. Periodontal ligament force

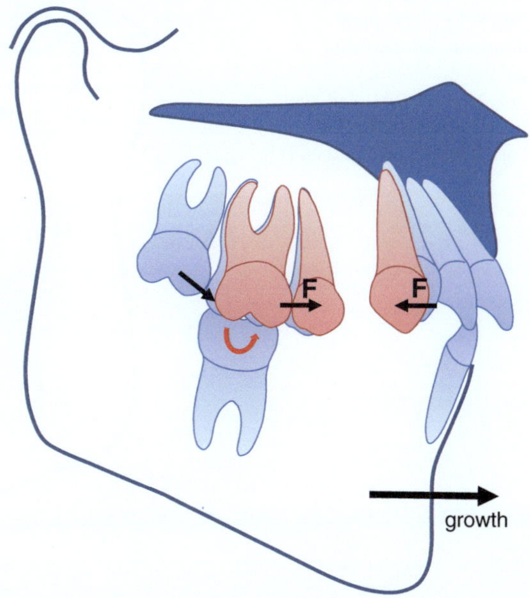

Fig. 8.11 Physiologic anchorage loss caused by mandible growth and U7 eruption

The PASS considers all above forces and moments in the treatment mechanics. When upper molar anchorage control is concerned, Class II is certainly more critical than Class I. So we take a Class II extraction case as an example to illustrate the mechanics of PASS technique (Fig. 8.11, 8.12, and 8.13).

Let's start with the extraction. From dentoalveolar compensation mechanism introduced by Prof. Johnston in Chap. 3 and teeth drift phenomena introduced in Chap. 7, we know that after premolars extraction, the original force equilibrium of dentition is broken. Upper posterior teeth tend to tip forward to lose anchorage, and canine tends to drift back toward extraction space (Fig. 8.11). So we advise you to bond molar XBT tube and anterior MLF brackets no later than 2 weeks after extraction. According to Chap. 7, teeth drifting were found as early as 10 days after extraction. When initial thin NiTi wires are engaged in −25° tip back tube on upper molar and −20° tip back "virtual tube" on lower molar, they give molars a tip back moment to prevent it from forward tipping (Fig. 8.12). When anchor molar occupies the dominant moment, canine usually gets the same direction moment in most cases except it tips back too much. Aided by transeptal fiber force and low-friction brackets, canines will "drift" back along the archwire to relieve anterior crowding. Our ongoing randomized clinical trial [17] comparing PASS and MBT technique in aligning stage showed upper canine tipped back 4.7° in PASS group without retraction force vs. 5.7° in MBT group with canine laceback force. Although the difference had no statistical significance, the laceback made anchor molar tip forward 2.4° significantly, while in PASS group it tipped back 0.9°. When canine moves back, the equilibrium force on incisors from back is interrupted too. The lip force will then tip incisors to lingual direction. Prof. Ko's FEM experiment in Chap. 5 tells us incisors may get lingual and extrusive force in PASS first-stage setting even

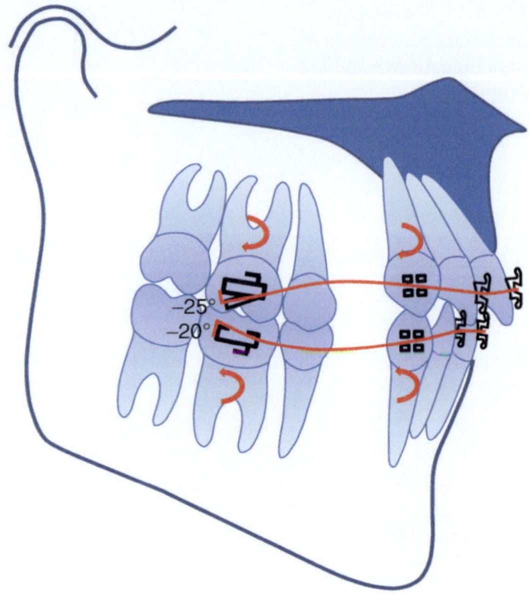

Fig. 8.12 Designed dominant moments on anchor molars may not only prevent PAL, but also facilitate canine backward "drifting" on first thin NiTi archwire

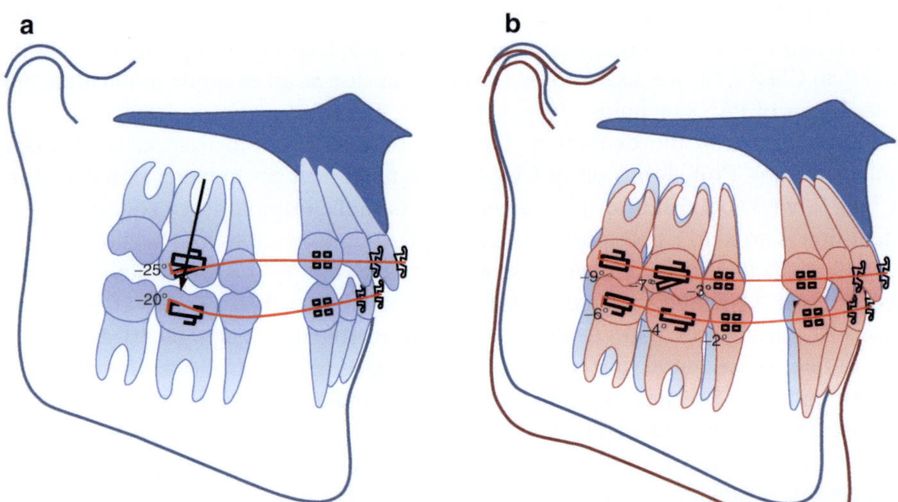

Fig. 8.13 (**a**) The forward-tipping compensation of upper first molar was resisted by first NiTi wire in aligning stage, although it may still erupt along its long axis to compensate jaw differential growth rotation, which is supposed to be good for upper molar apex moving downward and backward to increase arch length. (**b**) All posterior brackets or tubes are in tip back angle to resist the compensation of upper arch to mandible growth during whole treatment period. The upper archwires with normal or compensated curve of Spee are applied to avoid leveling upper posterior curve

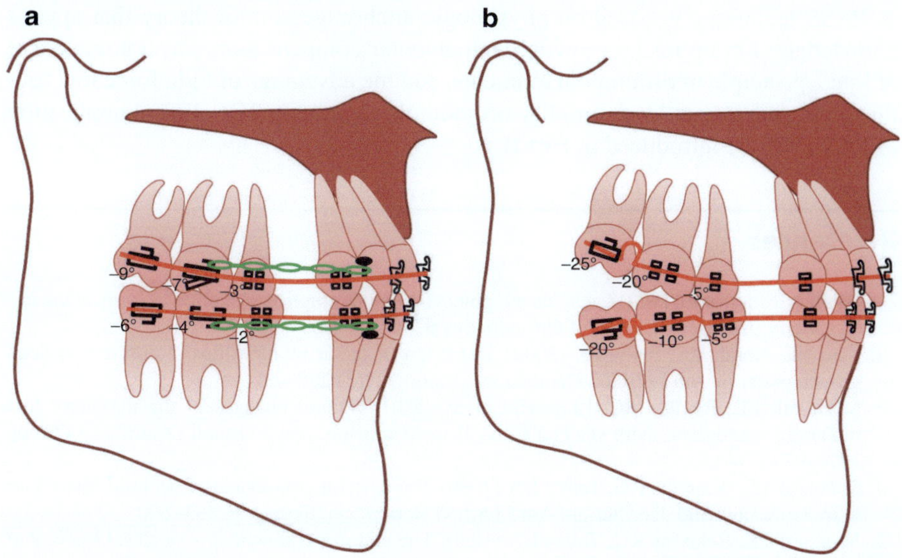

Fig. 8.14 (**a**, **b**) Gradually increased archwire sizes will tip all posterior teeth in relative backward angles, but much less than those in Tweed anchorage preparation

without lip force. Our randomized clinical trial showed upper incisor tipped back 3.5° while in MBT group it tipped back 2.4° with no statistical significance.

In vertical direction, although tip back mechanics give the molar an extrusion force and canine an intrusion force, the magnitude is quite small comparing to tip back bends on stainless steel wires in traditional Edgewise or Begg techniques. If vertical control is critical in some high-angle cases, TAP or TAD could be used. When canine is concerned, since intrusive force from NiTi wire coming from tip back tube is very light, it usually could not resist the natural eruption force of canine. Besides, canine may also get extrusion force from archwire mesial to it when pitting against occlusal positioned incisors (Fig. 8.12). So in clinic, canines will be extruded rather than being intruded.

When upper molars are stopped from forward tipping as in Fig. 8.12, the dento-alveolar compensation along with mandible growth starts to be interrupted from the first NiTi archwire. When malocclusion teeth are corrected to near normal or wire-slot angulation on all other teeth is less than 7°, we change to use −7° rectangular tube with the curve of Spee, always making the largest moment in backward direction on anchor molar, so they don't have a chance to tip forward during aligning and leveling stages. In this way, we reduce forward rotation of FOP comparing with contemporary straight wire mechanics.

For growing case, mandible will keep forward growth, and the upper molar will extrude to compensate the difference between maxilla and mandible rotation, although it is now resisted to tip forward by XBT tube (Fig. 8.13). When treatment progresses to space closing stage, backward inclined posterior teeth will provide more anchorage strength similar to Tweed anchorage preparation (Fig. 8.14).

PASS technique is based on physiologic anchorage control theory that applies knowledge of craniofacial growth, dentoalveolar compensation, physiologic curve of Spee, principle of differential moments, and the advantage of light force low friction to improve or at least simplify orthodontic treatment. The clinical application of PASS will be introduced in Part II.

References

1. Bjork A, Skieller V (1972) Facial development and tooth eruption. An implant study at the age of puberty. American Journal of Orthodontics 62(4):339–383
2. Kim YE, Nanda RS, Sinha PK (2002) Transition of molar relationships in different skeletal growth patterns. Am J Orthod Dentofacial Orthop 121(3):280–290
3. Martinelli FL, Ruellas AC, Lima EM et al (2010) Natural changes of the maxillary first molars in adolescents with skeletal Class II malocclusion. Am J Orthod Dentofacial Orthop 137(6):775–781
4. Southard TE, Behrents RG, Tolley EA (1989) The anterior component of occlusal force, Part 1: measurement and distribution. Am J Orthod Dentofacial Orthop 96:493–500
5. Southard TE, Behrents RG, Tolley EA (1990) The anterior component of occlusal force, Part 2: relationship with dental alignment. Am J Orthod Dentofacial Orthop 97:41–49
6. Su H, Han B, Li S et al (2014) Compensation trends of the angulation of first molars: retrospective study of 1403 malocclusion cases. Int J Oral Sci 6:175–181
7. Fu MK, Lin JX (2005) Orthodontics. Peking University Medical Press, Beijing
8. Liao CH, Yang P, Zhao ZH et al (2010) Study on the posterior teeth mesiodistal tipping degree of normal occlusion subjects among different facial growth patterns. West China Journal of Stomatology 28(4):377–377
9. Su H, Han B, Li S, Na B, Ma W, Xu TM (2014) Factors predisposing to maxillary anchorage loss: a retrospective study of 1403 cases. PLoS ONE 9(10):e109561
10. Johnston LE Jr (1986) A comparative analysis of Class II treatments. In: Vig PS, Ribbens KA (eds) Science and clinical judgment in orthodontics. Center for Human Growth and Development, Ann Arbor, pp 103–148
11. Osborn JW (1993) Orientation of the masseter muscle and the curve of Spee in relation to crushing forces on the molar teeth of primates. Am J Phys Anthropol 92:99–106
12. McKinney JR, Harris EF (2001) Influence of patient age and sex on orthodontic treatment: evaluations of Begg light wire, standard edgewise, and straight wire techniques. Am J Orthod Dentofacial Orthop 120(5):530–541
13. Braun S, Legan HL (1997) Changes in occlusion related to the cant of the occlusal plane. Am J Orthod Dentofacial Orthop 111(2):184–188
14. Xu TM, Zhang X, Oh HS et al (2010) Randomized clinical trial comparing control of maxillary anchorage with 2 retraction techniques. Am J Orthod Dentofacial Orthop 138(5):544.e1–544.e9
15. Zaher AR, Bishara SE, Jakobsen JR (1994) Posttreatment changes in different facial types. Angle Orthod 64(6):425–436
16. Glenn G, Sinclair PM, Alexander RG (1987) Nonextraction orthodontic therapy: posttreatment dental and skeletal stability. Am J Orthod Dentofacial Orthop 92(4):321–328
17. Su H (2002) Study on the correlation between first molar angulation growth pattern and anchorage control. Dissertation, Peking University

Part II

Clinical Application of PASS Technique

The Basic Treatment Procedures of PASS Technique

9

Tian Min Xu, Bing Han, Gui Chen, Fanfan Dai, and Mengjiao Ruan

Abstract

PASS technique is based on physiologic anchorage control theory introduced in Part I. It combines the classical treatment philosophy from Angle and Tweed and the modern self-ligating appliance's light force low friction correction with minimum wire bending. All the knowledge of fixed appliance orthodontists got from their training can be used. It is not a brand new technology. Technically, it is a modified straight wire based on physiologic characteristics of individual patient and classical anchorage control strategy. Theoretically, it aims at reduction of maxillary dentoalveolar compensation and shares the similar goal of Tweed when keeping the upper curve of Spee is concerned. Some wire bending is still needed considering the different compensation degrees for individuals. For very severe cases, headgear and TAD or even orthognathic surgery are still advised.

PASS technique is basically focusing on prevention or reduction of maxillary dentoalveolar compensation during Class I and Class II correction for adolescents and reversal of it for adults. Growth modification could not be finished by PASS itself, but headgear can be used with it if orthodontist sets the goal to inhibit maxilla growth.

Although treatment methods may differ for different malocclusions, the basic treatment procedure can help beginners to follow PASS mechanics.

T.M. Xu (✉) • B. Han • G. Chen • M. Ruan
Department of Orthodontics, Peking University School and Hospital of Stomatology, Beijing, China
e-mail: tmxuortho@163.com; orthohanks@sina.com; chengui723@163.com; relephant@163.com

F. Dai
Second Dental Center, Peking University School and Hospital of Stomatology, Beijing, China
e-mail: daifanfannihao@163.com;

T.M. Xu (ed.), *Physiologic Anchorage Control*,
DOI 10.1007/978-3-319-48333-7_9

PASS technique can be divided into three basic treatment stages; each has its own objective. Let us take Class II extraction treatment as an example to illustrate it.

Stage I: Alignment

Objectives:

1. Relieve crowding and correct rotation.
2. Prevent forward tipping of molar or upright forward tipped molar.
3. Start to open deep bite.
4. Start to correct midline.

Methods:

1. Bond upper and lower 3–3 MLF brackets. XBT on first molars. Upper and lower 0.014″ NiTi archwires engage in −25° round tube on upper molar and −20° "virtual tube" on lower molar (Fig. 9.1)

Bonding position for MLF is just like conventional straight wire appliance, but bonding XBT on first molar is a little bit tricky. Orthodontists used to orient the main tube direction parallel to occlusal rim of molar, which will make the −7° main tube a 0° tube just like conventional buccal tube. The correct way to orient it is to

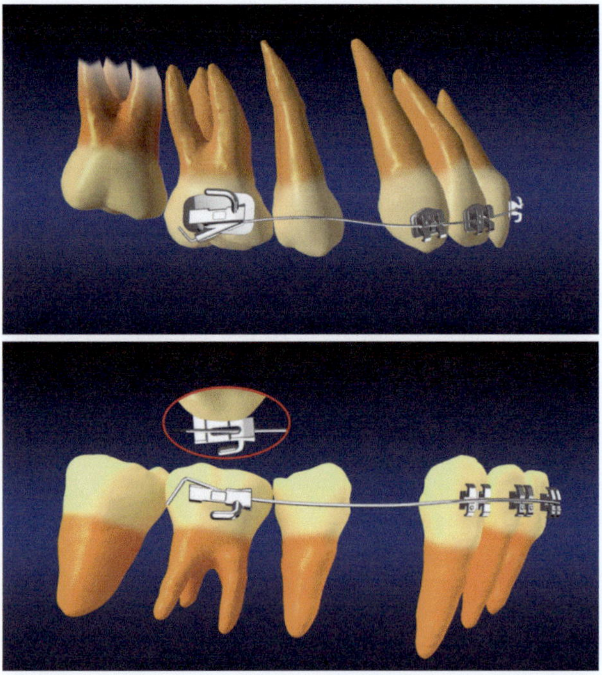

Fig. 9.1 Initial setting showing −25° tipback tube on *upper molar* and −20° "virtual tube" on *lower molar*

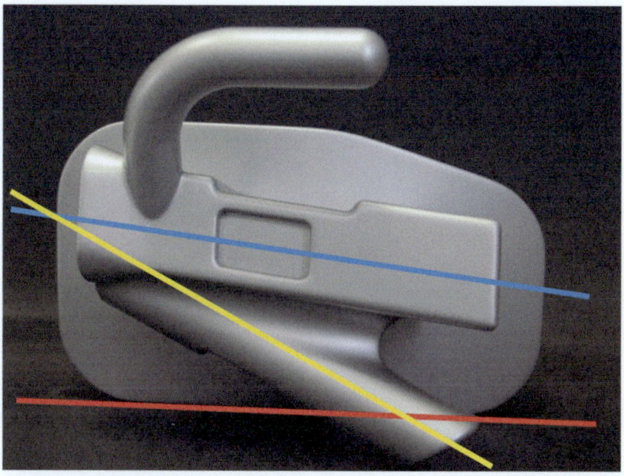

Fig. 9.2 The *red line* represents occlusal edge of the base of XBT, the *yellow line* is −25°, and the *blue line* is −7° relative to the *red line*

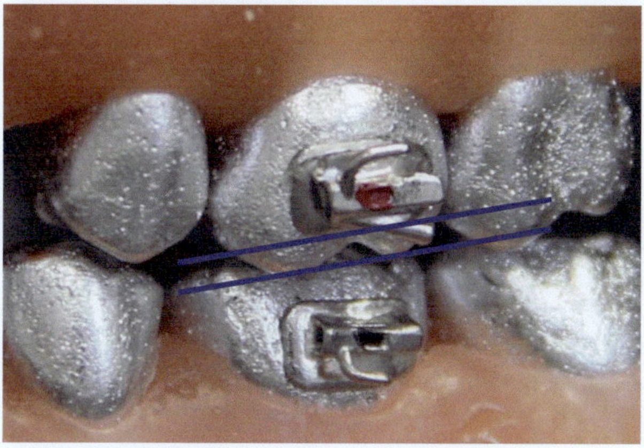

Fig. 9.3 The orientation of XBT on first molar

make the occlusal edge of the base parallel to molar cusps and the mesial entrance at the 1/2 crown height (Figs. 9.2 and 9.3).

When engaging NiTi wire in −25° upper XBT and −20° lower XBT tubes, dominant moment will be put on anchor molars for most cases, and this will also protect molar from forward drifting in aligning stage.

Orthodontists can adjust friction by selecting different ligatures and ligating methods. For example, selecting 0.2 mm, 0.25 mm, or 0.3 mm ligature wire based on severity of rotation of anterior teeth, single wing ligation can be used on rotated teeth and overhanging ligating on severely irregular tooth (Fig. 9.4). For canines, we advise you to select 0.2 mm ligature wire on distal wing to lower friction on it so that it can drift back more easily and gradually change to thicker ligature wires when anterior crowding is relieved. For midline-shifted cases, thin ligature wires on one side and thick ligatures on the other side will initiate midline correction earlier before changing to thick archwire.

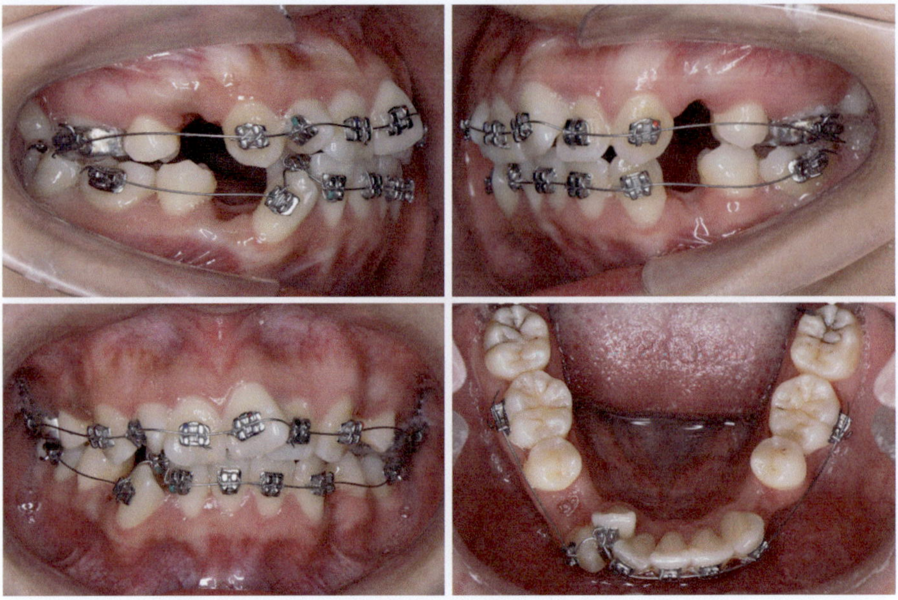

Fig. 9.4 Single wing ligature, diagonal ligature, and overhanging ligature

2. In deep overbite (OB) or forward tipped molar cases, a piggy back arch is used to tie on anterior segment (Fig. 9.5). It can be made of from 0.018″ SS round wire to 0.018×0.025″ SS rectangular wire depending on the tooth size and arch length, etc. To prevent flaring of anterior teeth, ligating on distal wing of lateral incisor or mesial wing of canine plus cinch back ligating on first molar will help. To tip molar back, ligating on canine wings combining with Class II elastics can be used (Fig. 9.6).

Stage II: Restore the Physiologic or Compensated Curve of Spee

1. Establish the curve of Spee for upper arch.

   Objectives:

1. Complete correcting rotation and midline deviation.
2. Establish the upper curve of Spee and a stable posterior anchorage unit.
3. Reduce the incisor proclination.
4. Level irregularity in the third-order direction.
5. Level the lower arch and finish deep bite correction.

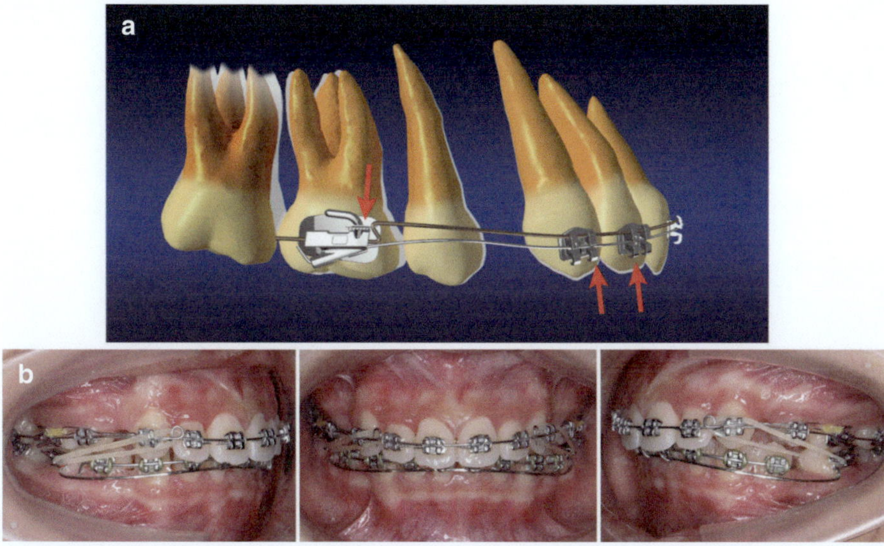

Fig. 9.5 Piggy back arch to tip molar back (**a**) or intrude anterior teeth (**b**). *Arrows* show cinch back ligating and ligating on distal wing of lateral incisor or mesial wing of canine

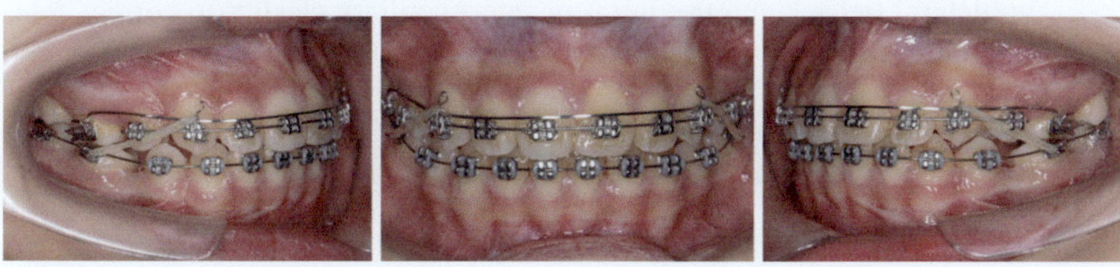

Fig. 9.6 Class II elastics on canine to facilitate upper molar backward tipping by piggy back arch

Methods:

1. Bond upper PM2 brackets and M2 tubes, gingivally a little bit on PM2 and occlusally on M2 (Fig. 9.7) in order to restore upper curve of Spee, which is crucial to prevent or reduce or even reverse functional occlusal plane as a strategy of dentoalveolar compensation correction suggested by Prof. Johnston in Chap. 3. In PASS technique, individualized curve of Spee can be realized by manually adjusting the curve size on archwire. There are three factors that determine the last formation of upper posterior curve of Spee: (1) the pre-adjusted backward tipping angles on posterior brackets or tubes, (2) the vertical positioning of brackets or tubes, and (3) the curve size on archwire. When less curve of Spee is desired, we can use PM1 bracket on PM2, position it closer to Andrews's FA point, and make a smaller curve on archwire. For PM2 extraction cases, the other side PM1 or PM2 brackets can be used to make PM1 a positive angle to enhance anterior anchorage if pulling posterior teeth forward after relieving crowding is planned.

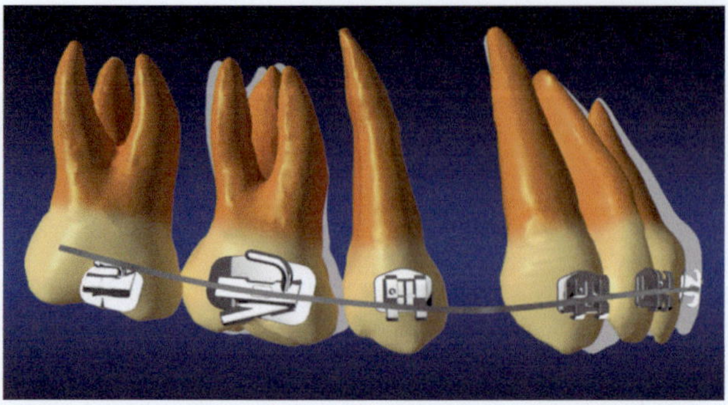

Fig. 9.7 Stage II set up. Notice the position of PM2 and M2. Archwire with curve of Spee before engagement is shown

2. Change to 0.016–0.018″ NiTi with normal curve of Spee into the main tube of upper first molar, continue midline correction by unlilateral canine laceback or tieback. For skeletal Class II, increase the curve for compensation.
3. After alignment with 0.018″ NiTi wire, choose the next wire according to:
   (a) If upper incisor is proclined apparently use 0.018″ stainless steel wire with helical loop and normal curve of Spee. Continue midline correction with unlilateral tieback and use intra- or intermaxillary elastics to correct anterior teeth inclination until they are uprighted to normal inclination and then change to 0.018×0.025″ NiTi archwire with normal curve of Spee.
   (b) If upper incisor inclination is almost normal, use 0.018×0.025″ NiTi archwire with normal curve of Spee to level irregularities in third-order direction.

The condition for a stable anchorage unit:

1. Upper first molar gets tipback moment (−7° tube).
2. Upper M1 and M2 have formed a normal curve of Spee, no steps in between.
3. Use thick stainless steel rectangular wire with normal curve of Spee, making the distal M2 and the mesial PM2 stable, so that they can prevent the middle M1 from forward tipping or mesial palatal rotation.

Note: round archwire can satisfy conditions (1) and (2), but not (3) when rotation is concerned, so do not retract anterior teeth on round archwire for too long time. Figure 9.8 shows the upper left first molar mesial-palatal rotation due to extended retraction of anterior teeth on 0.018″ SS round archwire.

2. Leveling of lower arch

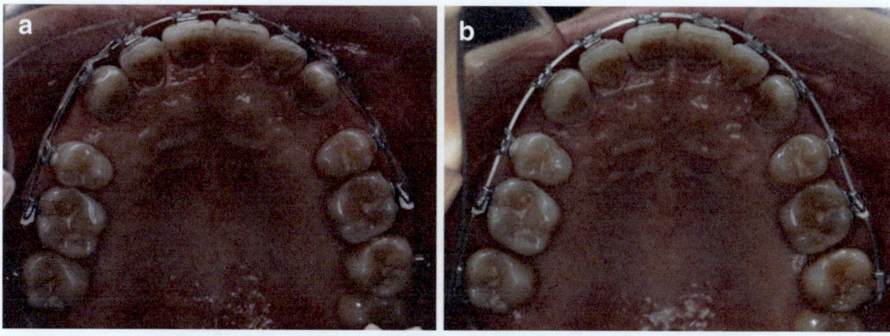

Fig. 9.8 Upper left first molar mesial-palatal rotation on round wire (**a**) and under correction by changing to rectangular wire (**b**)

Objectives:

1. Get teeth ready in third order for engaging SS rectangular wire.
2. Open the bite to normal.

Methods:

1. Bond lower PM2, change to 0.016–0.018″ NiTi with reverse curve of Spee, entering lower M1 main tube. Bond lower M2 if possible for deep overbite or maximum anchorage cases.
2. After correction of rotation, change to 0.018×0.025″ NiTi, make a reverse curve of Spee in deep overbite cases, and combine Class II elastics.
3. Change to 0.018×0.025″ rectangular stainless steel wire with necessary reverse curve of Spee especially in deep overbite cases.

Stage III: Space Closure and Refinement

Objectives:

Establish good occlusion according to skeletal jaw relationship.

Methods:

1. Upper 0.018×0.025″ SS with physiologic or compensated curve of Spee plus traction hooks (Fig. 9.9)

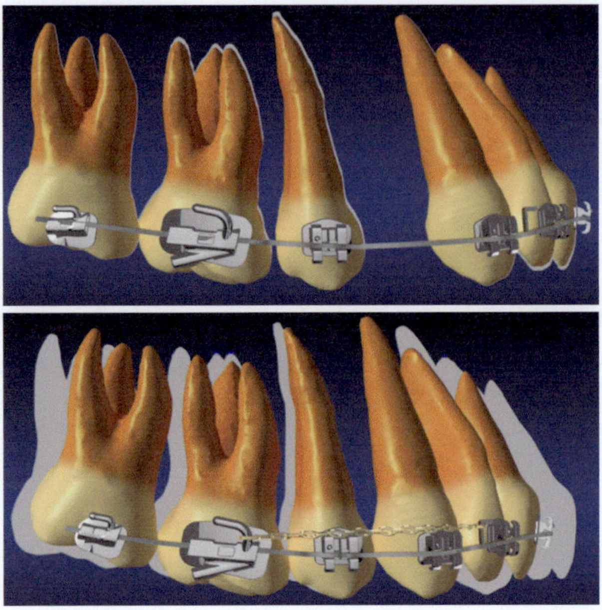

Fig. 9.9 Closing space on curved archwire

2. Lower 0.018×0.025″ SS with slight reverse curve of Spee plus traction hooks
3. Power chain to close space and intermaxillary elastics to adjust occlusion

The application of PASS appliance in different clinical situations will be shown in the next five chapters.

Class I Cases with Four First Premolars Extraction

10

Hong Su, Si Chen, and Gui Chen

Abstract

Crowded and bimaxillary protrusive cases are prevalent in Asian population, and the extraction treatment plan is often applied. Dental crowding is characterized by anterior crowding, malpositioned teeth, lack of space, and/or mesial shifting of molars, while bimaxillary protrusion is characterized by proclined anterior teeth and/or protrusive lips. Most of these patients seek orthodontic treatment for improving the appearance of their teeth or convex profile. Maximum anchorage is often required for these cases. To achieve a better treatment outcome, miniscrews and headgear are often used for anchorage reinforcement. The advent of PASS technique gives orthodontists another option, a simple solution that can reduce the usage of miniscrew anchorage in a large scale. Due to its innovative strategy of physiologic anchorage control and unique design of the appliance, PASS technique has many advantages in treatment of crowded or bimaxillary protrusive cases. In this chapter, we will introduce the application of PASS in crowded or protrusive Class I cases treated with four first premolars extraction.

H. Su (✉)
First Clinical Division, Peking University School and Hospital of Stomatology, Beijing, China
e-mail: suhong0309@qq.com

S. Chen • G. Chen
Department of Orthodontics, Peking University School and Hospital of Stomatology, Beijing, China
e-mail: elisa02chen@gmail.com; chengui723@163.com

T.M. Xu (ed.), *Physiologic Anchorage Control*,
DOI 10.1007/978-3-319-48333-7_10

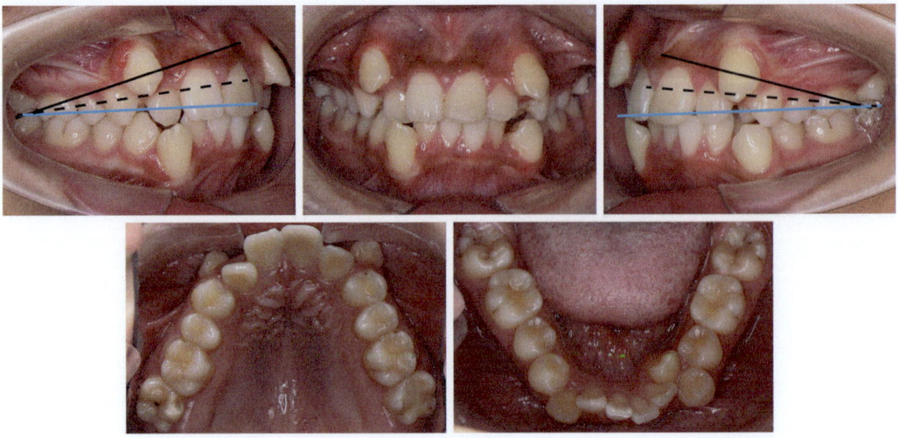

Fig. 10.1 The *blue line* parallels to the functional occlusal plane; the *black line* represents the engaged NiTi wire; the broken line shows a possible posterior occlusal plane after treatment with conventional straight wire appliance

Crowding

Two common causes of dental crowding are dento-skeletal discrepancy and abnormal displacements of the deciduous and permanent teeth. For example, deciduous tooth retention and early loss of deciduous molars could lead to the forward tipping and shifting of permanent molars and anterior crowding. Since upper canine is the last one to erupt in the dentition before first molar, it's often dislocated severely due to lack of space. As indicated in Chap. 2, if the canine is in high position, a straight NiTi archwire in initial aligning stage would cause the forward tipping of molars, early anchorage loss and change of functional occlusal plane (FOP) in counterclockwise direction as demonstrated in Fig. 10.1. Blue line in this figure represents the buccal tube plane, which is coincident with the pretreatment FOP. The black line shows the engage direction of the initial straight NiTi wire into the canine bracket and the conventional molar buccal tube. The posterior occlusal plane will end up somewhere in between (the broken line) according to the mechanics introduced in Chap. 6, which will reduce FOP/PP and increase the protrusion of upper arch.

The striking feature in PASS system is that a −25° tipback tube is designed on first molar buccal tube to overcome the above shortcoming [1, 2]. When a straight NiTi archwire is engaged in such a thin tipback round tube, the dominant moment will be on the anchor molar, which will usually result in a co-rotating moment on the canine according to Burstone's six geometric classes introduced in Chap. 2. This moment will tip the canine backward to relieve anterior crowding without using laceback or elastics so that there will be no anchorage burden on first molar which is crucial to maintain the FOP. Figure 10.2 shows when this case was treated with the PASS appliance, canines moved back into extraction space after engaging a 0.012″ NiTi in the tipback tube and the anterior teeth was aligned in just 3 months,

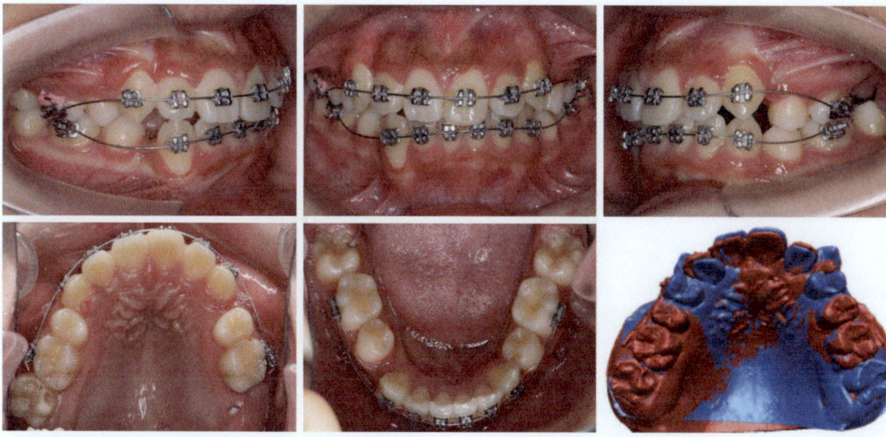

Fig. 10.2 The case was treated with the PASS technique. In only 3 months, the anterior teeth in this severe crowding case had been well aligned without anchorage loss

and the 3D superimposition shows good anchorage control (Fig. 10.2). PASS technique provides a novel and simplified way to align anterior teeth without stressing on anchor molar.

Case 1 Teenager, Class I, Severe Crowding

Figure 10.3 shows a 16-year-old girl, who sought orthodontic treatment because of the severe crowding.

Diagnosis: Angle Class I relationship and skeletal Class III relationship.
Treatment Plan: Extraction of four first premolars; PASS technique.
Duration: 18 months.

The first-stage PASS appliance as showed in Fig. 9.1 was put on and 0.012″ NiTi wires were used. After 3 months, canine moved back on low-friction MLF brackets without elastic force from molar. Anterior crowding was relieved, canines were aligned on the arch form and some spaces between anterior teeth appeared (Fig. 10.4). Upper molar tipped back a little bit showing good anchorage control. Figure 10.5 shows second premolars and second molars were bonded with brackets 4 months into the treatment. In the following stages, NiTi wires or stainless steel wires with normal curve of Spee were applied to space closure and occlusion adjustment.

With 18 months of treatment, the occlusion was greatly improved. Cephalometric film showed the normal curve of Spee was maintained. Superimposition of pretreatment (blue) and posttreatment (red) cephalometric tracings showed maximum molar anchorage and lip retraction (Fig. 10.6).

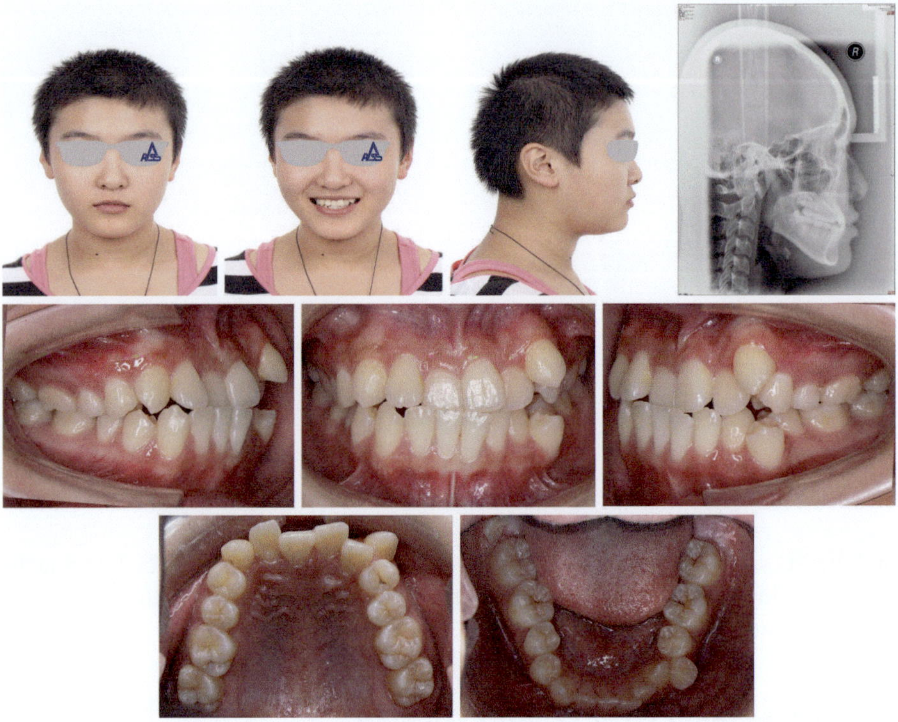

Fig. 10.3 The girl is Class I with severe crowding, anterior crossbite, and a mild skeletal Class III relationship

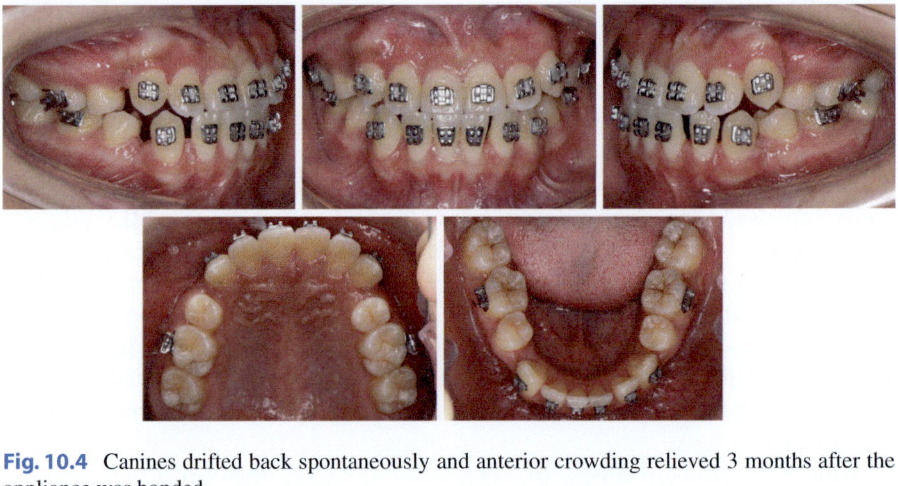

Fig. 10.4 Canines drifted back spontaneously and anterior crowding relieved 3 months after the appliance was bonded

Table 10.1 shows the cephalometric analysis of the case before and after treatment. FOP/PP increased by 1.7°, which reversed the forward rotation tendency of FOP in normal growth pattern instead of accelerating it as in conventional straight wire mechanics (Fig. 8.8).

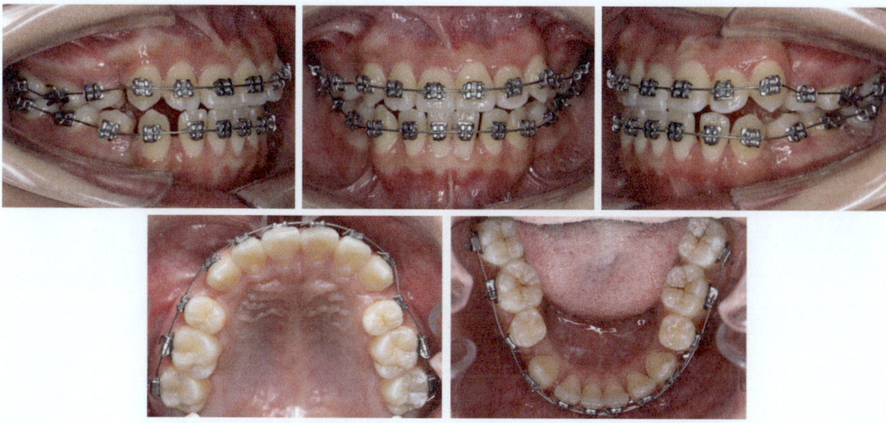

Fig. 10.5 Her PM2 and M2 were bonded, and 0.016″ NiTi wires were used 4 months after she started the treatment

Case 2 Adult, Class I, Severe Crowding, Periodontitis

Figure 10.7 showed a 33-year-old girl, who sought orthodontic treatment because of the severe crowding, gingival recession, and periodontitis.

Diagnosis: Angle Class I relationship and skeletal Class I relationship.
Treatment Plan: Extraction of four first premolars; PASS technique.
Duration: 24 months.

Intraoral photos show Class I molar relationship, severe crowding, and multiple gingival recession. The cephalometric radiograph shows a mild skeletal Class I jaw relationship and high mandibular angle (MP/SN 42.1°). The panoramic radiograph shows mild bone loss in multiple areas. The patient was bonded with XBTs on upper first molars and MLF brackets on anterior teeth after the first premolars had been extracted. The 0.012″ NiTi initial archwire was inserted into the −25° XBT tube on upper first molar (Fig. 10.8). When using 0.20 mm ligature wire, the friction was lower on anterior teeth so they can "drift" back to relieve crowding. Figure 10.9 shows canine tipped back without laceback or elastic force, and anterior crowding was relieved after 8 months of treatment, just like "driftodontics" along archwire. The difference is the upper molar tipped backward a little bit rather than tipped forward in noncontrol drifting. Lower second premolars were bonded after relieving lower anterior crowding, and 0.016 NiTi archwire was used to align premolars and upright canines. Figure 10.10 shows the treatment progress by using 0.018 × 0.025″ NiTi wires in upper dentition with normal curve of Spee and in the lower with reverse curve of Spee. Figure 10.11 shows 19 months into treatment, the space closure stage was proceeded with the 0.018 × 0.025″ rectangular stainless steel wires, with normal curve of Spee.

Figure 10.12 shows the posttreatment records. After 24 months of treatment, the alignment was fine, and the physiologic curve of Spee was maintained on lateral

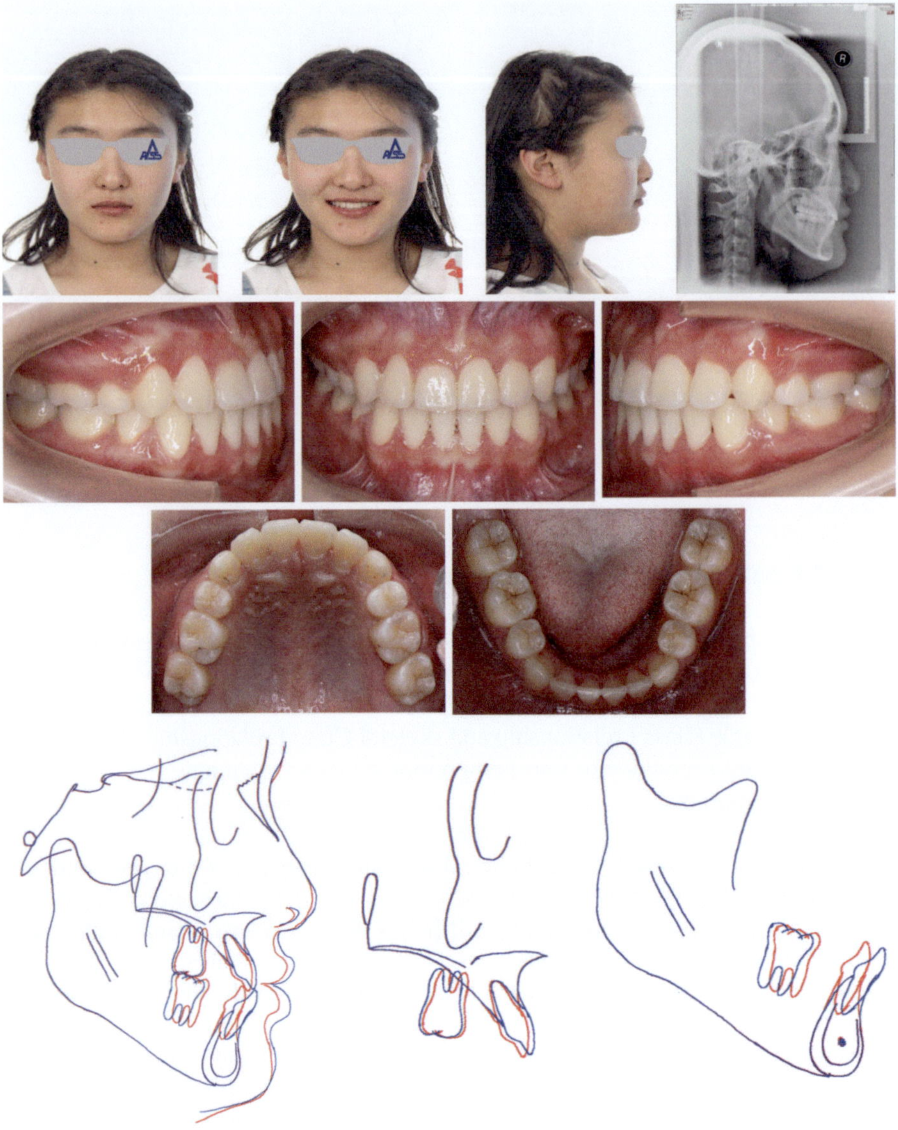

Fig. 10.6 The posttreatment alignment was good, and the physiologic curve of Spee was maintained

head film. Superimposition of pre- and posttreatment cephalometric tracings showed maximum molar anchorage and lip retraction [3].

Table 10.2 shows her cephalometric measurements before and after treatment. The FOP/PP increased by 1.7° indicating a good anti-tipping moment control of posterior segment. The MP/SN increased by 1.7° probably due to slightly extrusion and backward tipping of first molars. U1-AP and L1-AP decreased indicating anterior teeth retraction.

Table 10.1 Cephalometric analysis before and after treatment

Measurements	Norm. Mean	SD.	Pre.	Post.	Dif.
SNA (°)	82.8	4.0	80.1	80.6	0.5
SNB (°)	80.1	3.9	81.7	80.8	−0.8
ANB (°)	2.7	2.0	−1.5	−0.2	1.3
Wits appraisal (mm)	−1.1	2.9	−5.1	−2.3	2.8
PP/SN (°)	9.3	2.4	3.8	4.0	0.2
MP/SN (°)	32.5	5.2	32.5	32.1	−0.4
MP/PP (°)	27.6	4.6	28.8	28.2	−0.6
FOP/PP (°)	NA	NA	9.9	11.6	1.7
U1-AP (mm)	7.2	2.2	4.3	2.6	−1.8
L1-AP (mm)	4.9	2.1	4.6	0.2	−4.3
U1/PP (°)	115.8	5.7	116.2	115.2	−0.9
L1/MP (°)	93.9	6.2	87.5	84.9	−2.6

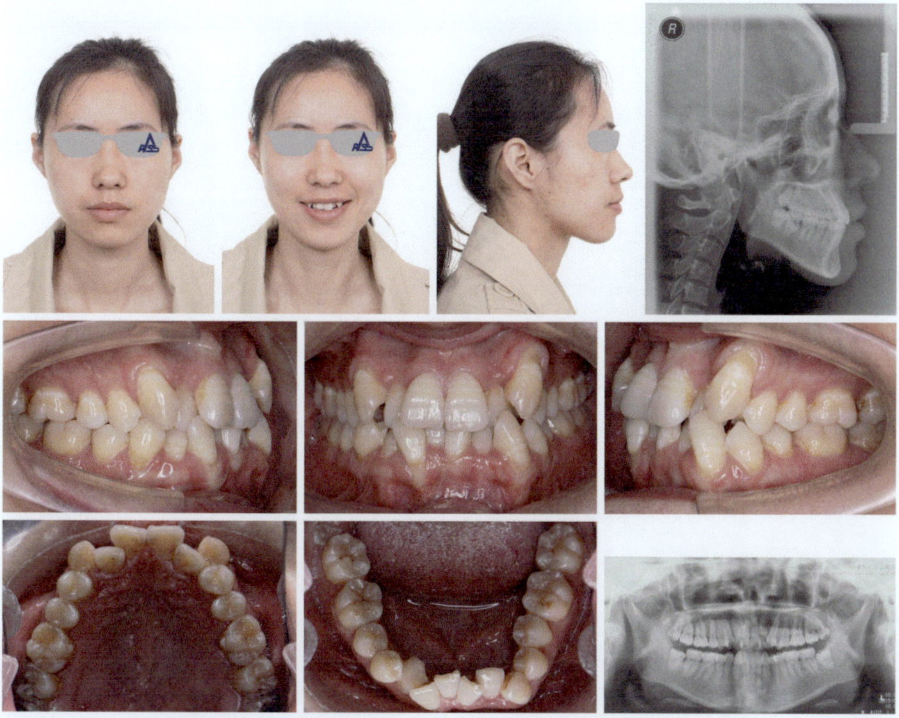

Fig. 10.7 The intraoral view and films show severe crowding, multiple gingival recession, and mild bone loss in multiple areas

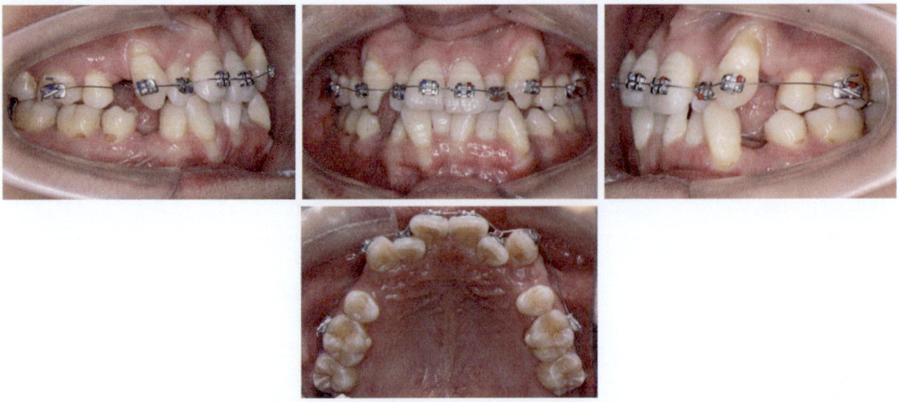

Fig. 10.8 The intraoral view of immediate bonding of upper appliance

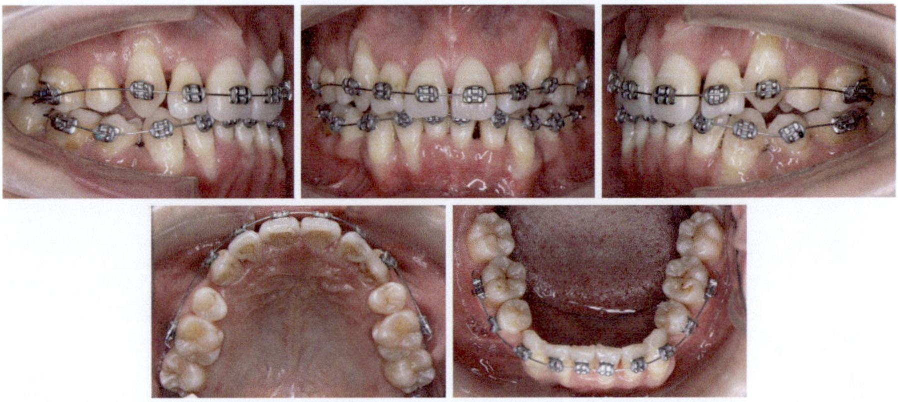

Fig. 10.9 The anterior crowding was relieved 8 months after bonding

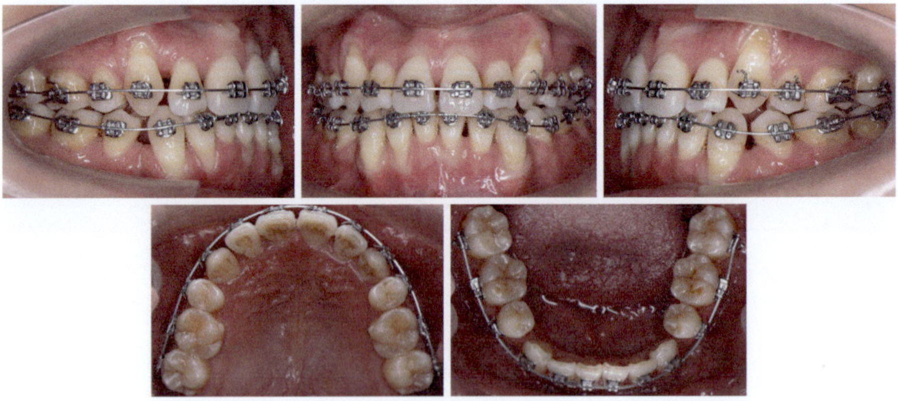

Fig. 10.10 All the teeth were bonded with appliances, and the aligning stage was almost finished

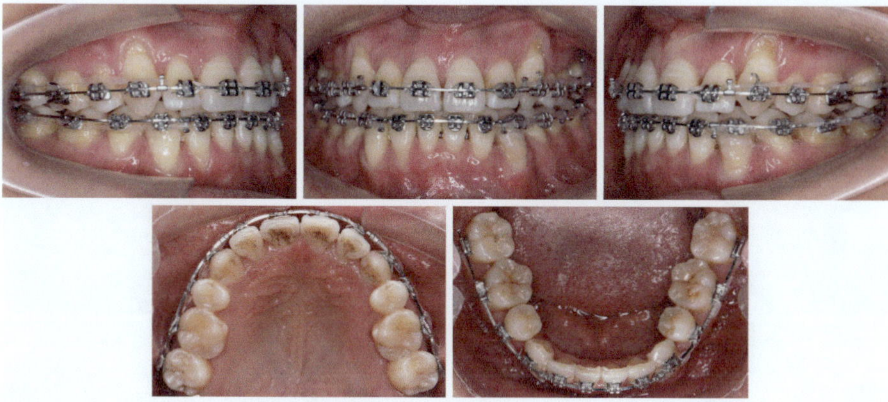

Fig. 10.11 The space closure stage was proceeding

Bimaxillary Protrusion

Bimaxillary protrusion is characterized by proclined anterior teeth, protrusive lips, and a convex lower facial profile. In our previous study [4], there was a positive correlation between the tipping of first molar and the torque of incisors, which seems to imply that if upper molar tipped forward, it might also squeeze forward all the teeth that are mesial to it. So the strategy of orthodontic correction of this type of malocclusion should involve retraction of all these teeth back with maximum anchorage, typically after extraction of the first premolars, thus correcting dentoalveolar protrusion [5, 6].

The advantages of PASS-treating bimaxillary protrusion involve XBTs to prevent molar forward tipping after premolar extraction and MLF brackets to facilitate anterior teeth "drifting" back along archwire when they got tipback moments, which may sometimes result in anterior scattered spacing as in Fig. 10.13. The backward tipping angles in all posterior brackets and buccal tubes also inhibit the forward tipping trend of the posterior teeth due to growth and extraction and maintain posterior curve of Spee that saves more spaces for anterior teeth retraction. Another advantage with PASS appliance is that incisor slot is 0.020 inch rather than 0.022 inch so that incisor torque control is strengthened even with 0.018 × 0.025″ SS retraction arch according to Chap. 7. And 0.018 × 0.025″ arch in 0.022 inch slots in posterior brackets or tubes also reduced the third-order friction in space-closing stage.

Case 3 Teenager, Class I, Bimaxillary Protrusion

Figure 10.14 shows a 15-year-old girl, who sought orthodontic treatment because of lip protrusion. Frontal view shows the patient had gummy smile. The whole dentition showed the typical characteristics of forward tipping canines and proclined incisors. Obvious curve of Spee could be seen from the lateral head film.

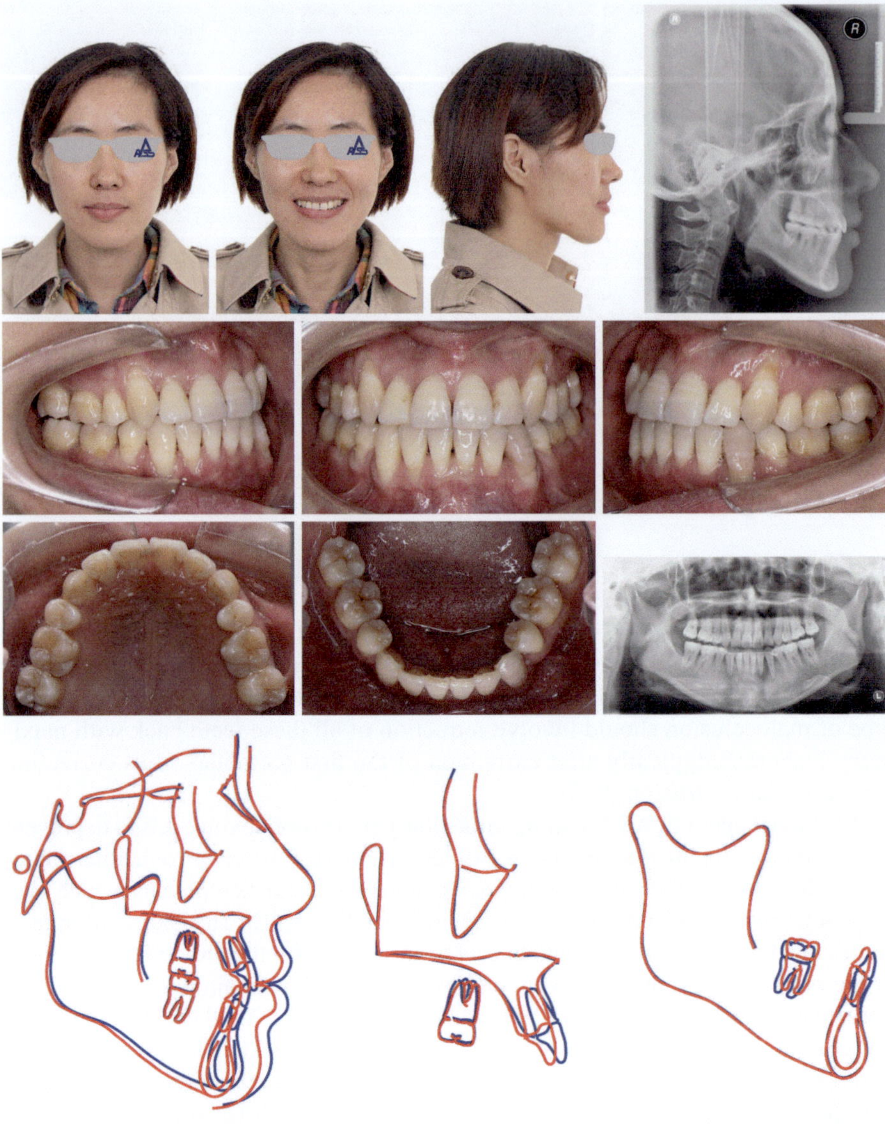

Fig. 10.12 The posttreatment records show good alignment. Superimposition of cephalometric tracings shows maximum molar anchorage and lip retraction (Reproduced from Chen et al. [3])

Diagnosis: Angle Class I and skeletal Class I with protrusion.
Treatment Plan: Extraction of four first premolars; PASS technique.
Duration: 19 months.

Figure 10.15 shows the intraoral view of 1 month after bonding XBTs on first molars and MLF brackets on anterior teeth. The initial archwire was 0.014″ NiTi round wire, inserted into the −25° round tube of XBT, using 0.20 mm ligature wire

Table 10.2 Cephalometric analysis before and after treatment

Measurements	Norm. Mean	SD.	Pre.	Post.	Dif.
SNA (°)	82.8	4.0	78.8	77.6	−1.2
SNB (°)	80.1	3.9	76.9	75.2	−1.7
ANB (°)	2.7	2.0	1.7	2.4	0.7
Wits appraisal (mm)	−1.1	2.9	−2.3	−1.1	1.2
PP/SN (°)	9.3	2.4	16.0	16.0	0.0
MP/SN (°)	32.5	5.2	42.1	43.8	1.7
MP/PP (°)	27.6	4.6	26.1	27.8	1.7
FOP/PP (°)	NA	NA	7.3	9.0	1.7
U1-AP (mm)	7.2	2.2	5.1	4.3	−0.8
L1-AP (mm)	4.9	2.1	2.4	1.3	−1.1
U1/PP (°)	115.8	5.7	115.8	113.4	−2.4
L1/MP (°)	93.9	6.2	80.6	78.3	−2.3

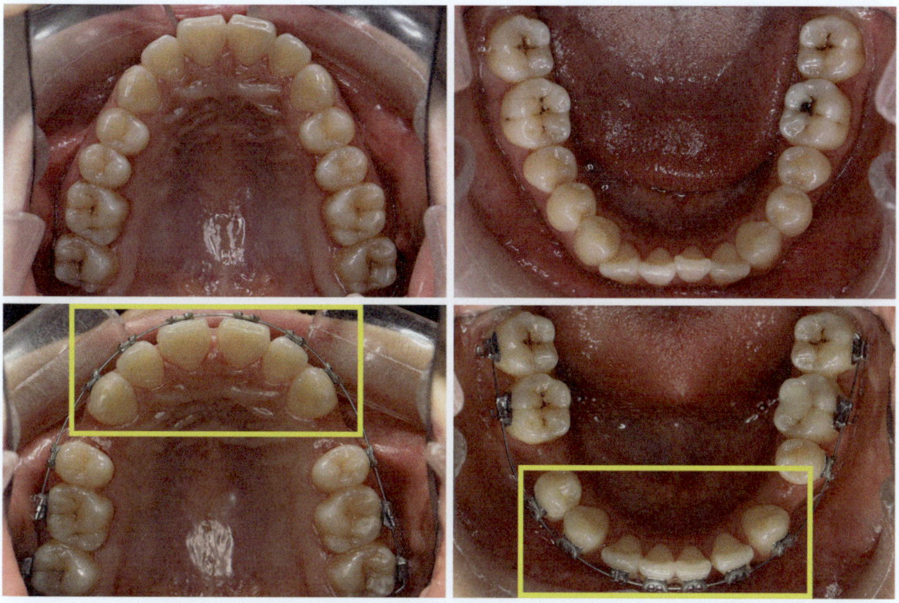

Fig. 10.13 A 24-year-old girl with bimaxillary protrusion. After 3 months alignment with the PASS appliance, scattered spaces appeared among the front teeth obviously

to reduce system friction. Two months later, her anterior crowding was relieved and we then bonded her upper PM2 and M2 and changed archwire to 0.016″ NiTi with the normal curve of Spee. The archwire was inserted into the −7° rectangular tube of XBT (Fig. 10.16). After aligning buccal segment teeth, 0.018 × 0.025″ NiTi archwire with normal curve of Spee in the upper arch and reverse curve of Spee in the lower were used to establish upper posterior curve that was crucial to stable the anchor molars; the following 0.018 × 0.025″ SS retraction archwire with the same curve of Spee as the preceding NiTi archwire were used to close the space as in Fig. 10.17.

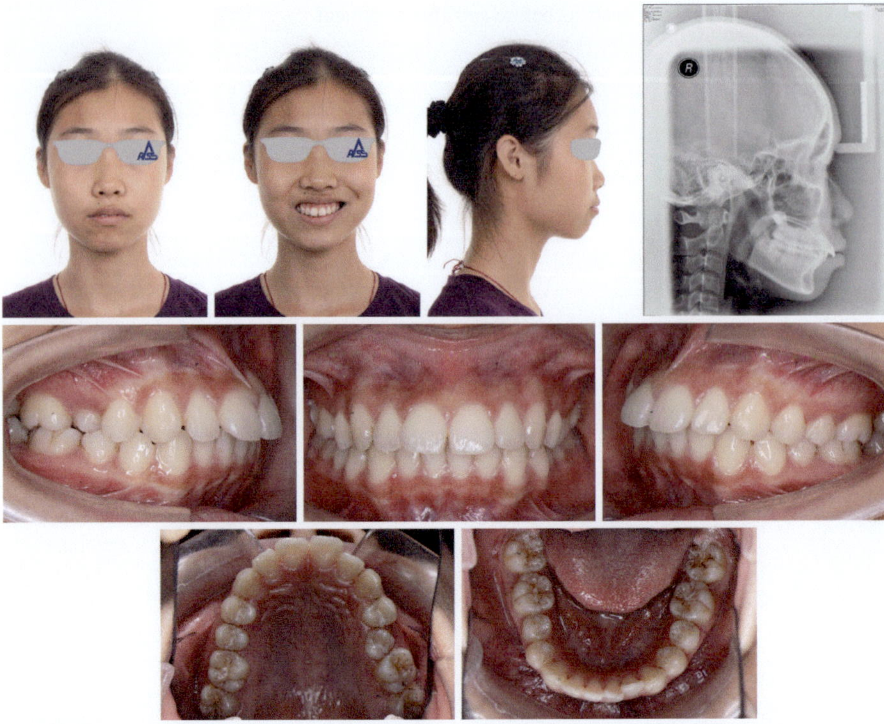

Fig. 10.14 There was a Class I molar relationship, II° overjet, labially proclined incisors, as well as apparent curve of Spee

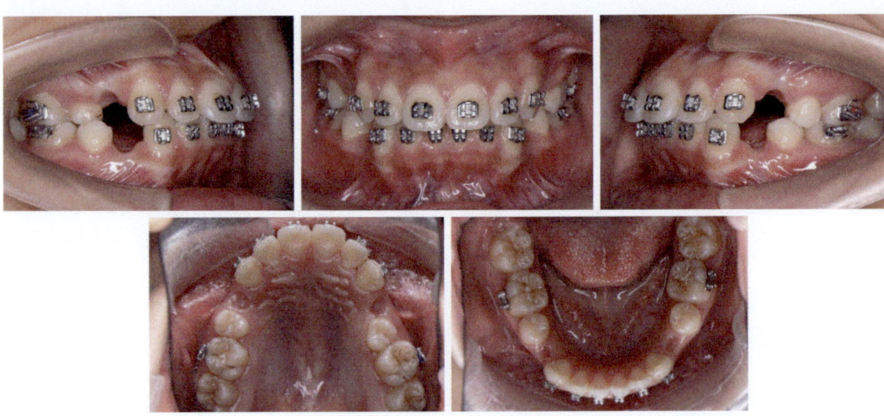

Fig. 10.15 The intraoral view of 1 month after bonding appliances

Both upper and lower incisors received intrusive force while being retracted back. Fig. 10.18 shows space just closed and the curve of Spee in upper archwire fully expressed itself comparing with elastic deformation of the archwire in Fig. 10.17.

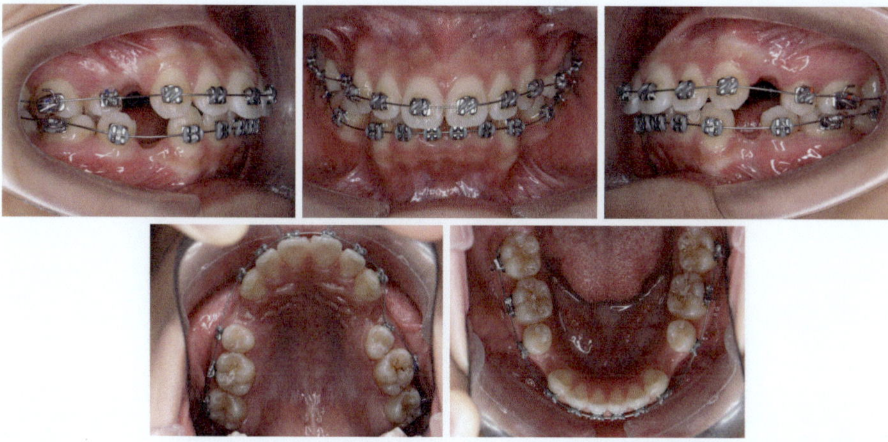

Fig. 10.16 All her teeth were bonded and we changed archwire to 0.016″ NiTi 2 months after starting treatment

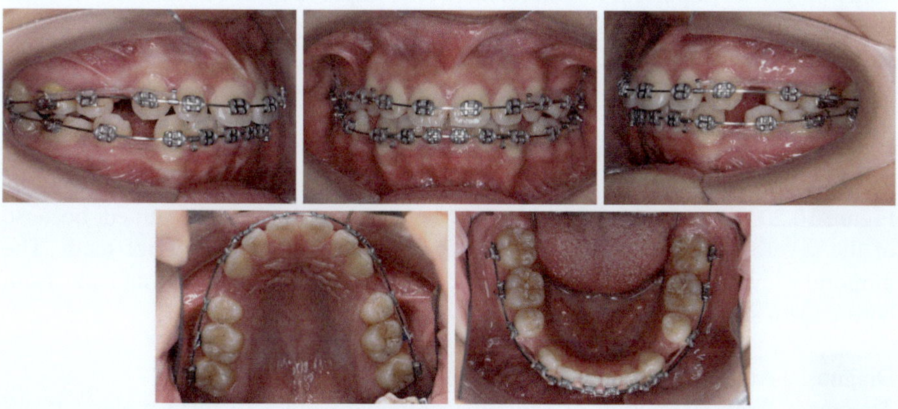

Fig. 10.17 The space-closing stage was proceeding

Fig. 10.19 is the posttreatment records. After 19 months of treatment, both the occlusion and appearance of the teeth were greatly improved. Cephalometric film shows the original posterior curve of Spee was maintained. Nevertheless, the inclinations of upper and lower incisors were pretty normal (Table 10.3). Superimposition of pre- and posttreatment cephalometric tracings shows great lip retraction and upper incisor intrusion. Gummy smile was disappeared. Also, both the upper molars showed a little distal tipping similar to but much less than Tweed occlusion.

Table 10.3 shows her cephalometric analysis before and after treatment. Her upper incisor protrusion and labial inclination were largely reduced (U1-AP decreased by 6.0 mm and U1/PP decreased by 14.8°) and lower incisor was more uprighted. The upper molar tipped back a little bit, reversed the dentoalveolar compensation. The FOP/PP increased 2.4°, contributing to the reduction of dental arch

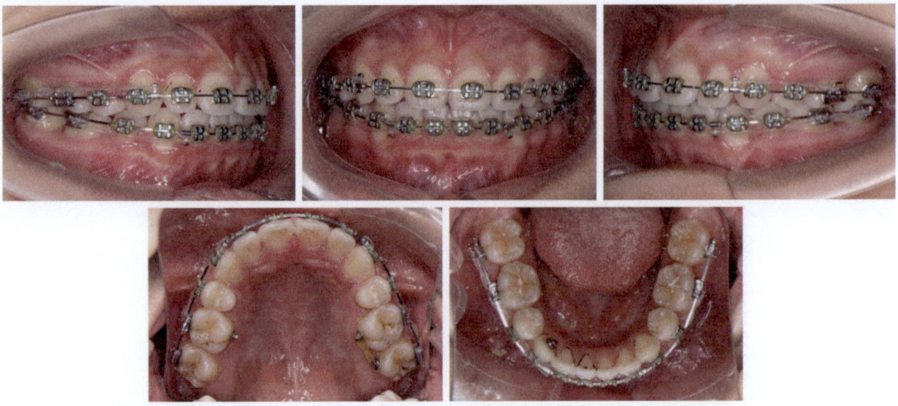

Fig. 10.18 The spaces were almost closed and the refinement was proceeding

protrusion, while not changing normal mandible forward growth pattern that certainly played an important role in facial profile improvement. Furthermore, we can see the intrusion of upper incisors, which indicates a good incisor control ability with 0.020 inch incisor slot.

Case 4 Adult, Class I, Bimaxillary Protrusion

Figure 10.20 showed a 21-year-old girl, who sought orthodontic treatment because of the severe lip protrusion, lip incompetence, and proclined anterior teeth. The intraoral view showed that all the third molars were well erupted and the teeth before them showed more forward tipping.

Diagnosis: Angle Class I and skeletal Class II relationship.
Treatment Plan: Extraction of four first premolars and four third molars; PASS technique.
Duration: 20 months.

The girl was bonded XBTs on first molars and MLF brackets on anterior teeth after the first premolars had been extracted. Figure 10.21 shows the intraoral view of first bonding of brackets after extraction. The 0.014″ NiTi wire was engaged in XBT −25° tipback tube that provide backward tipping moments not only on anchor molars but also on canines. We used 0.20 mm ligature wires to lower friction so that canine can "drift" back along the archwire. Figure 10.22 shows after 3 months of treatment, canines tipped back to relieve anterior crowding, incisors might also move lingually according to our research [7]. Therefore, openbite was reduced due to the pendulum effect. Considering the severe protrusive profile of the patient, a 0.018″ SS piggy back arch was used to tip upper first molars back to reinforce the anchorage. The auxiliary arch was inserted into the −7° tube and ligated on the lateral incisors while the thin NiTi archwire was inserted into the −25° tube to align anterior teeth.

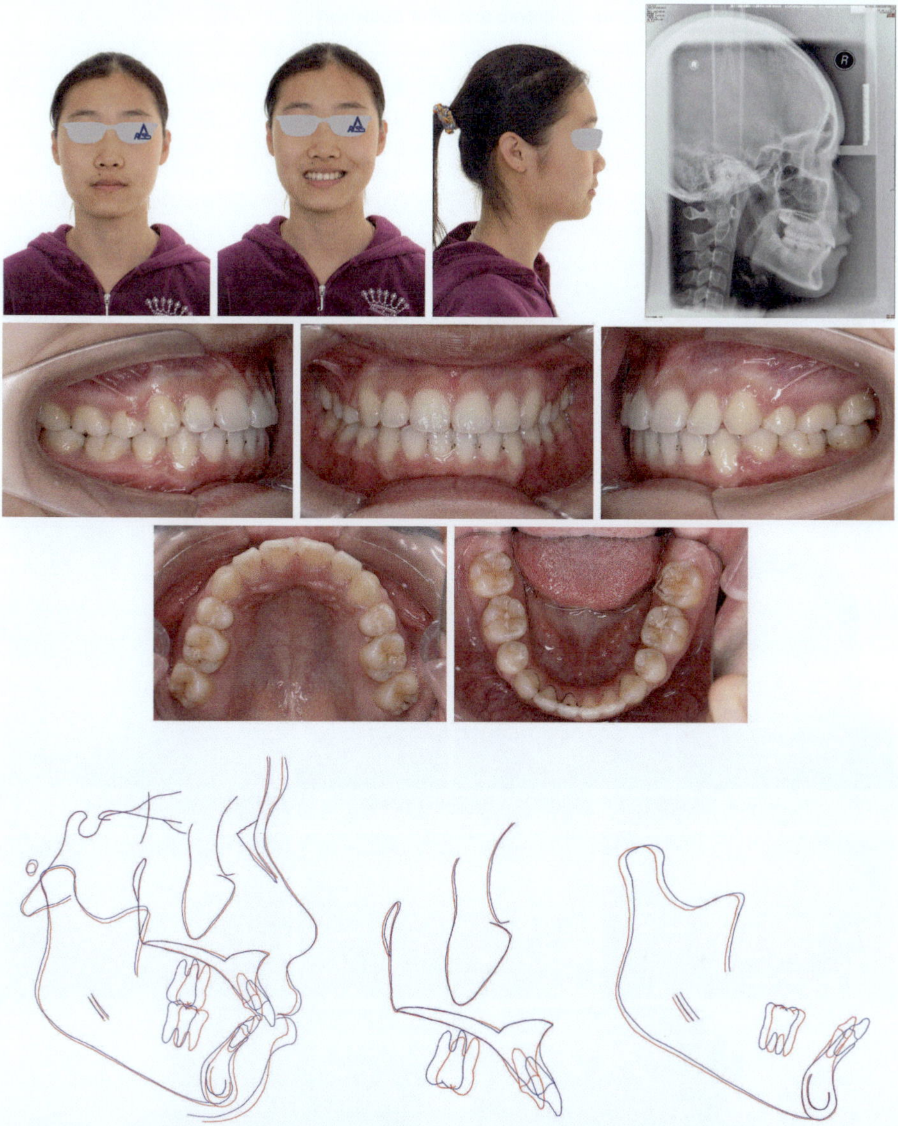

Fig. 10.19 The original posterior curve of Spee was maintained, and the incisor inclinations were pretty normal, as well as great lip retraction and upper incisor intrusion

After first molars being tipped back, PM2 and M2 were bonded, 0.018″ NiTi archwire with normal curve of Spee was then applied to align posterior teeth, followed by 0.018 × 0.025″ NiTi archwire to level the third-order irregularities and establish posterior curve of Spee. The retraction archwire was 0.018 × 0.025″ SS with crimple on hooks to close the spaces and improve occlusion. We finished the whole treatment of the severe bimaxillary protrusive woman in 20 months and

Table 10.3 Cephalometric analysis before and after treatment

	Norm.				
Measurements	Mean	SD.	Pre.	Post.	Dif.
SNA (°)	82.8	4.0	82.6	83.7	1.1
SNB (°)	80.1	3.9	78.7	79.5	0.7
ANB (°)	2.7	2.0	3.9	4.3	0.4
Wits appraisal (mm)	−1.1	2.9	1.4	1.8	0.5
PP/SN (°)	9.3	2.4	9.3	8.7	−0.6
MP/SN (°)	32.5	5.2	33.7	32.6	−1.1
MP/PP (°)	27.6	4.6	24.4	23.9	−0.4
FOP/PP (°)	NA	NA	1.4	3.8	2.4
U1-AP (mm)	7.2	2.2	10.8	4.8	−6.0
L1-AP (mm)	4.9	2.1	5.3	1.8	−3.5
U1/PP (°)	115.8	5.7	130.0	115.2	−14.8
L1/MP (°)	93.9	6.2	99.6	97.1	−2.5

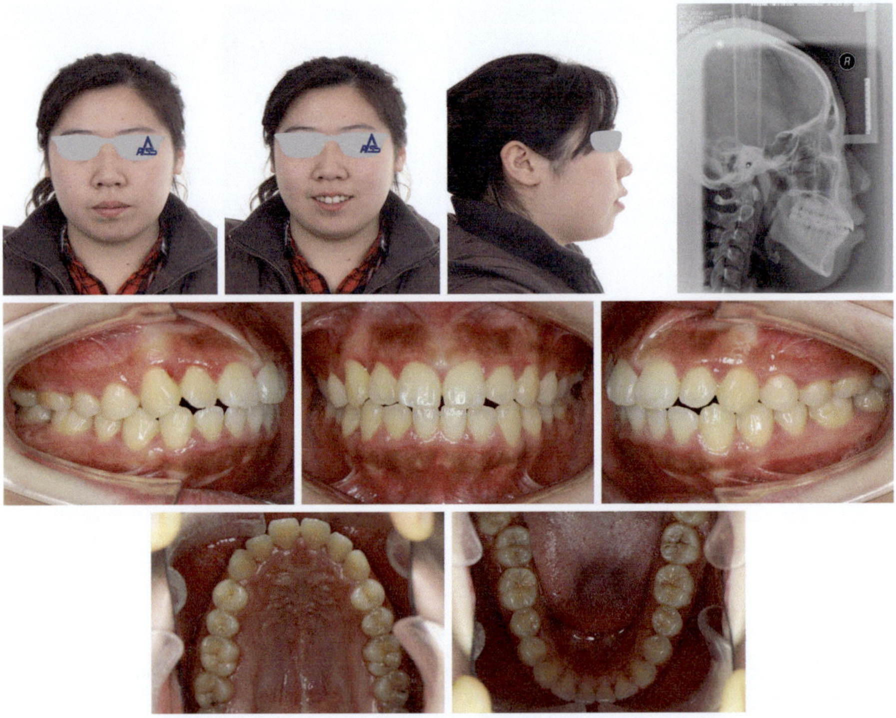

Fig. 10.20 The pretreatment view shows severely protruded upper jaw, partially open bite, and high mandibular plane angle

improved her profile apparently. Both her occlusion and appearance of the teeth were greatly improved (Fig. 10.23). Cephalometric superimposition shows obvious retraction of the upper and lower incisors and improved profile. The molars were tipped backward obviously which showed good anchorage control.

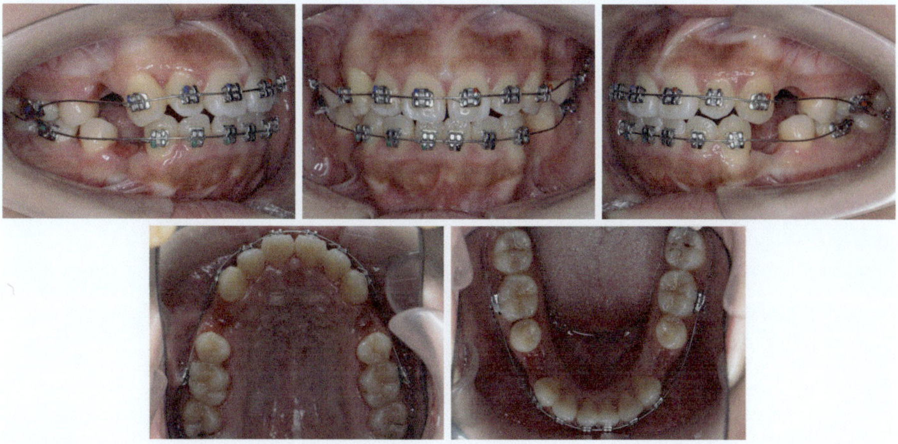

Fig. 10.21 The intraoral view of first bonding

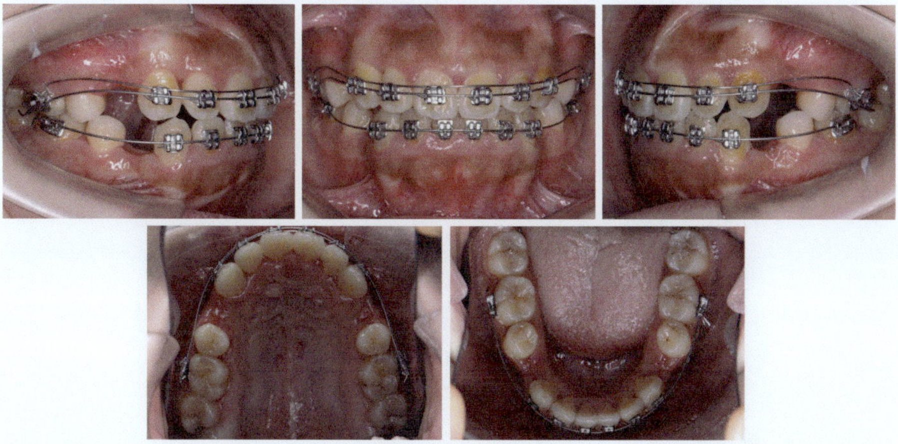

Fig. 10.22 A 0.018″ SS piggy back arch was added to tipback the first molars, being inserted into the −7° tube and ligated with the lateral incisors

Table 10.4 shows her cephalometric analysis before and after treatment. Her incisor protrusion and labial inclination were largely reduced (U1-AP decreased by 6.5 mm, L1-AP decreased by 5.8 mm), and the FOP/PP increased by 2.4°. The MP/SN was almost maintained.

Summary

For crowded cases, light-force correction is no doubt favorable and extensively used in conventional orthodontic treatment. The problem is how to prevent the labial inclination of anterior teeth and anchorage loss in the aligning stage of crowded

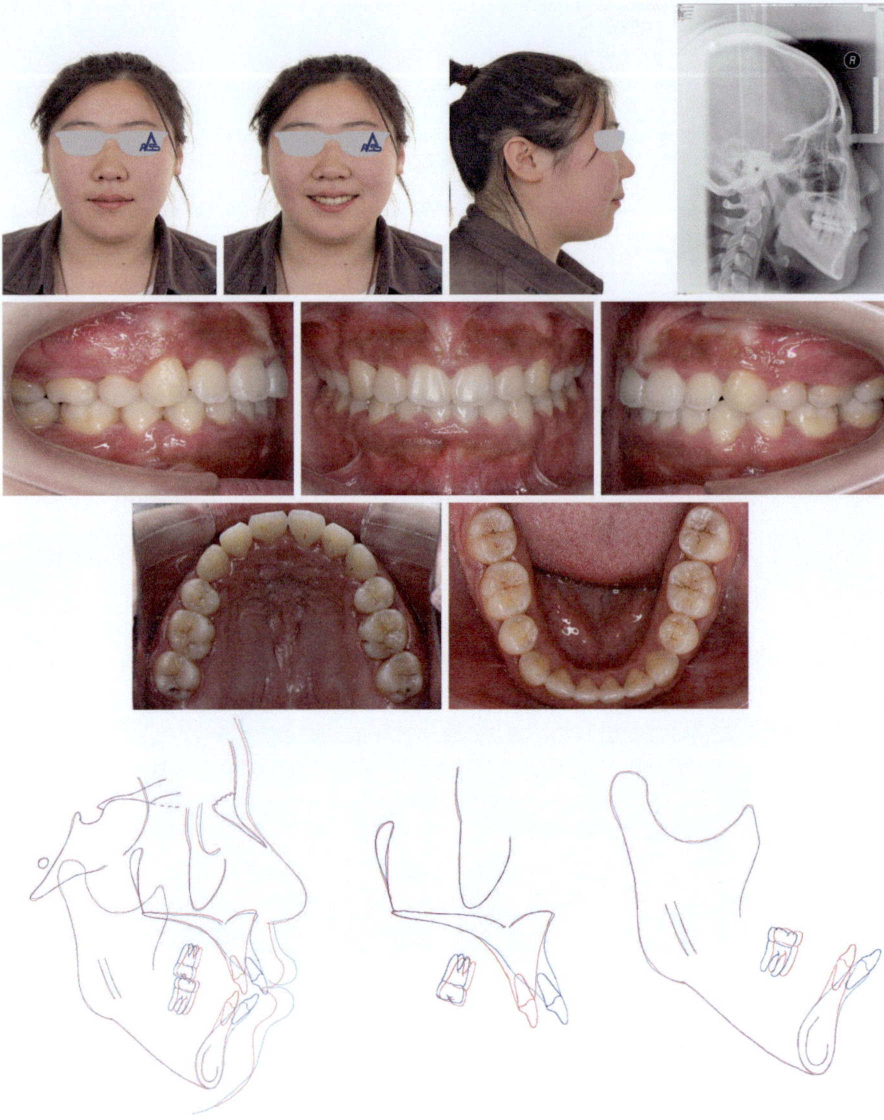

Fig. 10.23 The posttreatment records showed fine aligned teeth, Class I relationship, and a greatly improved facial appearance

cases. The low-friction mechanism of PASS system not only reduce the force to retract anterior teeth, but also lower the reaction acting on anchor molar so that the dominant moment on molar may resist it well enough instead of using heavy force anchorage auxiliaries. Meanwhile, when using the −25° tipback tube of XBT, the backward rotating moment on the canines will tip the canine distally to relieve anterior crowding without retraction force.

Table 10.4 Cephalometric analysis before and after treatment

Measurements	Norm. Mean	SD.	Pre.	Post.	Dif.
SNA (°)	82.8	4.0	87.1	84.3	−2.8
SNB (°)	80.1	3.9	81.8	80.6	−1.1
ANB (°)	2.7	2.0	5.4	3.7	−1.7
Wits appraisal (mm)	−1.1	2.9	−2.0	−5.7	−3.7
PP/SN (°)	9.3	2.4	11.4	11.5	0.1
MP/SN (°)	32.5	5.2	41.7	41.9	0.2
MP/PP (°)	27.6	4.6	30.4	30.4	0.1
FOP/PP (°)	NA	NA	9.4	11.8	2.4
U1-AP (mm)	7.2	2.2	12.7	6.2	−6.5
L1-AP (mm)	4.9	2.1	8.9	3.1	−5.8
U1/PP (°)	115.8	5.7	124.1	115.8	−8.3
L1/MP (°)	93.9	6.2	94.8	78.5	−16.4

When treating bimaxillary protrusion cases, the backward tipping design of XBT prevents the forward tipping of molars, while the piggy back arch can help in anchorage preparation for cases whose first molar has already tipped forward for any reasons. With the differential moment mechanism and low-friction design, canines can "drift" back along archwire relatively easier at early stage and trigger the drifting of the incisors. In the later stage, the upper archwire with normal curve of Spee can not only maintain the backward tipping of posterior teeth and prevent FOP forward rotation to reduce dental protrusion, but also help incisor torque control within 0.020 inch. slot, so that anchorage is saved, and treatment can be done with high efficiency and finished with great result.

References

1. Xu TM (2015) New concept of physiologic anchorage control. APOS Tends Orthod 5:250–254
2. Chen S, Du FY, Chen G et al (2013) Clinical research of the effects of a new type XBT buccal tube on molar anchorage control. Chin J Orthod 20:26–30
3. Chen S, Chen G, Xu TM (2015) Clinical application of the PASS technique. J Clin Orthod 49:508–515
4. Su H (2012) Factors influencing the mesiodistal tipping of first molars in malocclusion patients. Dissertation, Peking University. Beijing
5. Bills DA, Handelman CS, BeGole EA (2005) Bimaxillary dentoalveolar protrusion: traits and orthodontic correction. Angle Orthod 75:333–339
6. Solem RC, Marasco R, Guiterrez-Pulido L et al (2013) Three-dimensional soft-tissue and hard-tissue changes in the treatment of bimaxillary protrusion. Am J Orthod Dentofac Orthop 144:218–228
7. Su H (2015) Study on the correlation between first molar angulation growth pattern and anchorage control. Dissertation, Peking University. Beijing

Treatment of Class II Malocclusion with PASS Technique

11

Xiaoyun Zhang, Tian Min Xu, and Gui Chen

Abstract

Based on the fact reported by Prof. Johnston, for subjects with Class II malocclusion, dentoalveolar compensation characterized by upper molar forward migration movement during the growth tends to counteract favorable excessive mandible growth in pubertal spurt, which greatly reduced the chance of the spontaneous molar relationship correction; the strategy of Class II treatment with PASS technique focuses on upper dentition control by preventing upper first molars from forward tipping and maintaining the upper posterior curve of Spee, therefore reducing or even reversing the forward rotation of upper posterior occlusal plane and facilitating Class II correction, which are accomplished by the design of XBT tube and other knacks presented in this chapter.

Class II malocclusion is normally associated with Class II skeletal discrepancy, which is characterized by mandibular deficiency, maxillary excess, or both of them. Dentoalveolar compensation is usually observed in subjects with skeletal discrepancy. Our previous study disclosed the compensatory trends of mesiodistal angulation of first molars in malocclusion cases with different skeletal patterns [1]. For Class II malocclusion with relatively distally positioned mandibular first molars or retrognathic mandibles, maxillary first molars tended to be more distally inclined while the lower first molar more mesially tipped, and the opposite angulation compensation trend was found in Class III cases. Study also confirmed that the cant of the occlusal plane (OP) is significantly different in different skeletal patterns. The OP is much steeper in those with Class II malocclusions than that in the Class I occlusion group [2].

X. Zhang (✉) • T.M. Xu • G. Chen
Department of Orthodontics, Peking University School and Hospital of Stomatology, Beijing, China
e-mail: briskzhang@vip.sina.com; tmxuortho@163.com; chengui723@163.com

T.M. Xu (ed.), *Physiologic Anchorage Control*,
DOI 10.1007/978-3-319-48333-7_11

As indicated by Prof. Johnston in Chap. 3, four options could be used to the correction of a Class II malocclusion: retardant of maxillary growth, distalization of the maxillary dentition, enhancement of forward growth of the mandible, or mesial movement of the lower buccal segments. Although it is believed mandibular growth in pubertal spurt is usually favorable for the correction of Class II malocclusions, unfortunately, it has been noted that dentoalveolar compensation would prevent any excess—normal or even if in some way augmented—from having an effect on the molar relationship correction [3]. Within the four options, PASS technique focuses on upper dentition control by preventing upper first molars from forward tipping and maintaining the upper posterior curve of Spee, which is similar to classical Tweed mechanics, but different from contemporary straight wire mechanics when functional occlusal plane (FOP) control is concerned. According to Prof. Xu, leveling posterior curve of Spee of the upper arch may result in different FOP inclinations depending on the anchorage strength of teeth composing the curve (Fig. 8.5). Harris' study showed different treatment mechanics could cause different FOP [4]. Braun and Legan's study told us each degree of forward rotation of occlusal plane tends to increase 0.5 mm Class II molar relationship; therefore, for Class II correction, delaying or at least not accelerating FOP forward rotation during growth will be helpful for both distoclusion correction and upper arch protrusion reduction [5]. PASS technique for Class II treatment is established on the above theories and combines the advantages of simplicity of straight wire appliance and light force low friction of self-ligating appliance. It is reflected by the following four features.

First of all, the design of XBT tube, −25° auxiliary tube added into a maxillary molar tube, is the key to upper posterior anchorage control at the initial stage of the treatment, which aimed to act like a V- bend to prevent mesial tipping of upper molars which is a common finding when straight wire technique is applied.

Second, for cases with forward tipped upper molars, a piggy back arch can be inserted into the −7° tube; while initial NiTi wire can be used in the −25° tube for alignment, along with Class II elastics, upper molar will be uprighted and enhancement of the upper posterior anchorage can be achieved.

Third, pre-adjusted posterior brackets with tip-back angle and curved archwires used after initial alignment make posterior segment a strong anchorage unit as in Tweed mechanics. Meanwhile, before sliding technique is used to retract the upper anterior teeth, the curve of Spee of upper arch needs to be fully conserved or established by using NiTi rectangular wire with compensated curve of Spee according to the skeletal patterns, because we believe that it will help to prevent molar forward tipping and delay the counterclockwise rotation of occlusal plane rather than accelerate it.

The last but not the least, for cases with extremely proclined upper anterior teeth, round rather than rectangular stainless wire should be used for retraction of anterior teeth until the crown angulation of anterior teeth returns to normal. The reason for that is lighter force could be used to close the space with low friction because of the larger first-order clearance between 0.018″ round wire and the 0.022″ slots of posterior brackets as well as no third-order friction by contrast with rectangular wire, which is surely helpful to reserve upper molar anchorage.

In this section, four Class II cases are presented. Treatment mechanics and procedure are described in detail.

Case 1. Treatment of Angle Class II Division 1 Malocclusion with Growth Potential

A 13-year-old female's chief complaint was stuck-out front teeth and too full lips. Overjet was increased and anterior teeth were proclined on both arches. Full-step Class II molar relationship was presented on the left side. Increased lip prominence was observed. Cephalometric analysis indicated skeletal Class II discrepancy (Fig. 11.1). Treatment plan was extraction of four premolars to obtain the space to retract the anterior teeth and straighten the profile. Maximum upper posterior anchorage was demanded. Considering severe Class II molar relationship presented on the left side while neutral molar relationship on the right, upper PM1, lower left PM2, and right PM1 were extracted to facilitate correction of molar relationship.

Treatment procedure was illustrated in details in Fig. 11.2. Initially, only anterior teeth and first molars were bonded, and −25° tip-back tubes were used to prevent mesial drift of the upper molars (Fig. 11.2a). When anterior teeth were

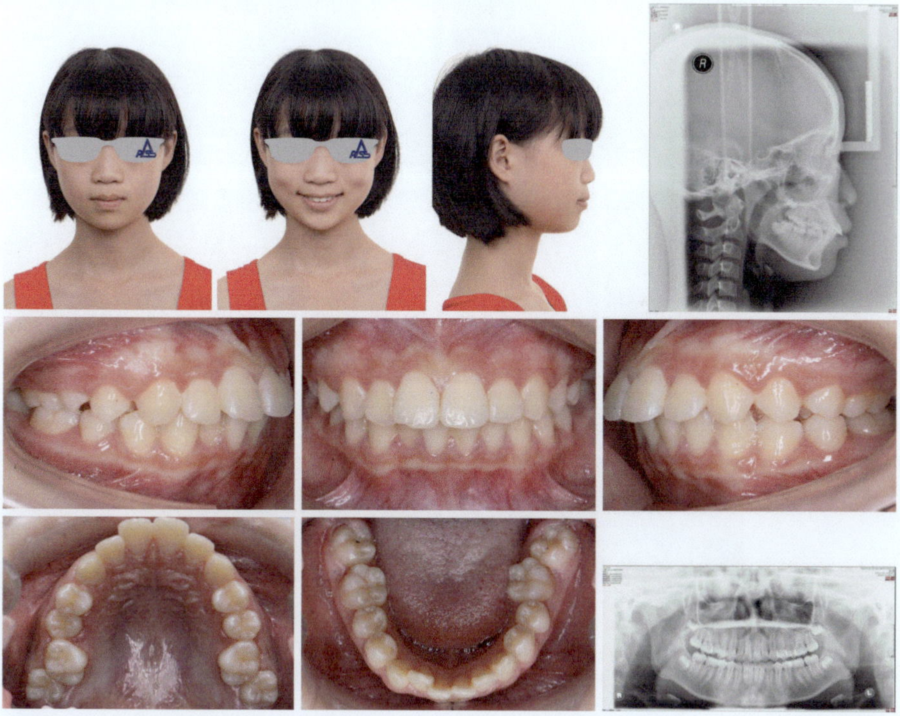

Fig. 11.1 Before treatment, a 13-year-old female patient presented with increased overjet, protruded incisors, and prominent lips

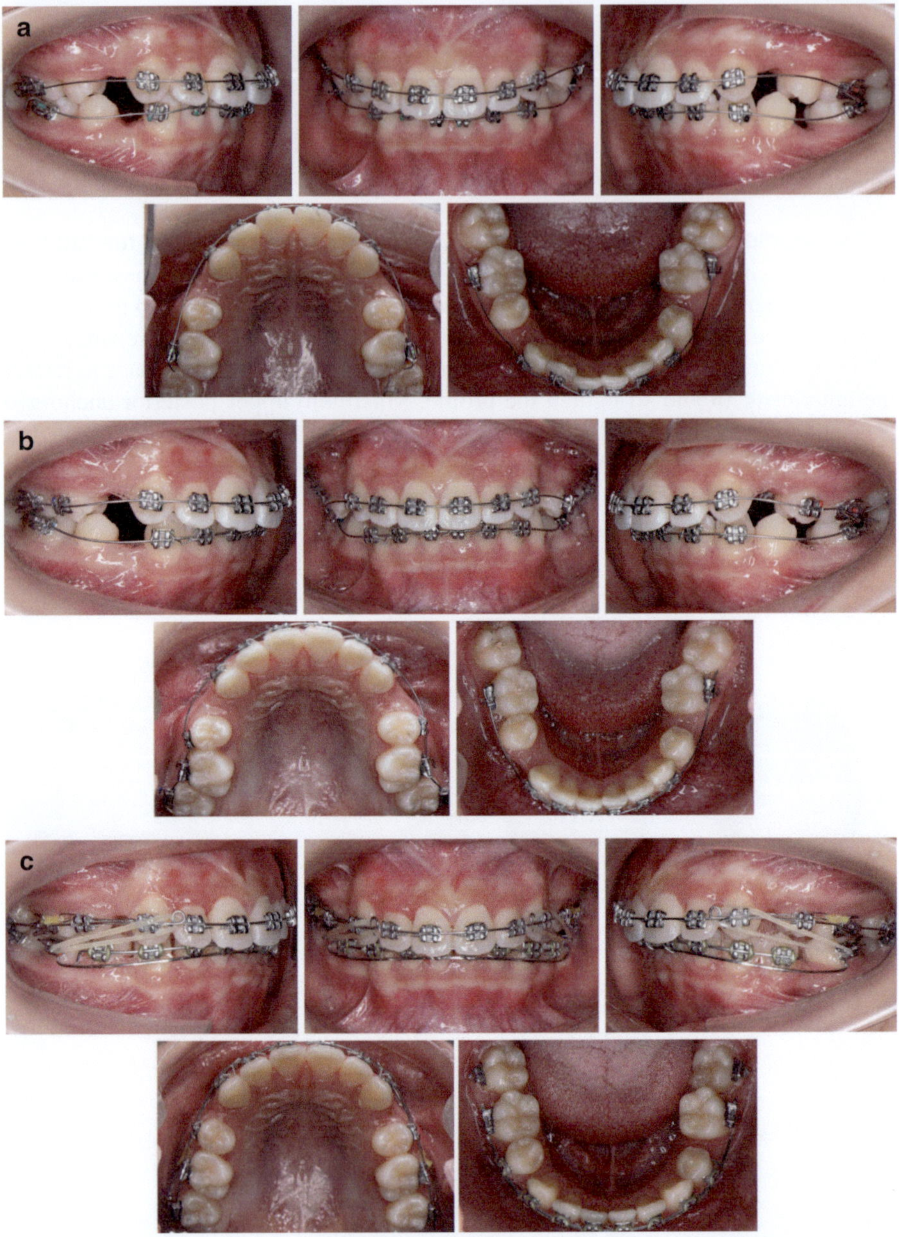

Fig. 11.2 Treatment procedure was displayed step by step. (**a**) Initially, only anterior teeth and first molars were bonded. (**b**) Upper second molars and premolars were bonded after upper anterior teeth were aligned. (**c**) 0.018″ stainless steel wire with helical loop and compensated curve of Spee combined with tieback and Class II elastics were used to correct anterior teeth inclinations. Piggy back arch was used to open the bite in the lower arch. Treatment procedure in details. (**d**) 0.018 × 0.025″ Ni-Ti wire with reversed curve of Spee, combining Class II elastics were used to correct the deep overbite in the lower arch. (**e**) Sliding mechanics using 0.018 × 0.025″ stainless rectangular wire was performed to close the residual space

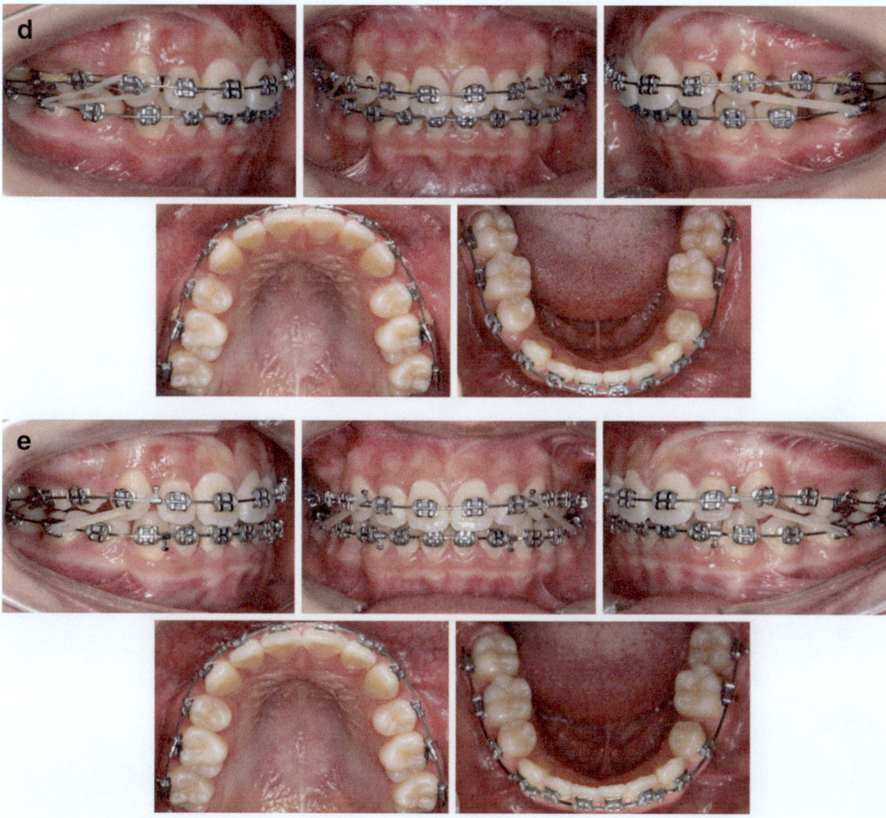

Fig. 11.2 (continued)

aligned, upper second molars and premolars were bonded, and 0.018″ NiTi wire with compensated curve of Spee was used to align the upper posterior teeth and maintain curve of Spee. Upper midline corrected itself by differential moments (Fig. 11.2b). Given the apparently proclined upper front teeth, 0.018″ stainless steel wire with helical loop and compensated curve of Spee combined with tieback, and Class II elastics were used to correct anterior teeth inclinations. Piggy back arch was used to open the bite in the lower arch (Fig. 11.2c). Nine months into treatment, the midline discrepancy and excessive overjet had been corrected; 0.018 × 0.025″ NiTi wire with reversed curve of Spee, combining Class II elastics, was used to correct the deep overbite in the lower arch (Fig. 11.2d). When the upper curve of Spee and a stable posterior anchorage unit are fully established, sliding mechanics using 0.018 × 0.025″ stainless rectangular wire was performed to close the residual space, and Class II elastics continued to correct the molar relationship (Fig. 11.2e).

After 20 months of active treatment, facial esthetic was greatly improved; teeth were well-aligned and a tight interdigitation was set up. Curve of Spee was not eliminated as conventional straight wire appliance; instead, compensated curve of

Spee was maintained. The angle between functional occlusal plane and palatal plane increased 5.0° after treatment (Fig. 11.3 and Table 11.1), indicating PASS technique reversed the compensation tendency of FOP, which is certainly beneficial to Class II correction.

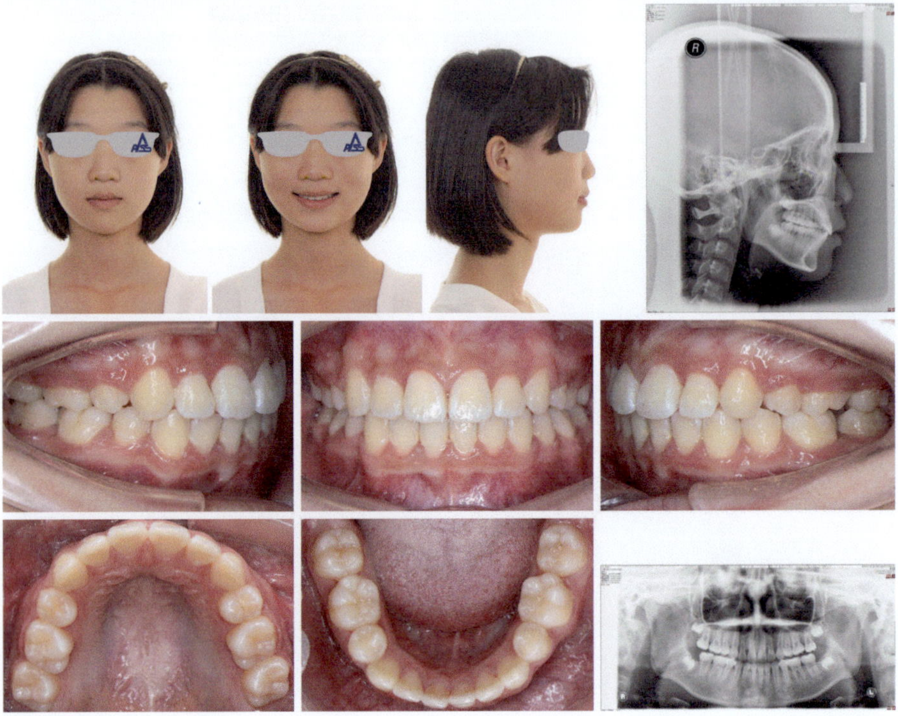

Fig. 11.3 Final treatment result is great and the improvement in facial appearance is due to marked retraction of lips

Table 11.1 Cephalometric analysis before and after treatment

Measurements	Norm		Pre	Post	Dif
	Mean	SD			
SNA (°)	82.8	4.0	83.3	81.0	−2.4
SNB (°)	80.1	3.9	76.3	76.4	0.1
ANB (°)	2.7	2.0	7.0	4.6	−2.4
Wits appraisal (mm)	−1.1	2.9	4.8	−2.4	−7.2
PP/SN (°)	9.3	2.4	8.5	8.7	0.2
MP/SN (°)	32.5	5.2	34.4	35.3	1.0
MP/PP (°)	27.6	4.6	25.8	26.6	0.8
FOP/PP (°)	NA	NA	8.4	12.6	4.2
U1-AP (mm)	7.2	2.2	10.1	5.7	−4.4
L1-AP (mm)	4.9	2.1	4.6	2.6	−2.0
U1/PP (°)	115.8	5.7	122.0	104.3	−17.7
L1/MP (°)	93.9	6.2	103.5	94.3	−9.2

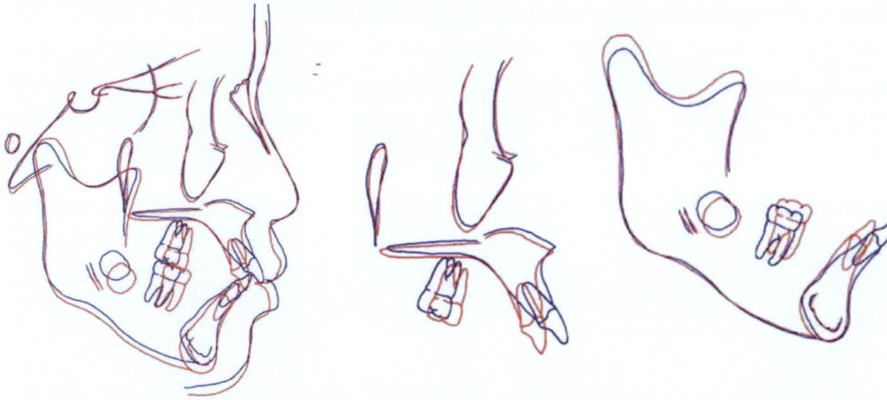

Fig. 11.4 Superimposition of pretreatment (*blue*) and posttreatment (*red*) cephalometric tracings (Reproduced from Xu [6])

Superimposition of pretreatment and posttreatment cephalometric tracings is displayed in Fig. 11.4. Structural superimposition of maxilla and mandible showed remarkable retraction of anterior teeth on both arches and excellent control of posterior anchorage.

Case 2. A Severely Crowded Class II Division 2 Malocclusion with Marked Skeletal II Discrepancy

An 11-year-old boy's chief complaint was crooked teeth. Upper lip was protrusive and everted. Retruded mandible and an ANB angle of 7.5° indicated skeletal II discrepancy (Table 11.2). A reduction of lower face height and flat mandibular plane angle confirmed it is a low angle case which means Class II intermaxillary traction and anterior bite plane were suitable for him. The overbite was increased and complete, and both arches were severely crowded. A full-unit Class II molar relationship was displayed on the right, and an end on Class II molar relationship was displayed on the left. Based on CVM analysis, great growth potential could be expected (Fig. 11.5). Given the degree of crowding, prominent upper lip and molar relationship, extraction of upper first and lower second premolar was performed. Upper anchorage should be carefully manipulated, because the extraction spaces need to be used to relieve the crowding and correct the molar relationship as well.

After extraction of upper first premolar, only upper anterior teeth and first molar were bonded, and NiTi wire was used to align the teeth, noticing that the wire was inserted into −25° tip-back tube to prevent mesial drift of upper molars (Fig. 11.6a). Two months later, upper anterior teeth were aligned, and deep overbite was partially corrected. Class II canine relationship on the right had changed into neutral due to the distalization of upper canine. Distal drift of upper canine is quite common when using PASS technique; it might be related to special biomechanics of −25° tip-back tube on upper molar which usually resulted in a tip-back moment on canine. Combined with transseptal fiber force and low-friction brackets, canines would drift

Table 11.2 Cephalometric analysis before and after treatment

Measurements	Norm		Pre	Post	Dif
	Mean	SD			
SNA (°)	82.8	4.0	79.9	79.3	−0.6
SNB (°)	80.1	3.9	72.5	74.1	1.6
ANB (°)	2.7	2.0	7.5	5.2	−2.2
Wits appraisal (mm)	−1.1	2.9	8.1	3.2	−4.9
PP/SN (°)	9.3	2.4	6.8	6.8	−0.1
MP/SN (°)	32.5	5.2	28.1	32.4	4.3
MP/PP (°)	27.6	4.6	21.3	25.6	4.4
FOP/PP (°)	NA	NA	0.4	4.0	3.6
U1-AP (mm)	7.2	2.2	1.4	3.1	1.7
L1-AP (mm)	4.9	2.1	5.1	0.8	−4.3
U1/PP (°)	115.8	5.7	76.6	105.8	29.2
L1/MP (°)	93.9	6.2	94.7	93.7	−1.1

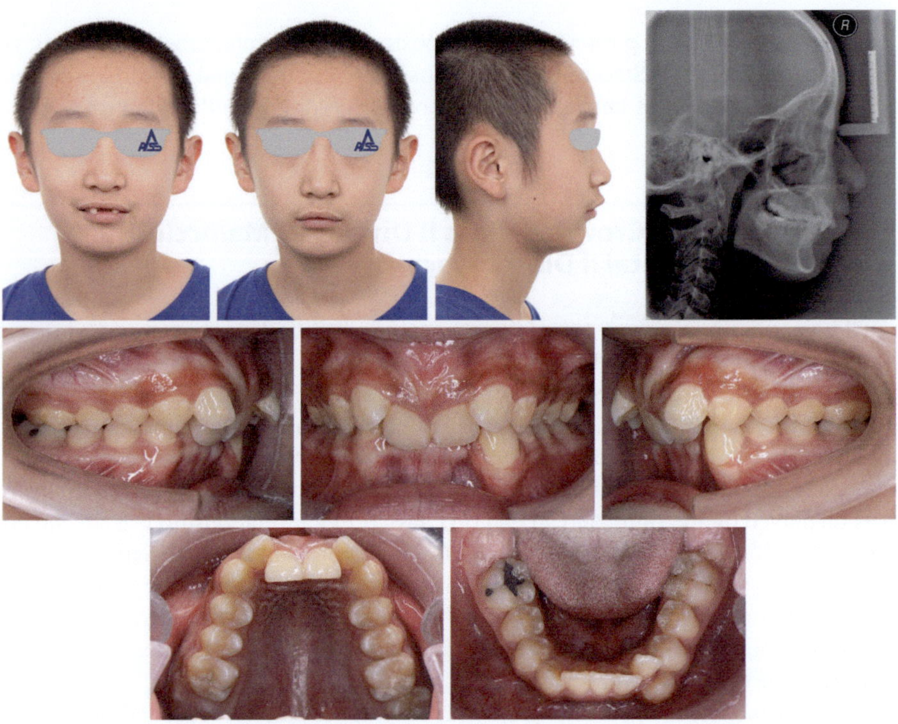

Fig. 11.5 An 11-year-old boy presented with severely crowed Class II division 2 malocclusion and marked skeletal II discrepancy

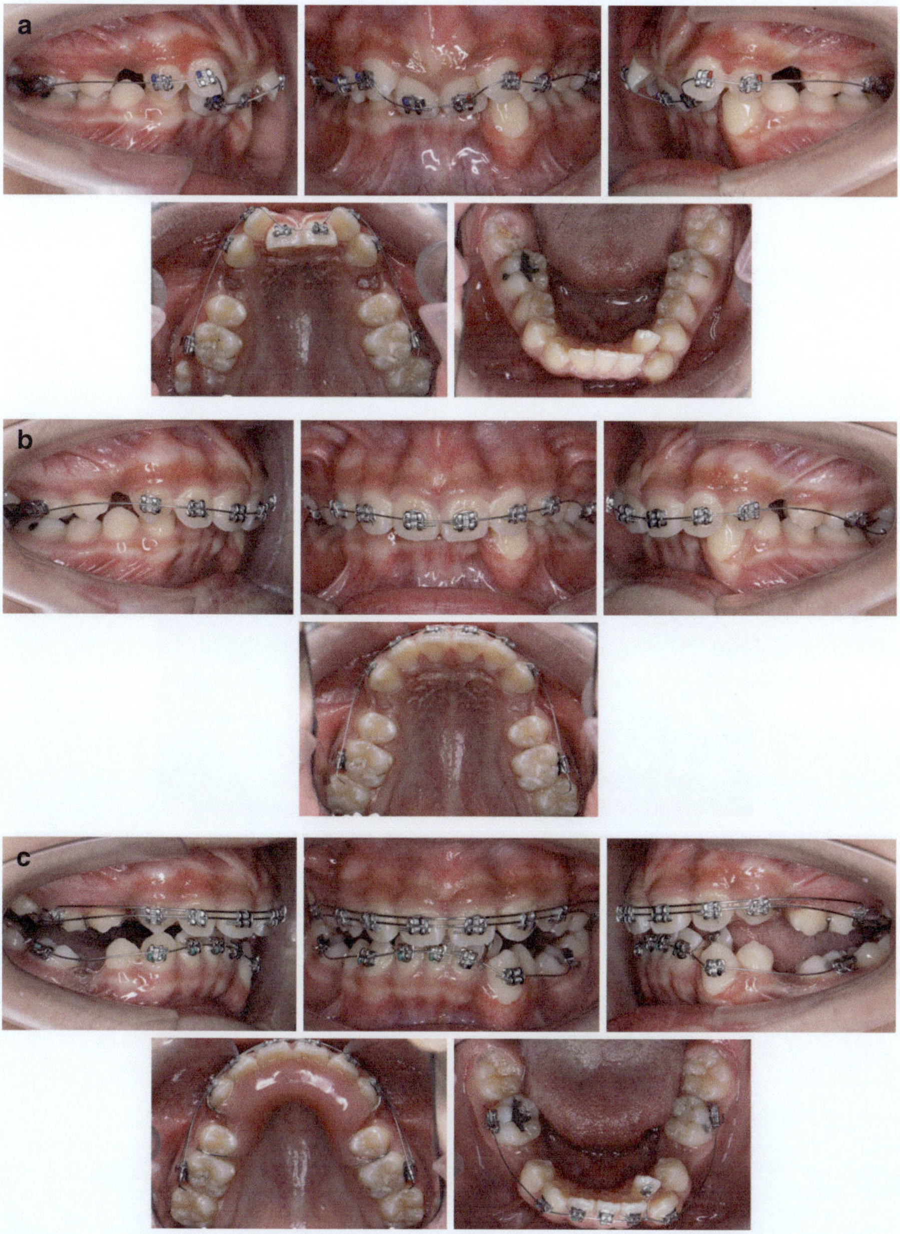

Fig. 11.6 Treatment procedure is presented here in detail. (**a**) After initial bonding, 0.014″ NiTi wire was used to align the upper anterior teeth. (**b**) Two months later, upper anterior teeth was aligned and canine relationship on the right side changed into Class I due to distalization of upper canine. (**c**) A piggy back arch and anterior bite plate were used to open the bite. (**d**) Second premolar and second molar were bonded when anterior teeth wee aligned. Main buccal tube with -7° tip were used to sustain the distal angulation of upper molar. (**e**) Less than 3 months later, rectangular nickel-titanium wire with compensated curve of Spee for the upper arch and reversed curve of Spee for the lower arch furthered the alignment and leveling. (**f**) 0.018 × 0.025″ Stainless rectangular wire with physiologic or compensated curve of Spee and Class II elastics were used to close the space, reduce the overjet and correct the molar relationship. (**g**) Space were fully closed 9 months later

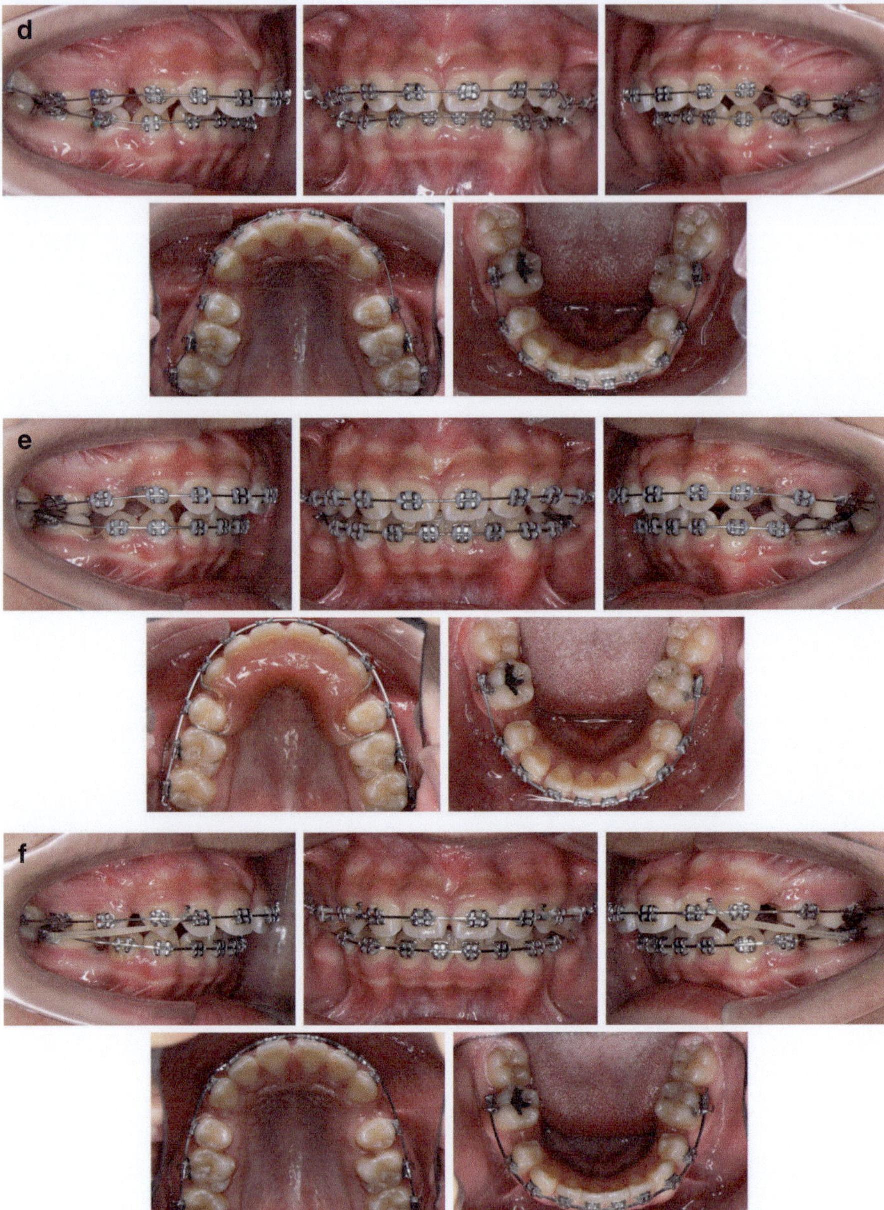

Fig. 11.6 (continued)

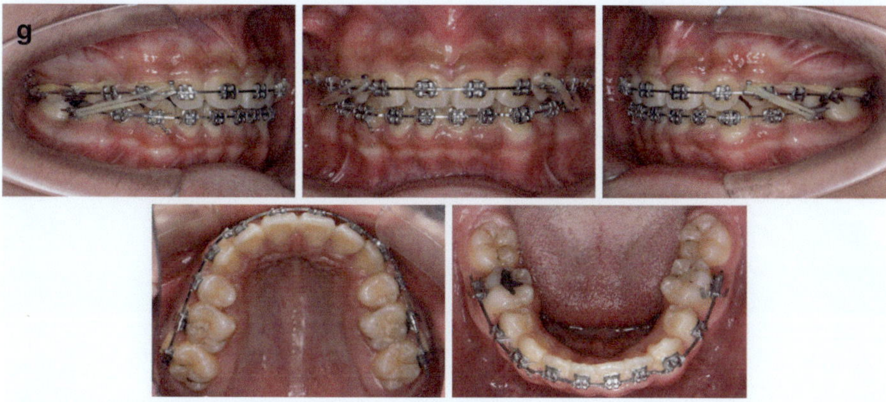

Fig. 11.6 (continued)

distally along the archwire to relieve anterior crowding (Fig. 11.6b). Later on, a piggy back arch and an anterior bite plate were used to open the bite. Lower anterior teeth and molar were bonded to relieve the crowding (Fig. 11.6c). When lower teeth were aligned, the upper second premolar and second molar were bonded. One should keep in mind that, for facilitating the maintenance of curve of Spee, the brackets of upper second premolar should be placed gingivally a little bit while brackets of upper second molar closer to occlusal rim. Instead of −25° tip-back auxiliary buccal tube, −7° main buccal tube was used to sustain the distal angulation of upper molar (Fig. 11.6d). In less than 3 months, posterior teeth were also aligned; rectangular nickel-titanium wire with compensated curve of Spee for the upper arch and reversed curve of Spee for the lower arch furthered the alignment and leveling (Fig. 11.6e). Two months later, 0.018 × 0.025″ stainless rectangular wire with physiologic or compensated curve of Spee and Class II elastics were used to close the space, reduce the overjet, and correct the molar relationship (Fig. 11.6f). It took another 9 months to close the residual space (Fig. 11.6g).

With 39 months of treatment, the patients got balanced face and solid Class I molar and canine relationship, noticing that the curve of Spee was maintained, while deep overbite was completely corrected. Reversal of functional occlusal plane as mechanics of dentoalveolar compensation for Class II skeletal discrepancy was detected in this case too. See Fig.11.7 and Table 11.2.

Pre- and posttreatment cephalometric superimpositions show remarkable skeletal growth occurred during the treatment, especially obvious vertical growth of maxilla. Although there was significant amount of condyle growth, the forward displacement of the mandible was limited due to the backward remodeling of mandibular fossa and condyle (Fig. 11.8).

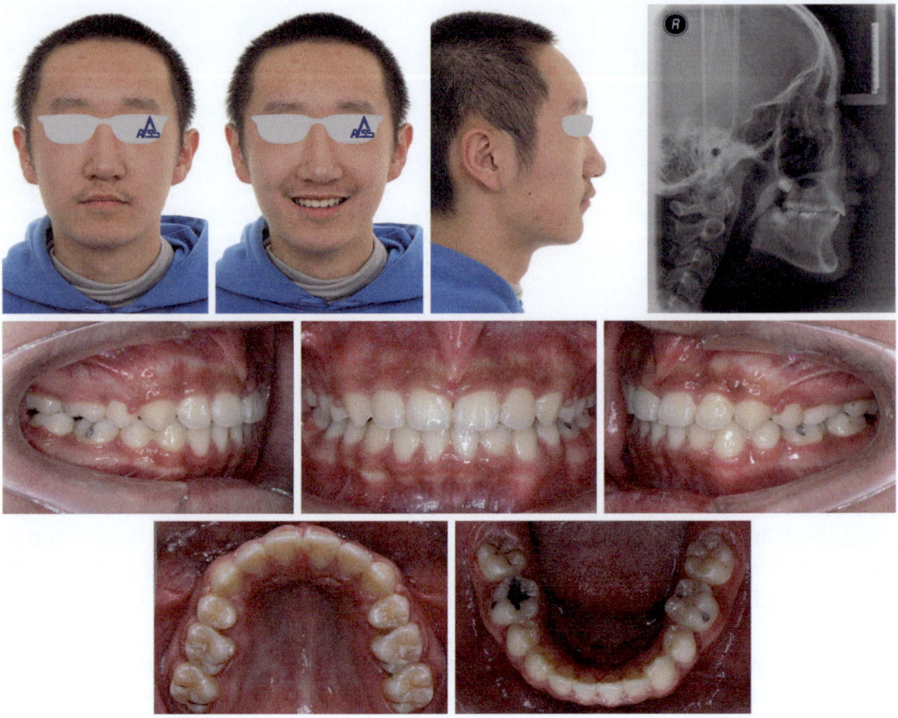

Fig. 11.7 Final result showed balanced face and solid Class I molar and canine relationship; the curve of Spee was maintained while deep overbite was completely corrected

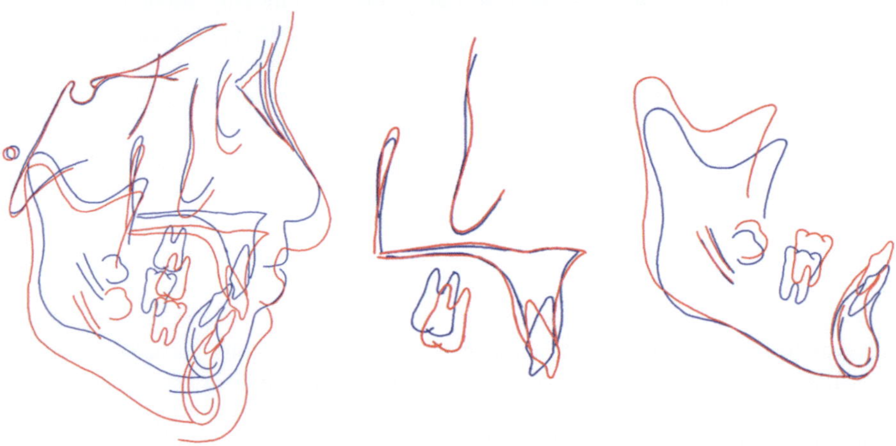

Fig. 11.8 Superimpositions of pretreatment (*blue*) and posttreatment (*red*) cephalometric tracings

Case 3. A Severely Crowded Class II Division 1 Malocclusion with Marked Skeletal II Discrepancy

A 13-year-old boy presented with protruded incisors, excessive overjet, 100 % of deep overbite, severe crowding, and extremely retruded mandible. From lateral view of his face, we could barely identify his chin (Fig. 11.9). Since his father showed the same pattern of profile, his mandibular dysplasia is clearly inherited. Lateral cephalogram disclosed severe skeletal II deformity with remarkable mandibular deficiency (SNB = 72.4°, ANB = 9.7°), steep mandibular plane (FH/MP = 31.7°), and apparently distal tipped upper molars as a dental compensation for skeletal II discrepancy (Table 11.3). The parents did not accept orthognathic surgery for their son.

Given the fact that his skeletal deformity is hereditary, we could not expect too much growth of mandible; how could we handle the problem of sagittal discrepancy? According to Prof. Johnston, mandibular excess and upper molar movement during the growth tend to balance, even for patients who showed quite amount of mandibular excess growth but not intervened orthodontically; the intercuspated

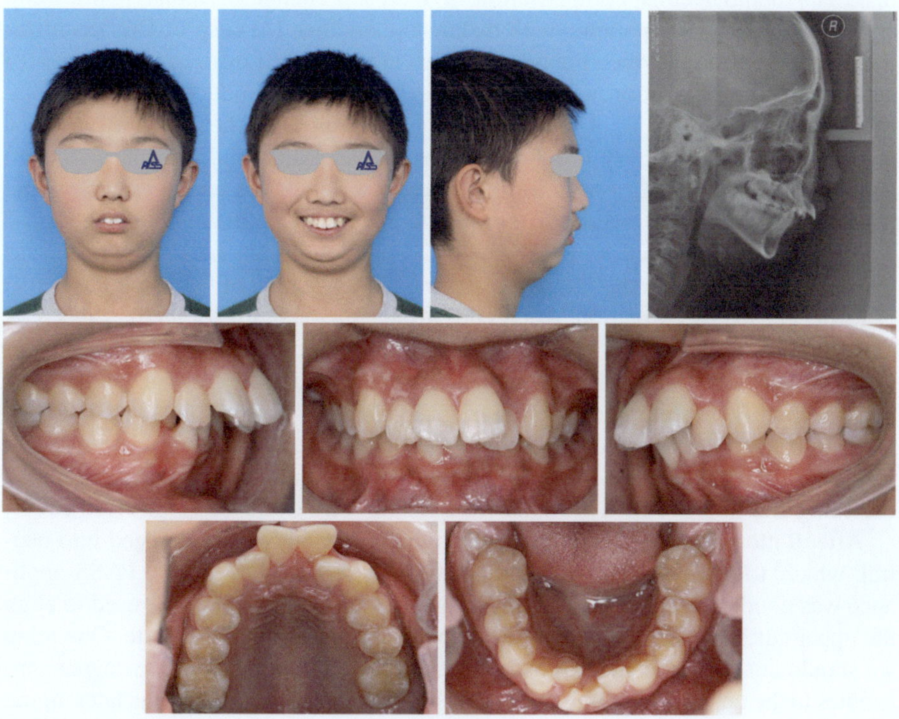

Fig. 11.9 Pretreatment photos and lateral cephalogram

Table 11.3 Cephalometric analysis before and after treatment

Measurements	Norm		Pre	Post	Dif
	Mean	SD			
SNA (°)	82.8	4.0	82.1	78.7	−3.4
SNB (°)	80.1	3.9	72.4	74.5	2.1
ANB (°)	2.7	2.0	9.7	4.2	−5.5
Wits appraisal (mm)	−1.1	2.9	12.9	−0.7	−13.6
PP/SN (°)	9.3	2.4	3.0	6.6	3.6
MP/SN (°)	32.5	5.2	34.7	33.9	−0.8
MP/PP (°)	27.6	4.6	31.7	27.4	−4.4
FOP/PP (°)	NA	NA	14.0	10.0	−4.0
U1-AP (mm)	7.2	2.2	13.2	5.7	−7.6
L1-AP (mm)	4.9	2.1	2.3	2.7	0.5
U1/PP (°)	115.8	5.7	119.8	107.7	−12.2
L1/MP (°)	93.9	6.2	104.6	97.9	−6.6

Class II cannot change to Class I spontaneously. But when maxillary holding devices (Nance button, pendulum, Distal Jet, headgear, etc.) were used to prevent maxillary dentoalveolar compensation, a 1/2 cusp change of molar relationship could be obtained; for patients with distal step, another 1/2 cusp of U6 "distalization," plus a period in which the upper molars are prevented from compensating for additional 1/2 cusp of normal mandibular excess, would produce a Class I molar relationship (Fig. 11.9) [3]. Therefore, for this case, high-pull headgear was applied at first to inhibit maxillary growth, distalize upper molar, and prevent unwanted extrusion of molars; four PM1s were extracted to relieve the severe crowding and retract protruded upper incisors. Anterior bite plate was applied to open the bite.

Treatment was started with headgear and extraction, but fixed appliance was intentionally delayed in the thought of taking the advantage of "physiological drift of teeth" caused by extraction. Apparently, "physiological drift of teeth" caused by extraction of premolar will drive the posterior teeth moving forward except upper molars because of usage of headgear, distalize the cuspid and retrocline the incisors, which certainly benefit the correction of Class II molar relationship and alleviation of crowding in the lower arch; this phenomenon has been documented in numerous studies [7–11] and discussed in Chap. 7. Within several months, relief of lower arch crowding and improvement of molar relationship were observed (Fig. 11.10).

After 9 months of headgear, molar relationship on both sides changed into neutral, which, to a large extent, make the rest of treatment much easier. PASS appliance was bonded on the upper molar and anterior teeth, NiTi wire was used to align the upper anterior teeth, and anterior bite plate was used to open the bite. One thing we should not neglect is that anchorage loss of lower dentition to some degree contributes to the correction of molar relationship (Fig. 11.11). Four months later, upper front teeth were aligned and bonding of lower front teeth initiated (Fig. 11.12).

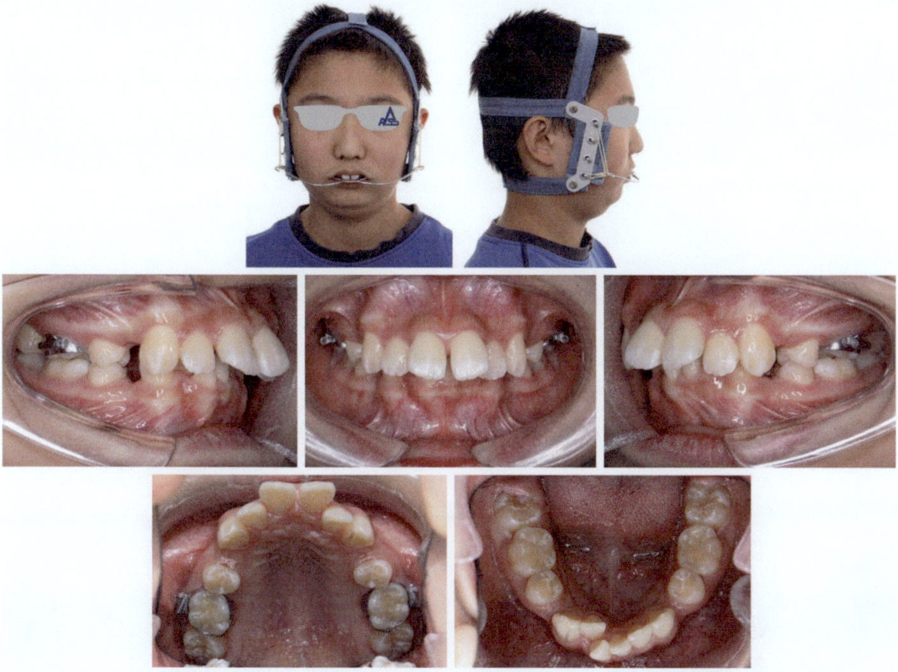

Fig. 11.10 Headgear was used at first to inhibit maxillary growth and distalize upper molar, noting that the Class II molar relationship had been partly corrected and lower incisor crowding was relieved

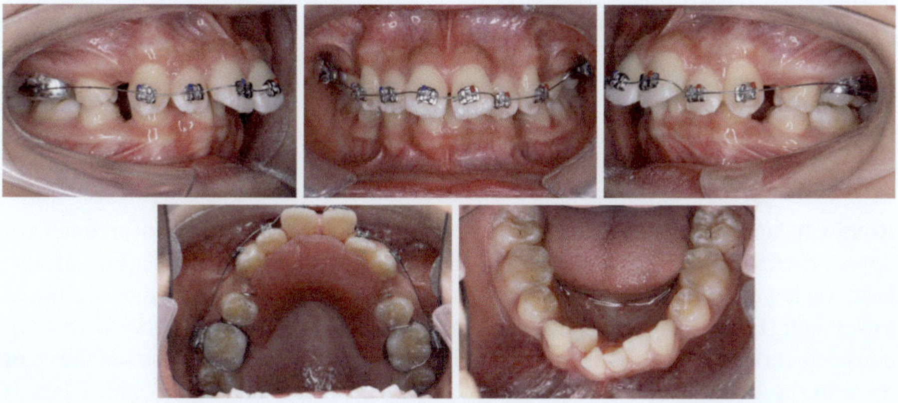

Fig. 11.11 After 9 months of headgear wearing, PASS appliance was bonded on the upper molar and anterior teeth, 0.014 NiTi wire was engaged in −25° tip-back tube to align the upper anterior teeth, and anterior bite plate was used to open the bite

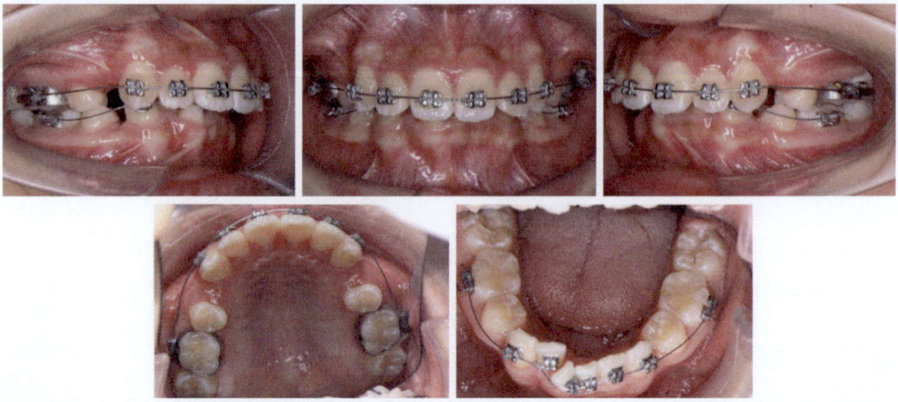

Fig. 11.12 Lower anterior teeth were bonded 4 months later, when we could find that the upper anterior teeth had been aligned

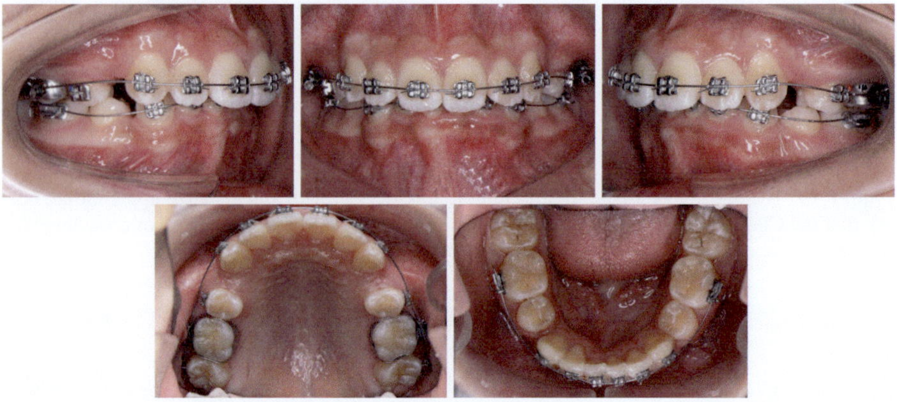

Fig. 11.13 Upper second molar and premolar were bonded for the purpose of aligning posterior teeth and establishing compensated curve of Spee

Routinely, upper second molar and premolar were engaged to help reinforcement of upper posterior anchorage and establish the compensated curve of Spee (Fig. 11.13). Later on lower second molar and premolar were engaged to facilitate the leveling of lower arch (Fig. 11.14). In the stage of space closure, 0.018 × 0.025″ SS with compensated curve of Spee in upper arch and 0.018 × 0.025″ SS with reversed curve of Spee in the lower arch were used, respectively. Elastic chain along with Class II elastics was used to close the space and adjust occlusion (Fig. 11.15).

Totally 45 months elapsed when perfect alignment and occlusion were obtained (Fig. 11.16). Even though the patient's profile is not quite pleasing due to the big nose and underdevelopment of the chin, the boy is very happy for no one mocked

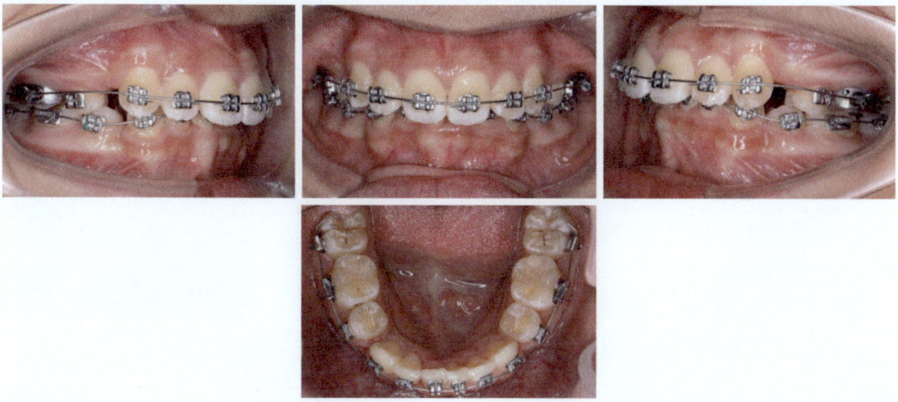

Fig. 11.14 When anterior teeth were aligned, lower second molar and premolar were engaged to facilitate the leveling of lower arch

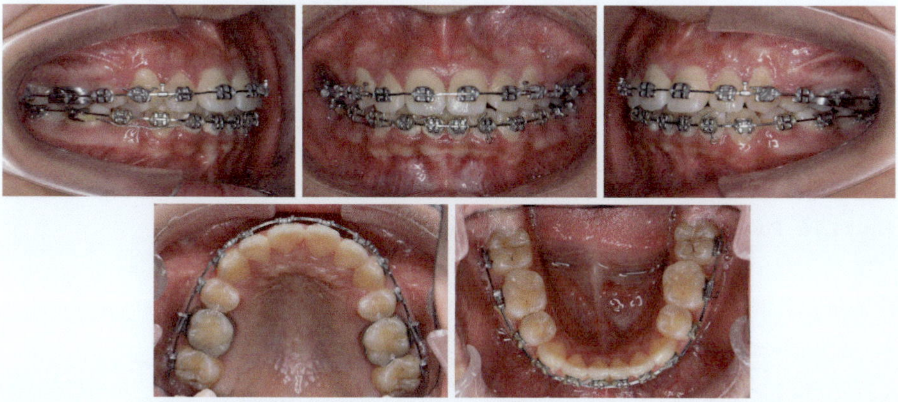

Fig. 11.15 In the end, stainless rectangular wire was used to close the space and thoroughly open the bite

at his stuck-out front teeth anymore. Moreover, advancement genioplasty could be performed in adulthood to further improve facial esthetic. Significant retraction of upper incisors contributes the most for correction of increased overjet. Remarkable extrusion of lower molars and relative intrusion of lower incisors are responsible for correction of deep overbite. Little forward and downward displacement of upper molar indicates great anchorage control (Fig. 11.17). The curve of Spee was maintained. However the FOP/PP decreased in this case (Table 11.3), probably due to the growth that happened during the long treatment time and the direction of extra-oral force.

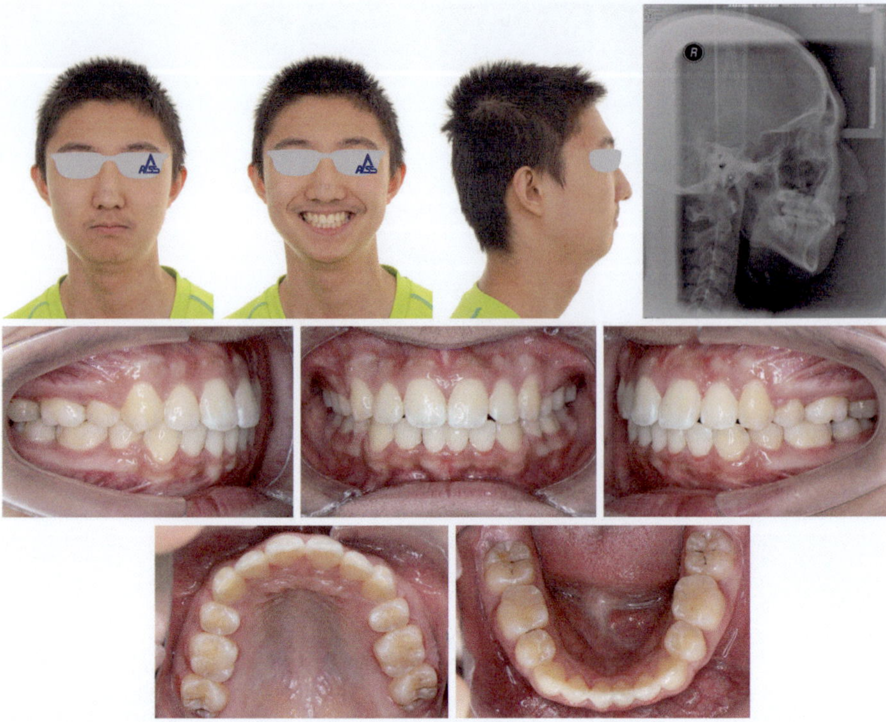

Fig. 11.16 Posttreatment photos and lateral cephalogram

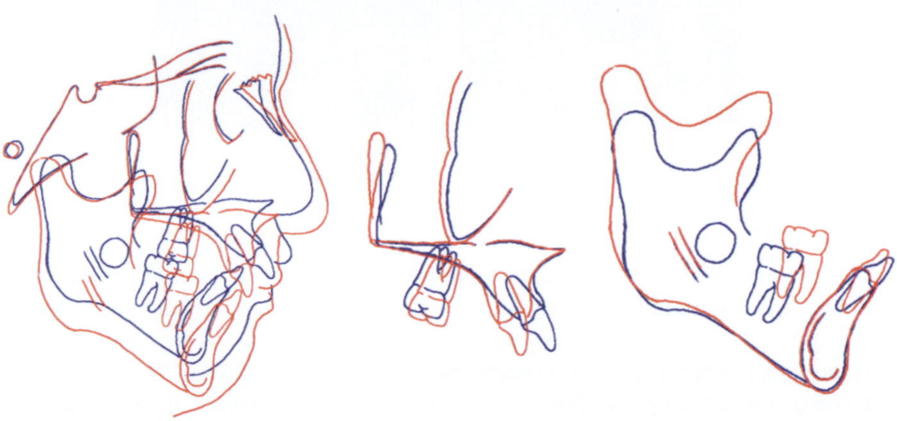

Fig. 11.17 Superimpositions of pretreatment (*blue*) and posttreatment (*red*) cephalometric tracings

Case 4. Treatment of an Adult with Severe Skeletal Class II Relationship and Convex Profile

A 23-year-old female's chief concern was her profile and lip incompetence. Although molar relationship remained Class I due to forward tipping of lower first molars, increased overjet and distal canine relationship indicated existence of sagittal discrepancy. Mandible was severely retruded and marked lip incompetency presented (Fig. 11.18). According to pretreatment cephalometric analysis (Table 11.4), ANB angle is 9.9°, and SN/MP angle is 51.7°. Obviously, this is an extremely tricky skeletal Class II and high angle case! Orthognathic surgery was recommended at first, but was rejected by the patient. Orthodontic camouflage treatment had to be adopted; therefore, upper first and lower second premolars were extracted. There is no doubt that absolute upper posterior anchorage is mandatory to improve facial appearance.

Remarkable mandibular deficiency and maxillary excess are easily identified from the lateral cephalogram, so does the distal tipped upper molars. Steep

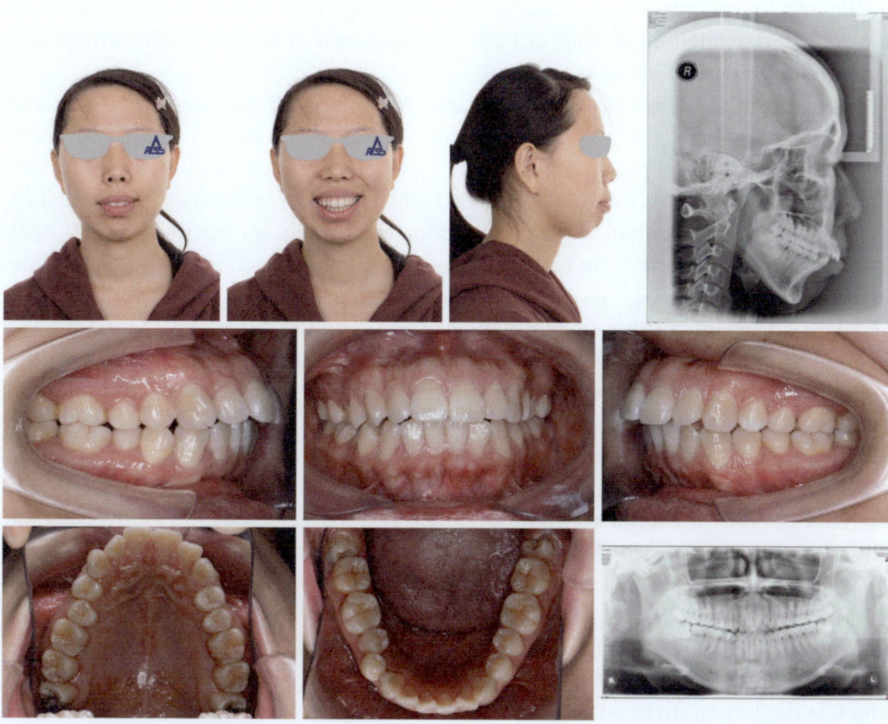

Fig. 11.18 Pretreatment photos, lateral cephalogram, and panoramic radiograph

Table 11.4 Cephalometric analysis before and after treatment

	Norm				
Measurements	Mean	SD	Pre	Post	Dif
SNA (°)	82.8	4.0	81.3	80.8	−0.5
SNB (°)	80.1	3.9	71.4	72.9	1.5
ANB (°)	2.7	2.0	9.9	7.9	−2.0
Wits appraisal (mm)	−1.1	2.9	6.7	−1.7	−8.4
PP/SN (°)	9.3	2.4	10.1	10.5	0.5
MP/SN (°)	32.5	5.2	52.0	52.4	0.4
MP/PP (°)	27.6	4.6	42.0	41.9	−0.1
FOP/PP (°)	NA	NA	0.4	4.7	4.3
U1-AP (mm)	7.2	2.2	13.8	10.2	−3.6
L1-AP (mm)	4.9	2.1	6.8	7.9	1.1
U1/PP (°)	115.8	5.7	120.6	97.1	−23.5
L1/MP (°)	93.9	6.2	96.7	95.8	−0.9

mandibular plane and long face indicate the vertical discrepancy. Apparent convex profile and lip incompetence made her quite a tough case which did need absolute upper posterior anchorage control both sagittally and vertically when orthodontic camouflage treatment alone is adopted.

Soon after extraction of upper first and lower second premolar, bonding and alignment of anterior teeth started to prevent the possible mesial tipping of upper posterior teeth due to “physiological drift” caused by extraction (Fig. 11.19a). One month after bonding, crowding of upper front teeth was obviously relieved (Fig. 11.19b). In order to enhance upper posterior anchorage, an auxiliary piggy back arch was applied to further tip back the upper first molar which is in some way similar to the mechanics of “anchorage preparation” used in Tweed technique (Fig. 11.19c). Afterward, further consolidation of the curve of Spee for upper arch and leveling of the lower arch was achieved with NiTi rectangular wire, which is a crucial step for reinforcement of upper posterior anchorage before retraction of front teeth starts (Fig. 11.19d).

Satisfied final result was obtained after 27 months of active treatment. Prominent upper lip and protruded front teeth were retracted significantly without usage of any auxiliary device for anchorage reinforcement. Deep overjet was fully corrected and Class I canine relationship was established. Compensated curve of Spee was sustained, and the cant of functional occlusal plane was reversed, which is certainly helpful to correction of Class II relationship of dentition (Fig. 11.20 and Table 11.4). Structural superimposition of the maxilla confirmed that the absolute upper posterior anchorage was obtained both sagittally and vertically even without using TADs, which is the key to successful treatment of this tough case (Fig. 11.21).

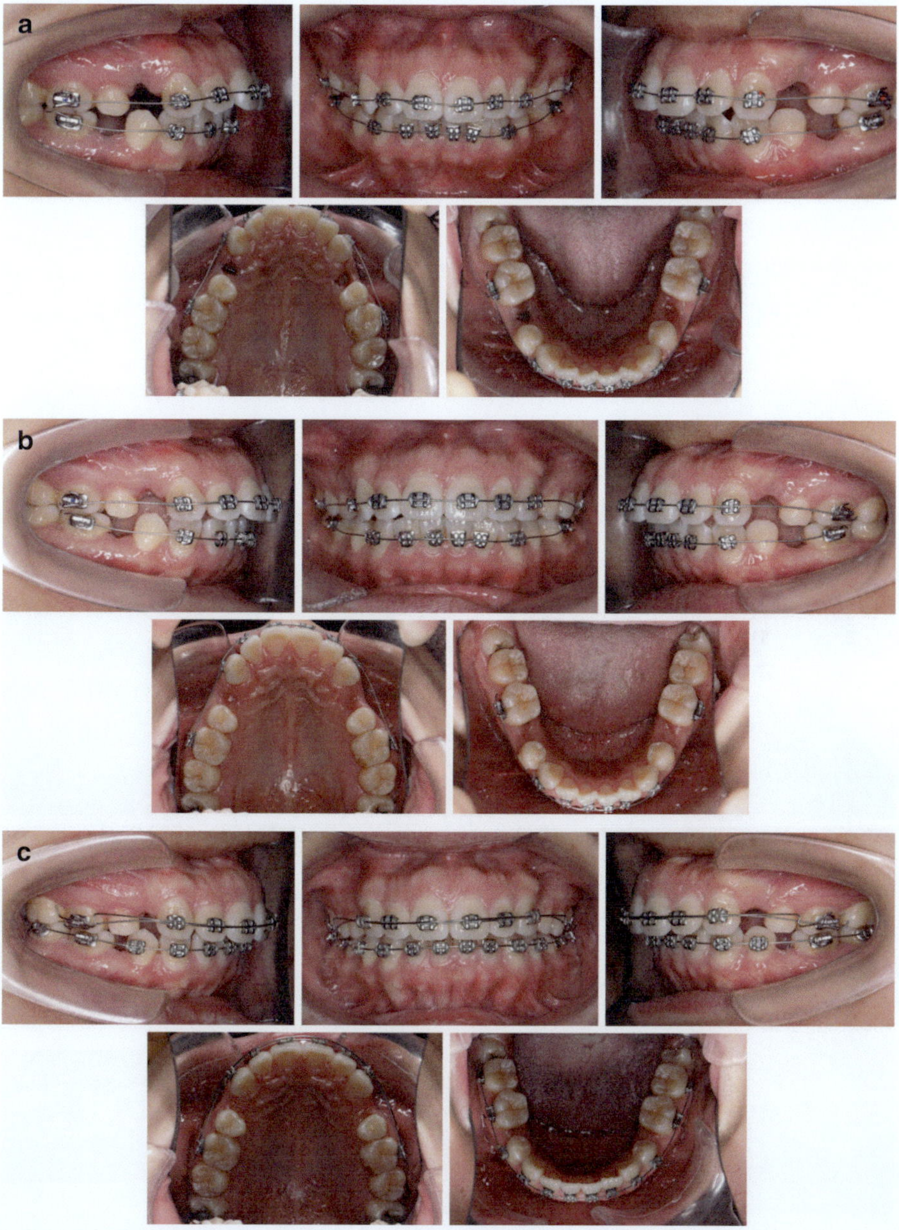

Fig. 11.19 Treatment procedure for this case with PASS technique is demonstrated in steps (**a**) Bonding and alignment of anterior teeth started shortly after the extraction to prevent the possible mesial tipping of upper posterior teeth due to "physiological drift" caused by extraction. (**b**) Crowding of upper front teeth was obviously relieved in one month. (**c**) An auxiliary piggy back arch was applied to further tip back the upper first molar for the enhancement of upper posterior anchorge. (**d**) Further consolidation of the curve of Spee for upper arch and leveling of the lower arch was achieved with Ni-Ti rectangular wire, which is a crucial step for reinforcement of upper posterior anchorage before retraction of front teeth start

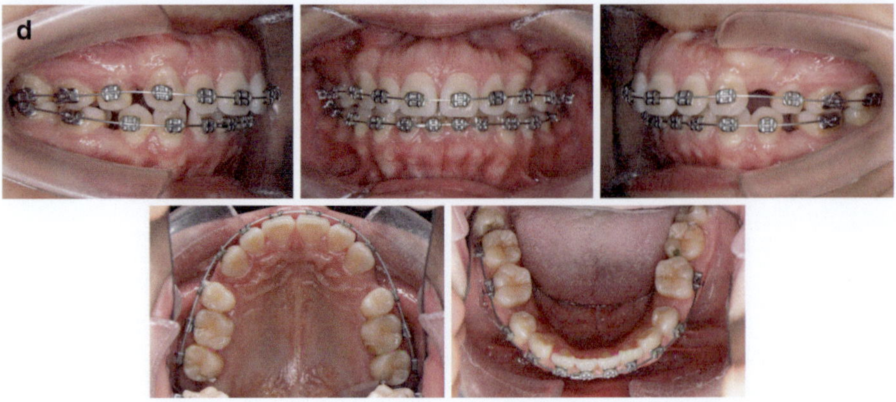

Fig. 11.19 (continued)

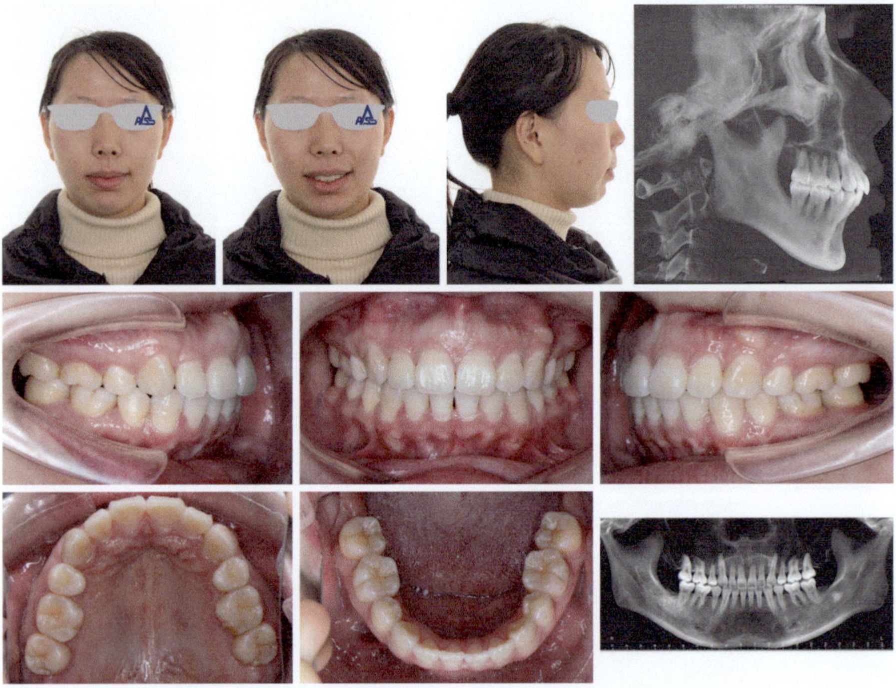

Fig. 11.20 Posttreatment photos revealed remarkable improvement on facial appearance and occlusion

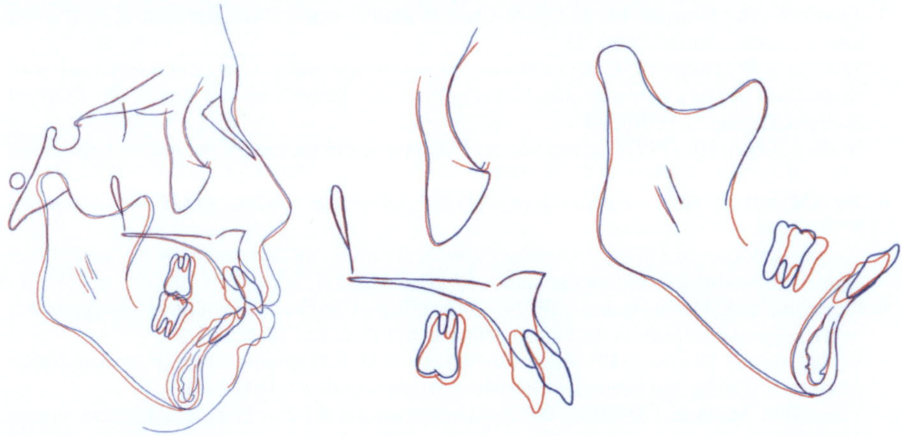

Fig. 11.21 Superimpositions of pretreatment (*blue*) and posttreatment (*red*) cephalometric tracings

Summary

Strategy of Class II treatment with PASS technique focuses on upper dentition control by preventing upper first molars from forward tipping and maintaining the upper posterior curve of Spee. The design of XBT tube, −25° auxiliary tube added into a maxillary molar tube, is the key to upper posterior anchorage control at the initial stage of the treatment. Simultaneously, a piggy back arch can be inserted into the −7° tube to upright the forward tipped upper molar just like "anchorage preparation" used in Tweed technique. Pre-adjusted posterior brackets with tip-back angle and archwires with compensated curve of Spee used after initial alignment could not only make posterior segment a strong anchorage but also reduce or reverse the tendency of flattening of functional occlusal plane during the growth which is beneficial to the correction of Class II molar relationship. For cases with extremely proclined upper anterior teeth, round rather than rectangular stainless wire is recommended to retract anterior teeth until the crown angulation of anterior teeth returns to normal. Knowing the regulation of dentoalveolar compensation is the key to successful treatment.

References

1. Su H, Han B, Li S et al (2014) Compensation trends of the angulation of first molars: retrospective study of 1403 malocclusion cases. Int J Oral Sci 6:175–181
2. Tanaka EM, Sato S (2008) Longitudinal alteration of the occlusal planeand development of different dentoskeletal frames during growth. Am J Orthod Dentofac Orthop 134:602 e1–11

3. Tsourakis AK, Johnston LE Jr (2014) Class II Malocclusion: The aftermath of A "Perfect Storm". Semin Orthod 20:59–73
4. McKinney JR, Harris EF (2001) Influence of patient age and sex on orthodontic treatment: Evaluations of Begg lightwire, standard edgewise, and straightwire techniques. Am J Orthod Dentofac Orthop 120:530–541
5. Braun S, Legan HL (1997) Changes in occlusion related to the cant of the occlusal plane. Am J Orthod Dentofac Orthop 111:184–188
6. Xu TM (2015) New concept of physiologic anchorage control. APOS Trends Orthod 5:250–254
7. Campbell-Wilson M (1975) Preliminary investigation into the movement of the lower labial segment following loss of first premolars. Br J Orthod 2(1):25–28
8. Robertson NAE, Cavina R, Moss JP (1979) The effect of the extraction of lower first premolars on the migration of teeth in the human dental arch. J Dent Res 58:1252
9. Papandreas SG, Buschang PH, Alexander RG et al (1993) Physiologic drift of the mandibular dentition following first premolar extractions. Angle Orthod 63(2):127–134
10. Swessi DM, Stephens CD (1993) The spontaneous effects of lower first premolar extraction on the mesio-distal angulation of adjacent teeth and the relationship of this to extraction space closure in the long term. Eur J Orthod 15(6):503–511
11. Jia QL, Gao XM, Fu MK (1995) Physiological drift of the mandibular dentition after first premolar extractions. Chin J Stomatol 30(1):23–25

Treatment of Class III Malocclusion with PASS Technique

12

Si Chen and Guangying Song

Abstract

Class III malocclusion, in spite of its relatively low prevalence, presents big challenges to orthodontists around the world. Different dental and skeletal patterns as well as development stages need to be taken into account when making the individualized treatment plans. Though facemask therapy is well understood and widely used in mixed dentition patients with deficient maxilla, fixed appliance therapy is usually performed to solve the dental discrepancy and to improve facial profile in early permanent dentition and adult Class III patients. Due to its unique treatment philosophy and appliance design, PASS technique provides a new way to correct Class III malocclusion based on patients' specific dental-skeletal characteristics. In this chapter, three Class III cases treated by PASS technique were presented. Treatment details and possible mechanics for the correction were discussed based on individual case.

Class III malocclusion is characterized by anterior crossbite and mesial molar relationship, which might be associated with or without skeletal discrepancy. The prevalence of Class III malocclusion is significantly higher in Chinese (4–14 %) than in Caucasians (1–4 %). A concave profile is commonly found in Class III patients and most frequently to be the reason why patients seek orthodontic treatment.

Though it remains controversial that whether severe skeletal Class III malocclusion could be treated by conservative orthodontic approaches, mild to moderate cases are more likely to be the candidates for nonsurgical orthodontic treatment, which is also the preference of the patients, at least in China.

S. Chen (✉) • G. Song
Department of Orthodontics, Peking University School and Hospital of Stomatology, Beijing, China
e-mail: elisa02chen@gmail.com; songguangying@gmail.com

T.M. Xu (ed.), *Physiologic Anchorage Control*,
DOI 10.1007/978-3-319-48333-7_12

The craniofacial characteristics of Class III subjects involve retrusive maxillary positions, protrusive mandibular positions, prominent mandible, and proclined maxillary incisors [1]. Therefore extraction and Class III elastics are usually applied in orthodontic camouflage treatment to use dentoalveolar compensation and inter-maxillary position adjustment to correct anterior crossbite and establish Class I canine and molar relationship.

In addition, according to our previous study [2, 3], the maxillary first molars distally inclined the least and the mandibular first molars distally inclined the most in Class III cases. At the meantime, Spee's curve of Class III cases is relatively flat when compared with Class I cases. These physiological characteristics should be born in mind and made the best use of in the treatment of Class III cases.

Case 1. Treatment of Dental and Skeletal Class III Malocclusion in an Adolescent Patient

A 15-year-old female presented with the chief complaint of crossbite (Fig. 12.1). She had a Class III malocclusion with anterior crossbite and crowding. The patient and her parents also addressed the concave profile with protruded lower lips.

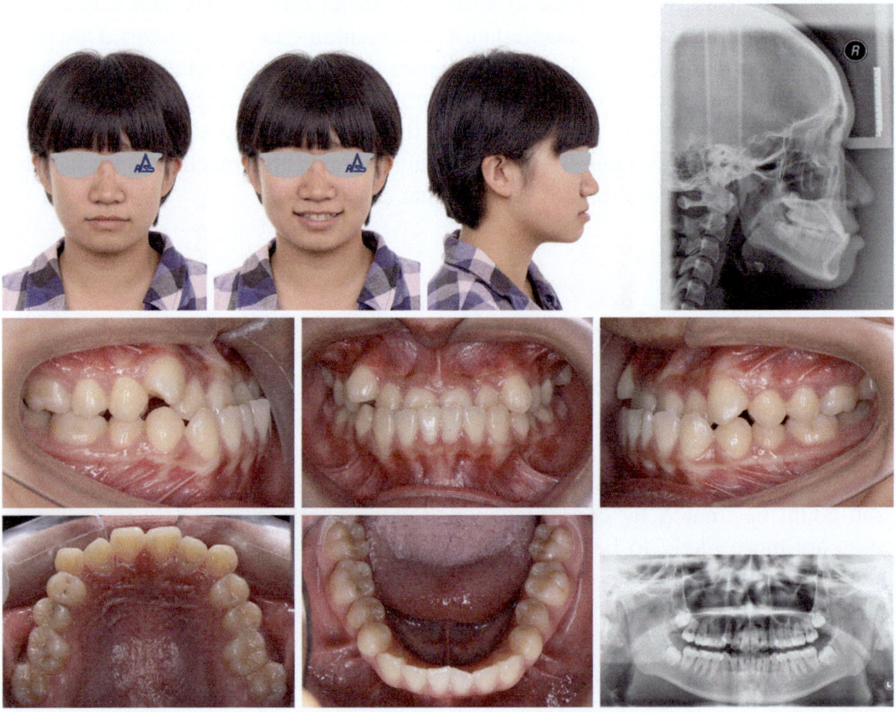

Fig. 12.1 Fifteen-year-old female patient with anterior crossbite, crowding, and protruded lower lips before treatment

Cephalometric analysis revealed it was a moderate skeletal Class III (ANB: −3.6°, see Table 12.1) with teeth compensation. Mild curve of Spee could be noticed as well. Since the patient and her parents didn't consider orthognathic surgery as option, orthodontic camouflage treatment was applied using PASS technique.

Upper 2nd and lower 1st premolars were extracted to provide space for alignment and retraction of lower anterior teeth.

The first step was to align the upper arch. MLF brackets were bonded from canine to canine in the upper arch, and XBT buccal tubes were bonded on the upper 1st molars. Upper 1st premolars were not bonded at the beginning of the treatment. 0.014–0.016″ NiTi wires were inserted into the −25° tip-back molar tube sequentially during alignment. Since the moment created on the molar was the dominant one (see Chap. 2), canine alignment was achieved without extra distal retraction force (i.e., laceback). In the lower arch, the 2nd premolars were bonded at the beginning, and 0.016″ NiTi wire was engaged in the main tube of XBT since there was no apparently inclined teeth in lower dentition. Due to the deep anterior crossbite, glass ionomer cement (GIC) was temporarily placed on the lower 1st molars to open the anterior deep bite and facilitate bracket placement.

After alignment, 0.018″ SS arch wires were placed into the main tubes in both arches. Omega loop with a tip-back molar bend was added to the upper arch wire. Power chain was used in the lower arch from the helical loop distal to the lateral incisor to the hook on the molar buccal tube to close the lower extraction space. At the meantime, Class III elastics were applied to assist space closure and anterior crossbite correction as well as molar relationship adjustment (Fig. 12.2).

After partial space closure, posterior occlusion was also improved (Fig. 12.3). Then lower 2nd molars were bonded and aligned. Continuous ligature from 6 to 6 was used to maintain the anterior space closure during alignment of the 2nd molars. Upper 1st premolars and 2nd molars were bonded on the next appointment. 0.016″, 0.017 × 0.025″ and 0.019 × 0.025″ NiTi wires with compensated Spee's curve were sequentially used to achieve the complete alignment in the upper arch.

Table 12.1 Cephalometric analysis before and after treatment

	Norm.				
Measurements	Mean	SD.	Pre.	Post.	Dif.
SNA (°)	82.8	4.0	78.5	80.2	1.7
SNB (°)	80.1	3.9	82.1	81.5	−0.6
ANB (°)	2.7	2.0	−3.6	−1.3	2.3
Wits appraisal (mm)	−1.1	2.9	−9.1	−5.9	3.2
PP/SN (°)	9.3	2.4	12.9	12.6	−0.3
MP/SN (°)	32.5	5.2	34.8	34.0	-0.8
MP/PP (°)	27.6	4.6	21.9	21.4	−0.5
FOP/PP (°)	NA	NA	3.9	2.9	−1.0
U1-AP (mm)	7.2	2.2	3.6	6.0	2.4
L1-AP (mm)	4.9	2.1	7.4	1.5	−5.9
U1/PP (°)	115.8	5.7	117.9	127.1	9.2
L1/MP (°)	93.9	6.2	88.7	75.1	−13.6

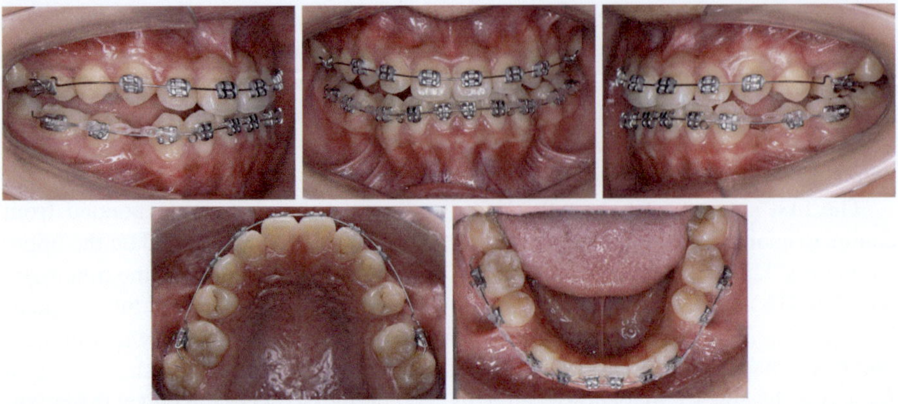

Fig. 12.2 Nine months into treatment

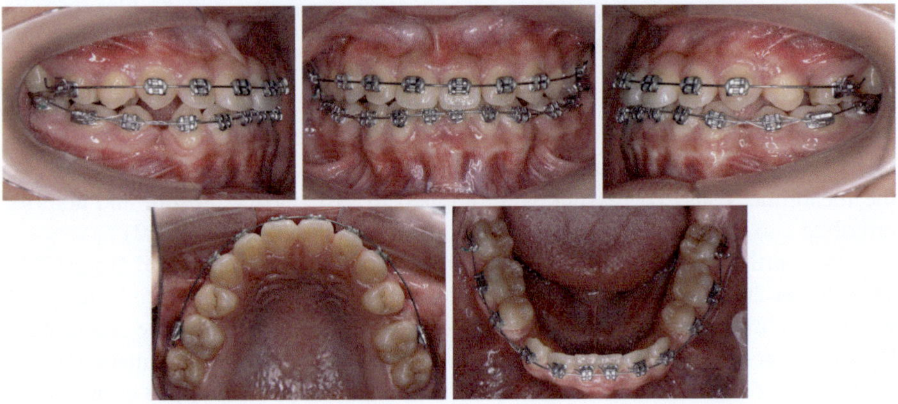

Fig. 12.3 Thirteen months into treatment

Seventeen months later, 0.019 × 0.025″ SS arch wires with compensated Spee's curve were placed in both arches for the final space closure (Fig. 12.4). Reinforcement of upper molar anchorage from the beginning of the treatment ensured both the efficient use of the extraction space for anterior alignment and enough anchorage to be provided for intermaxillary Class III elastics.

A well-aligned dentition and a harmonious facial balance were achieved after 24-month's treatment. A stable Class I canine and molar relationship with good interdigitation and ideal overjet and overbite were obtained.

Superimposition of pretreatment (blue) and posttreatment (red) cephalometric tracings shows good molar anchorage control and remarkable lower incisor and lip retraction (Fig. 12.5). Cephalograms show the mild curve of Spee which fits the Class III skeletal pattern was reserved after the treatment. Table 12.1 shows her lower incisor retroclined 13.6° and upper incisor proclined 9.2°. The sagittal dental compensation position of the upper incisors was generally maintained. Functional

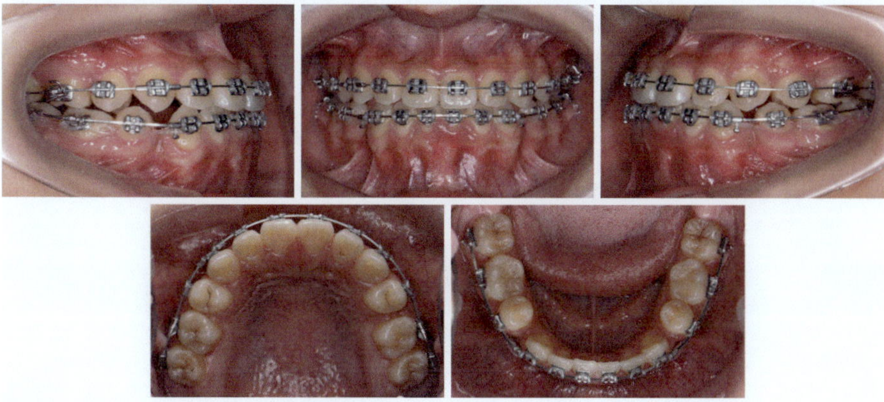

Fig. 12.4 Seventeen months into treatment

occlusal plane decreased 1.0°, while mandibular plane decreased 0.8°. The post-treatment panoramic radiograph shows good root parallel with no root resorption. Extraction of the 3rd molars was suggested.

After two years' retention, the treatment results including good alignment, nice occlusion and balanced profile were well maintained. The mild curve of Spee stayed the same as the end of the treatment (Fig. 12.6).

Case 2. Treatment of a Class III Adult Patient with Protruded Profile

A 24-year-old male presented with the chief complaint of crossbite and crowding (Fig. 12.7). Intraoral examination showed Class III molar relationship, anterior crossbite, crowding and 90° rotated lower 2nd premolars. Cephalometric analysis revealed it was a skeletal Class I (ANB: 0.7°, see Table 12.2) with protrusive profile. Orthodontic camouflage treatment using PASS technique was applied with the aim to deliver maximum anchorage in lower dentition to retract lower anterior teeth and moderate anchorage in upper dentition to relieve crowding and establish Class I molar relationship.

Upper 2nd and lower 1st premolars were extracted. Though lower 2nd premolars were about 90° rotated, they were retained in consideration of maximum anterior teeth retraction. Lower 3rd molars were also extracted before treatment to release posterior crowding and provide space for possible whole lower dentition distalization.

Since no apparently mesial-distal inclined teeth (especially the canines) were presented in both arches, MLF brackets were bonded on all teeth from premolars to premolars (except the extracted ones), and XBT buccal tubes were bonded on the 1st molars at the beginning of the treatment. GIC was temporarily placed on the lower molars to open the anterior deep bite and facilitate bracket placement. In the upper arch, a piggy back wire (0.018″ SS) with 30° tip-back bend was inserted into the

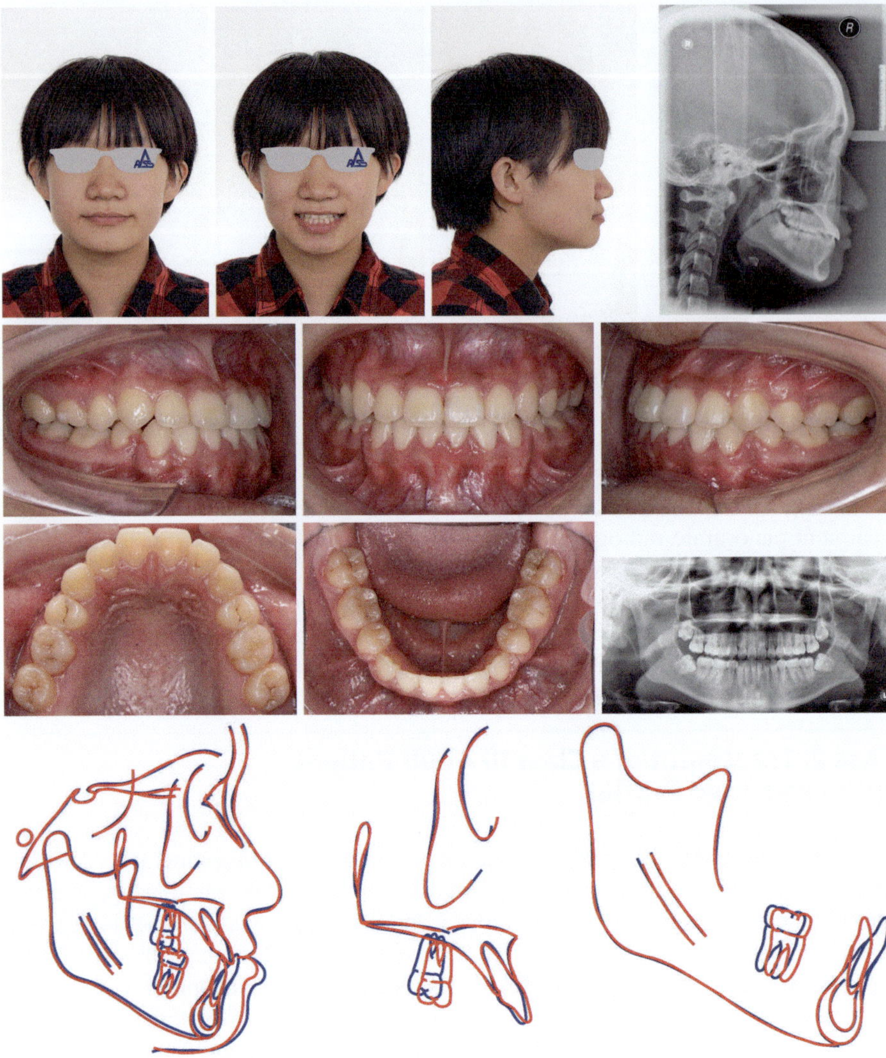

Fig. 12.5 Patient after 24 months of treatment

main tube to control the upper incisor vertical position and assist bite opening, while alignment could be achieved simultaneously by the underneath NiTi wire engaged in the −25° tip-back tube. After initial alignment, 0.018″ SS arch wire with helical loops was placed in the lower dentition, and light Class III elastics (3/8″) were applied (Fig. 12.8).

Eight months later, upper dentition was initially aligned. Anterior teeth were edge to edge. Power chain was used in the lower arch to close the scattered space. GIC was gradually grinded to allow occlusal adjustment of the posterior teeth (Fig. 12.9).

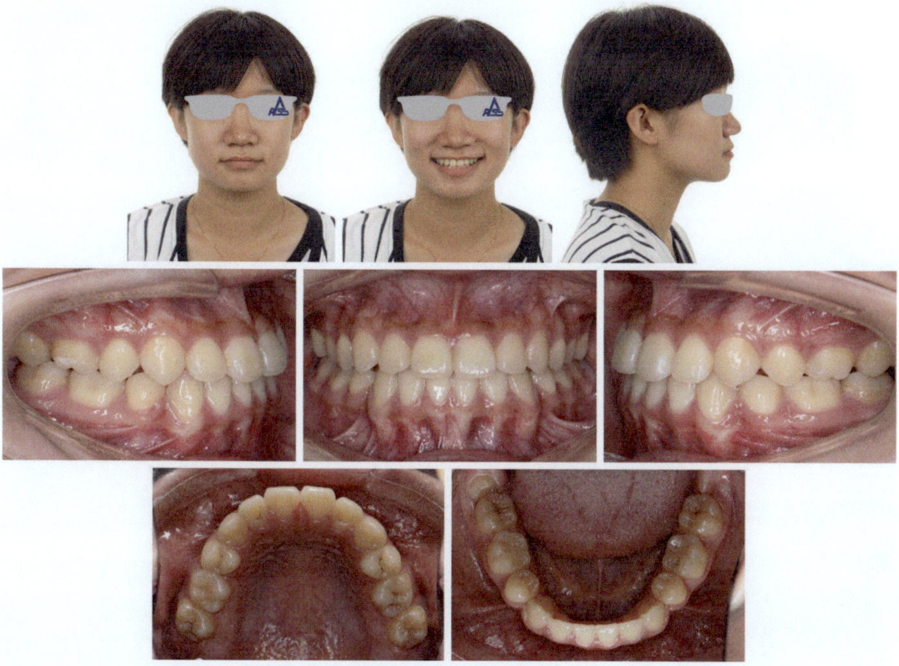

Fig. 12.6 Patient after 2-year retention (night only)

Twelve months later, normal anterior overbite and overjet were established. Then the 2nd molars were bonded and aligned (Fig. 12.10).

Sixteen months later, 0.019 × 0.025″ stainless steel arch wires with compensated Spee's curve were placed in both arches for the final space closure (Fig. 12.11). Due to the double-slot size bracket design (0.20″ for anterior teeth and 0.22″ for the posterior teeth), good anterior torque control resulted from better expression of the prescribed data, and more efficient space closure with less friction in the posterior section during sliding could be achieved.

Good treatment result was achieved in 24 months. Besides well-aligned dentition and good occlusion, the facial profile was improved by retracting the lower anterior teeth. Superimposition of pretreatment (blue) and posttreatment (red) cephalometric tracings shows maximum molar anchorage control (especially the lower one) and significant lower incisor and lip retraction. The upper incisors maintained the same dental compensation position (Fig. 12.12). Table 12.2 shows his lower incisor retroclined 13.5° and upper incisor proclined 4.5°. The sagittal dental compensation position of the upper incisors was well maintained. Functional occlusal plane decreased 3.0°, while mandibular plane increased 0.6°. The posttreatment panoramic radiograph shows good root parallel with no root resorption. The height of the alveolar bone stayed the same. Extraction of the upper 3rd molars was suggested.

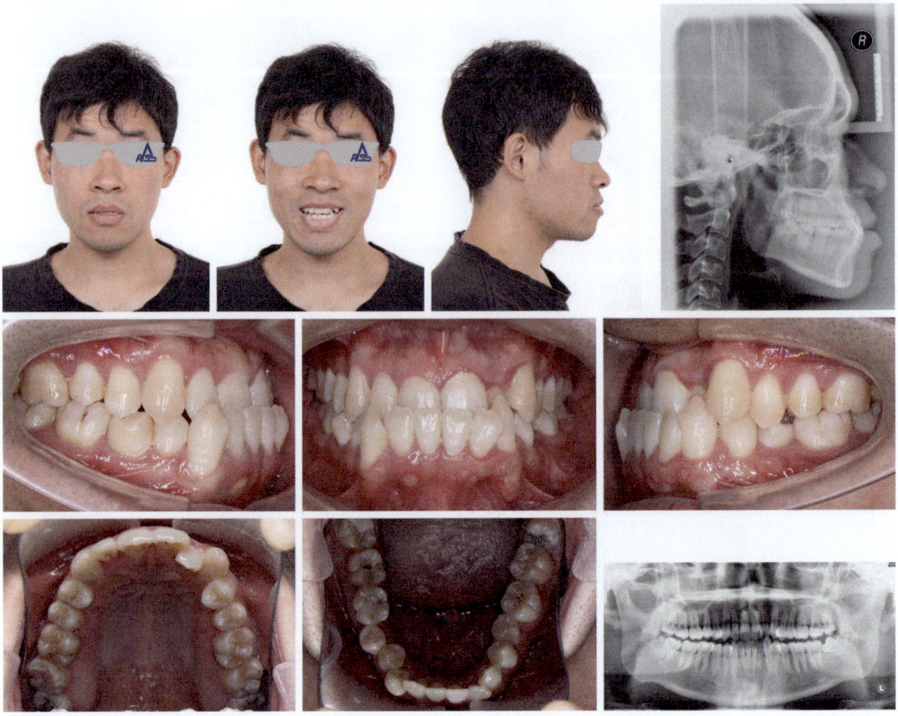

Fig. 12.7 Twenty-four-year-old male patient with anterior crossbite, crowding, and Class III molar relationship before treatment

Table 12.2 Cephalometric analysis before and after treatment

	Norm.				
Measurements	Mean	SD.	Pre.	Post.	Dif.
SNA (°)	82.8	4.0	89.3	88.7	−0.6
SNB (°)	80.1	3.9	88.5	87.2	−1.3
ANB (°)	2.7	2.0	0.7	1.5	0.8
Wits appraisal (mm)	−1.1	2.9	−4.5	−5.1	−0.6
PP/SN (°)	9.3	2.4	8.9	8.9	0.0
MP/SN (°)	32.5	5.2	25.9	26.5	0.6
MP/PP (°)	27.6	4.6	17.0	17.6	0.6
FOP/PP (°)	NA	NA	6.5	3.5	−3.0
U1-AP (mm)	7.2	2.2	5.5	5.3	−0.2
L1-AP (mm)	4.9	2.1	6.8	2.1	−4.7
U1/PP (°)	115.8	5.7	117.4	121.9	4.5
L1/MP (°)	93.9	6.2	84.0	70.5	−13.6

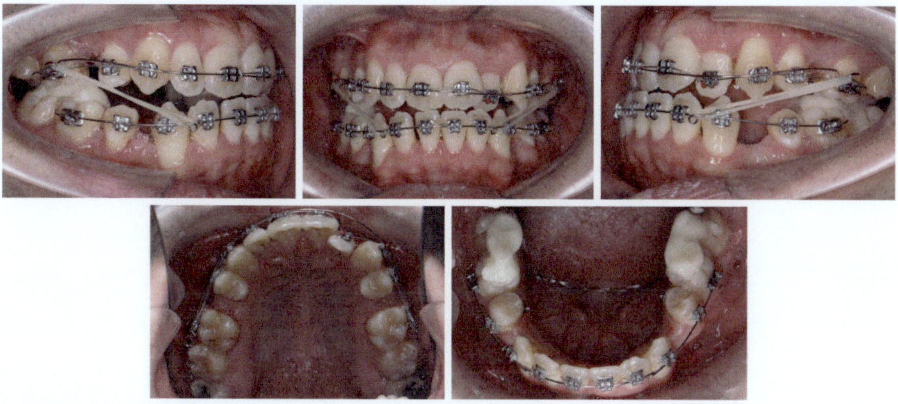

Fig. 12.8 Four months into treatment

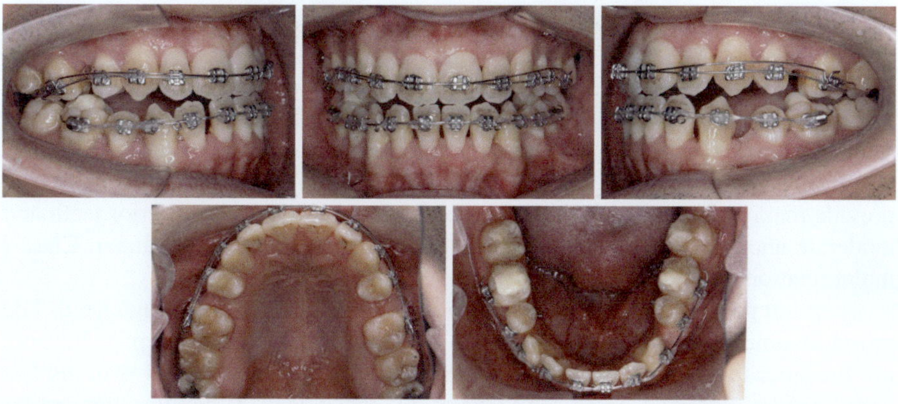

Fig. 12.9 Eight months into treatment

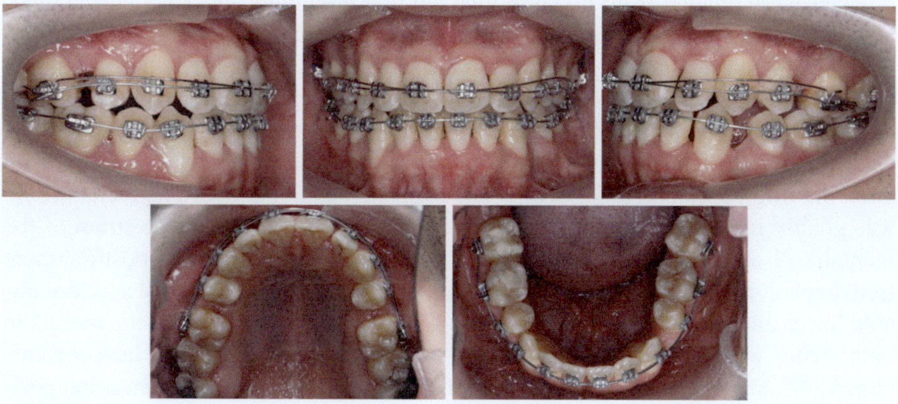

Fig. 12.10 Twelve months into treatment

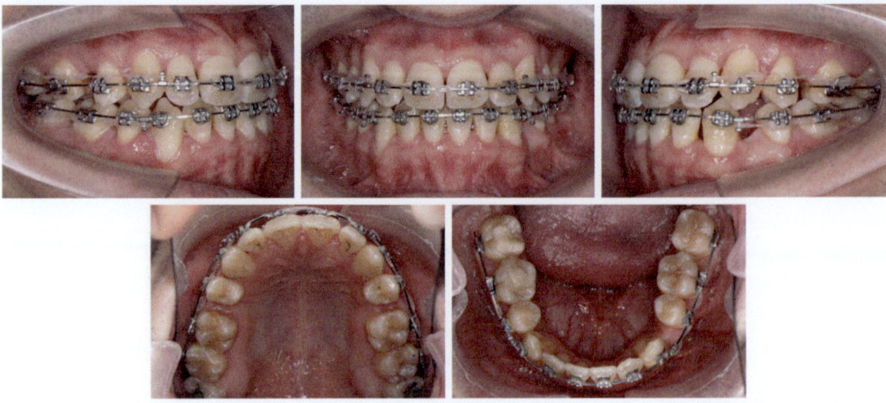

Fig. 12.11 Sixteen months into treatment

Case 3. Treatment of Anterior Crossbite in an Adult Patient

A 26-year-old female presented with the chief complaint of crossbite (Fig. 12.13). Intraoral examination showed Class I molar relationship, anterior crossbite, and mild crowding. Cephalometric analysis revealed it was a mild skeletal Class III (ANB: −1.8°, see Table 12.3) with concave profile. PASS technique was used to provide maximum anchorage in lower dentition to retract lower anterior teeth and moderate anchorage in upper dentition to relieve crowding and maintain Class I molar relationship.

Four 2nd premolars were extracted to meet the moderate anchorage need. The crossbite anterior teeth was mainly due to the mild crowding of upper incisors not the anteroposterior discrepancy. Therefore, the treatment aim was to moderately retract anterior teeth and maintain the Class I canine and molar relationship.

Since there was no apparently mesial-distal inclined teeth in both arches, MLF brackets were bonded from first premolars to first premolars and XBT buccal tubes were bonded on the 1st molars and upper 2nd molars at the beginning of the treatment. 0.014″ NiTi wire was inserted into the −7° main tube for the initial alignment. 6 months later, anterior crossbite was corrected and the upright position of the 1st molars was maintained (Fig. 12.14).

After 30 months of treatment, a stable Class I canine and molar relationship with good interdigitation and ideal overjet and overbite were obtained. The facial profile was greatly improved to a more balanced and esthetic status. Muscle strain of the mentalis disappeared. Superimposition of pretreatment (blue) and posttreatment (red) cephalometric tracings shows maximum molar anchorage control and remarkable lower anterior teeth retraction. Good mesial-distal inclination of the molars in both arches was maintained (Fig. 12.15). Table 12.3 shows her lower incisor retroclined 2.9° and upper incisor proclined 2.6°. The sagittal dental compensation position of the upper incisors was well maintained. Functional occlusal plane decreased 1.1°, while mandibular plane remained the same. The posttreatment CBCT reconstructed panoramic radiograph shows good root parallel with no root resorption.

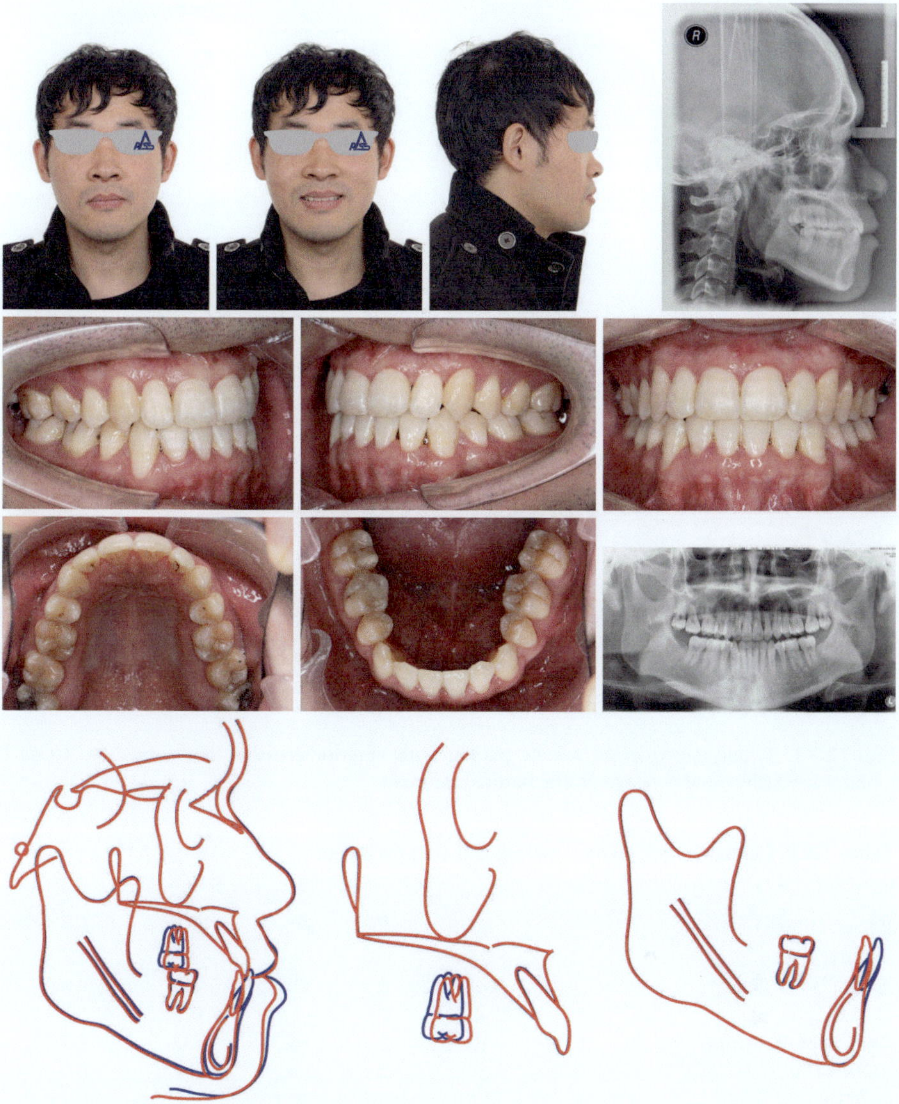

Fig. 12.12 Patient after 24 months of treatment

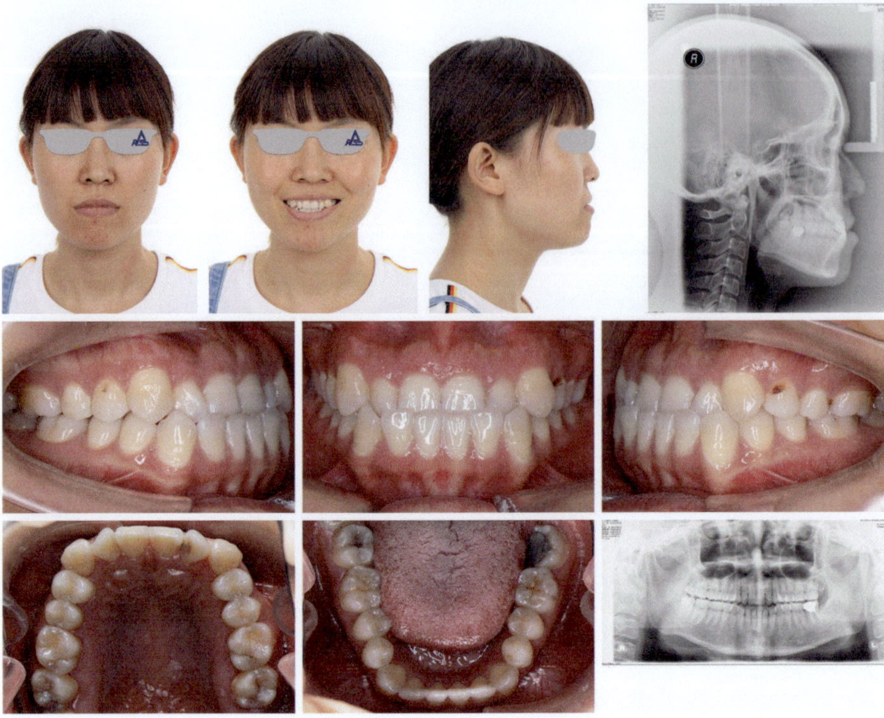

Fig. 12.13 Twenty-six-year-old female patient with anterior crossbite and crowding, Class I molar relationship, and concave profile before treatment

Table 12.3 Cephalometric analysis before and after treatment

Measurements	Norm. Mean	Norm. SD.	Pre.	Post.	Dif.
SNA (°)	82.8	4.0	79.1	80.5	1.4
SNB (°)	80.1	3.9	80.9	80.2	−0.6
ANB (°)	2.7	2.0	−1.8	0.3	2.0
Wits appraisal (mm)	−1.1	2.9	−6.7	-3.0	3.7
PP/SN (°)	9.3	2.4	5.4	5.4	0.0
MP/SN (°)	32.5	5.2	28.9	29.0	0.1
MP/PP (°)	27.6	4.6	23.5	23.6	0.1
FOP/PP (°)	NA	NA	8.8	7.7	−1.1
U1-AP (mm)	7.2	2.2	4.4	5.0	0.6
L1-AP (mm)	4.9	2.1	5.6	1.9	−3.7
U1/PP (°)	115.8	5.7	113.0	115.6	2.6
L1/MP (°)	93.9	6.2	90.8	87.9	−2.9

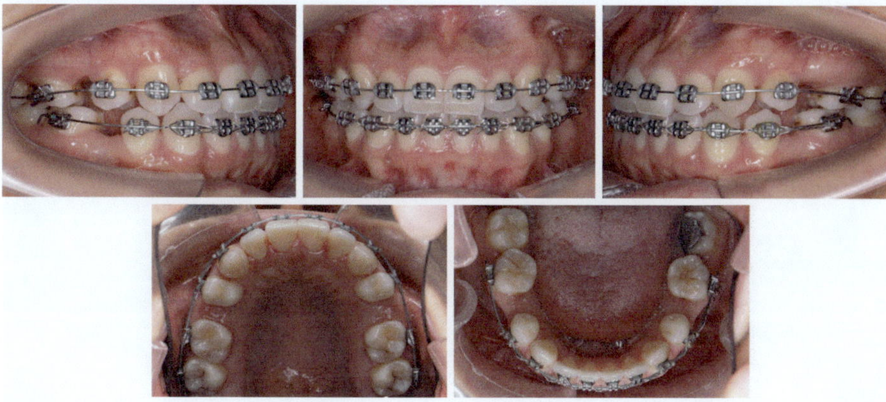

Fig. 12.14 Six months into treatment

The height of the alveolar bone indicates good periodontal status. Extraction of the upper right 3rd molar was suggested.

Summary

Class III elastics were extensively used in conservative orthodontic treatment for Class III malocclusion. It might result in mild extrusion of upper molars and lower incisors and therefore lead to counterclockwise rotation of the occlusal plane. In order to retain its perpendicular direction to the occlusal plane, lower molars need to be tipped backward to maintain the intermolar inclination, which is required for efficient bite force transfer from masticatory muscles. The tip-back angle designed in the lower posterior teeth in PASS appliance could facilitate this adjustment. In the meanwhile, lower molar anchorage would be reinforced in this tip-back position to ensure maximum anterior retraction in lower dentition, which usually plays an important role in significant profile improvement in Class III cases.

Besides lower teeth retraction, backward and downward rotation of the mandible was considered to be a contributory factor in profile improvement in Class III nonsurgical treatment. Mild extrusion of upper molars will result in clockwise rotation of the mandible. Therefore the chin projection can be decreased.

Though maximum upper molar anchorage is not usually needed in Class III treatment, reinforcement of upper molar anchorage still has three benefits:

1. At the stage of alignment – Moderate to severe crowding is commonly found in the upper anterior teeth in Class III cases; however, in consideration of molar relationship adjustment and anchorage requirement, upper 2nd premolars are most commonly extracted. Prevention of mesial tipping of upper 1st molars can ensure efficient use of the extraction space for anterior alignment.

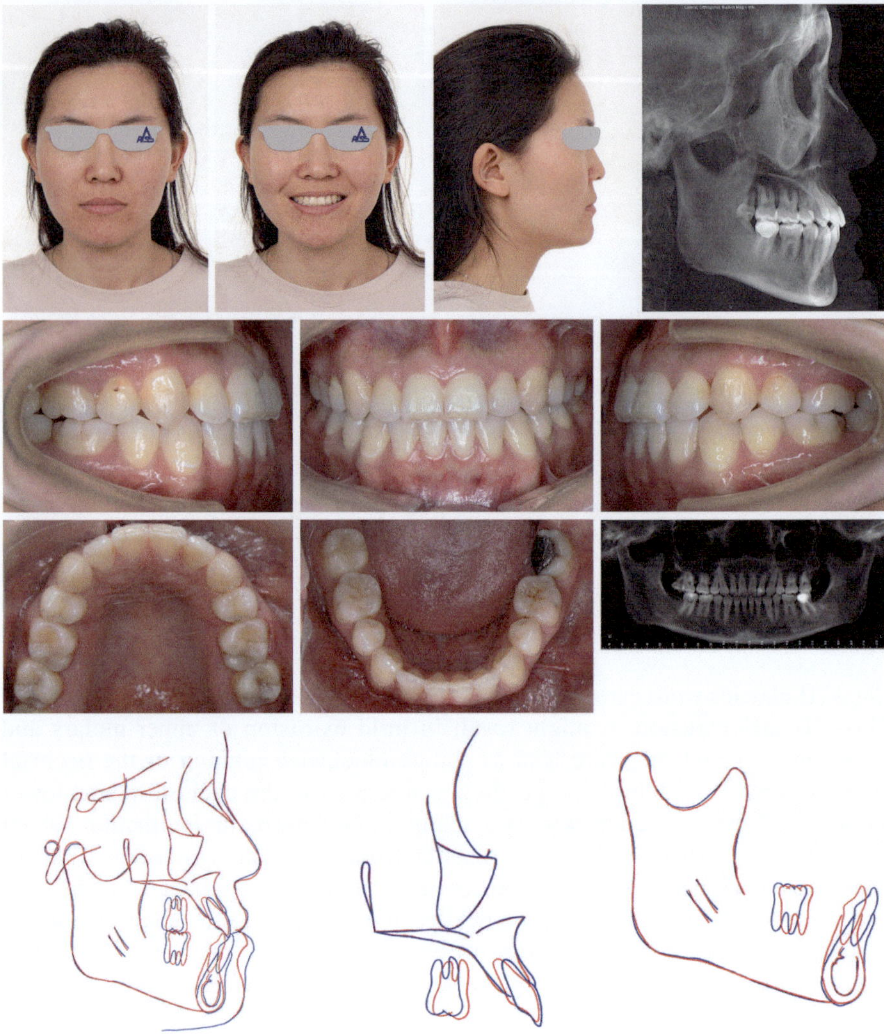

Fig. 12.15 Patient after 30 months of treatment

2. At the stage of space closure – Extra anchorage can be provided for intra-maxillary Class III elastics.
3. At the stage of Class III elastics – Less horizontal pressure will be transmitted to the upper incisors; hence the original dental compensation position of these teeth can be maintained, which is important to a balanced profile.

References

1. Battagel JM (1993) The aetiological factors in Class III malocclusion. Eur J Orthod 15(5):347–370
2. Su H, Han B, Li S et al (2014) Compensation trends of the angulation of first molars: retrospective study of 1403 malocclusion cases. Int J Oral Sci 6(3):175–181
3. Yu Y, Xu TM (2015) Spee's curve measurement based on least square curve fitting method. Chin J Orthod 22(2):78–82

Vertical Control in PASS 13

Gui Chen, Jingjing Zeng, Fanfan Dai, Guangying Song, Kaifan Xu, and Tian Min Xu

Abstract

In high-angle cases, both sagittal and vertical anchorage control are important to achieve a successful treatment. How to control the sagittal anchorage has been fully discussed and demonstrated in our previous chapters. In this chapter, a unique vertical control device named TAP (tongue anchorage pad) will be introduced. It is a member of physiologic anchorage control system. The procedure of making a TAP as well as its clinical use will be depicted.

In the previous chapters, we have discussed about the sagittal problems and how to treat them by PASS. Our previous study proved that the compensation of molar angulation varied among different vertical jaw relationships [1]. Both upper and lower first molars are more distal tipping in high-angle cases than in low-angle cases, which means they are easier to be tipped forward to lose anchorage when using contemporary straight wire appliance. So sagittal anchorage control is challenging in high-angle extraction cases.

Orthodontic treatment is always about tooth movement in three dimensions. Therefore, not only sagittal anchorage reinforcement needs careful treatment

G. Chen (✉) • G. Song • T.M. Xu
Department of Orthodontics, Peking University School and Hospital of Stomatology, Beijing, China
e-mail: chengui723@163.com; songguangying@gmail.com; tmxuortho@163.com

J. Zeng • F. Dai
Second Dental Center, Peking University School and Hospital of Stomatology, Beijing, China
e-mail: today-forever@qq.com; daifanfannihao@163.com

K. Xu
Guanghua School and Hospital of Stomatology, Sun Yat-sen University, Guangdong, China
e-mail: capricorn1987@sina.cn

T.M. Xu (ed.), *Physiologic Anchorage Control*,
DOI 10.1007/978-3-319-48333-7_13

planning, but change of vertical dimensions is also an important issue to be controlled in order for a successful treatment of high-angle or anterior open bite cases. In these cases, clockwise rotation of the mandibular plane, which also means an increased anterior facial height, is the last thing an orthodontist wishes to see. In growing patients, the clockwise rotation of mandible is probably due to backward condylar growth [2] or a result of more posterior alveolar vertical growth than condyle growth [3]. In adult patients, however, the backward rotation is believed to be caused by extrusion of molars during orthodontic treatment. Previous studies revealed that molars tended to be extruded during fixed appliance treatment [4–6]. Therefore, it comes very naturally that PASS system tries to resolve this common issue by exploring ways to restrict molar extrusion. This time, just as PASS gets its inspiration to treat sagittal problem from the curve of Spee, the answer once again comes from human physiologic features, which is the power of the tongue.

Nowadays, various auxiliary devices have been designed to inhibit molar extrusion or intrude the molar, such as high-pull headgear, transpalatal arch (TPA), bite blocks, and temporary skeletal anchorage devices, which can be used separately or in combination [7, 8]. Of course, any of the above devices could be integrated into PASS system to achieve vertical control. Since utilization of physiological force is more emphasized in physiologic anchorage control system, a unique vertical control device named TAP (tongue anchorage pad) was invented. It is developed from TPA and designed to transmit continuous tongue pressure that comprised of upward and backward component to adjust the molar position both vertically and sagittally (Fig. 13.1). This feature exhibits special advantages in treating high-angle case. The manufacture method is introduced as below.

The Procedure of Making a TAP

The movement of the tongue during deglutition is believed to be upward and backward toward the hard palate, sweeping the fluid backward down the pharynx. To find the appropriate height between tongue and palate that bore this kind of tongue force well, we took impression for each individual patient because large individual variation existed in tongue pressure exerted both on the hard palate and on the TPA among

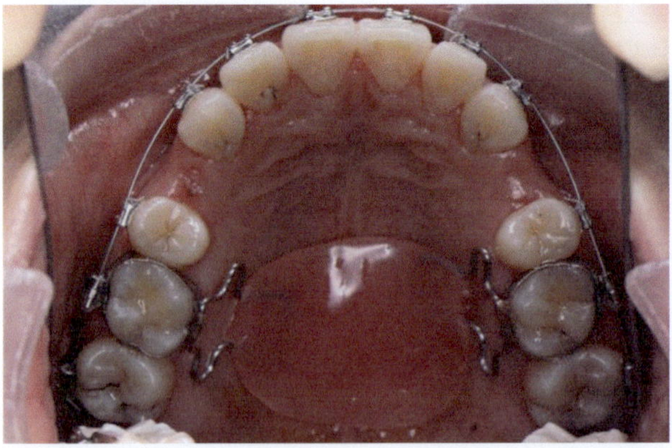

Fig. 13.1 TAP used in clinic

different subjects. Tongue surface morphology during swallowing exercises was also different. So firstly, we created individual silastic swallowing tongue records to reflect individual differences in muscle strength and functional tongue morphology during swallowing, which was proved to be a repeatable and reliable method by a recent study [9]. Palatal pads fabricated according to individual swallowing tongue records might be more comfortable when used in the clinic because they were in accordance with physiologic movement of individual tongues. We had the patients seated on the chair in a 45° oblique position, where a defined amount (a spoon) of silastic impression material (Betasil-putty soft, Germany) was placed on their hard palate to obtain an impression of the tongue during dry swallowing. Thus, we recorded the morphologic feature and position of the tongue during the swallowing exercise in that condition. Negative molds were made with plaster using these silastic records (Fig. 13.2).

Molar bands were used as the retention part of the TAP, and the XBT tubes were welded to the bands. A framework for the acrylic pads was constructed out of 0.9 mm stainless steel wire. The palatal acrylic pads were created by occluding the negative plaster mold of the swallowing tongue record with the maxillary cast to shape the resin before it polymerized. This allowed the distance from the mucosa to the lingual surface of the acrylic pad to be identical to the thickness of the swallowing tongue records. In addition, the lingual surface of the pad was made in accordance to the functional morphologic feature of the tongue. Increasing the distance of the acrylic pads to the palatal mucosa based on the swallowing tongue records would dramatically augment the pressure exerted on the pads. Tongue pressure decreased significantly when the pads were positioned somewhat closer to the mucosa. Next, the pads were trimmed to an appropriate and individualized size. The

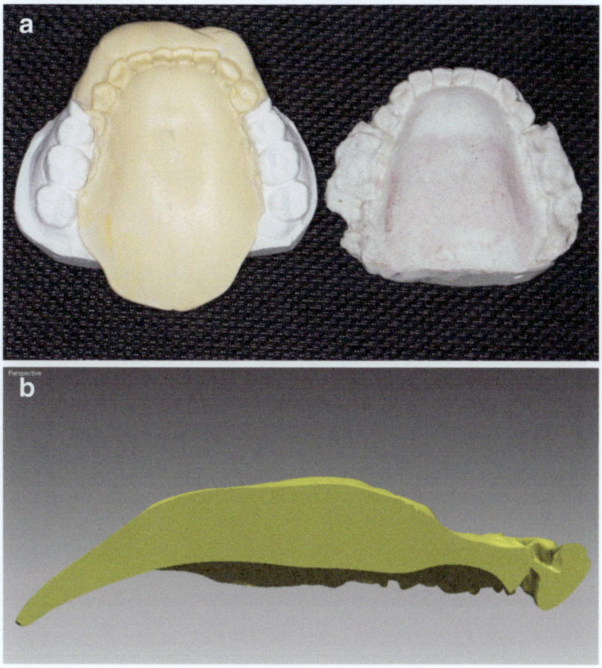

Fig. 13.2 (**a**) Swallowing tongue record and negative mold. (**b**) A sagittal vertical section of the silastic record on the mid-palatal plane (Reproduced from Xu et al. [9])

width of the pads was about two thirds of the molar-to-molar distance. The anterior edge of the pad was at the level of the mesial aspect of the first molars, and the posterior edge extended to the distal aspect of the second molars. To note, the distance from the palatal surface of the framework and the acrylic pads to the mucosa should be more than 2 mm to prevent mucosa from being impinged while the molars were intruded. This appliance, presented in Fig.13.1, would transmit an upward and backward force originated from the tongue to upper molars both in rest and functional state, which aided in the intrusion and backward tipping of upper first molars [9, 10]. Its application will be introduced in the following part.

Case 1. Angle's Class I Adult Case with Anterior Open Bite

This 20-year-old female came to the office complaining about her malfunctioning anterior teeth and protrusive lips. She had Class I malocclusion with 3 mm anterior open bite and mild crowding in both arches. Curve of Spee was apparent in the upper arch and relative flat in the lower. Cephalometric analysis indicated a skeletal Class II (ANB 7.8°) and hyper-divergent (MP/SN 44.6°) skeletal pattern with protrusive incisors (Fig. 13.3 and Table 13.1).

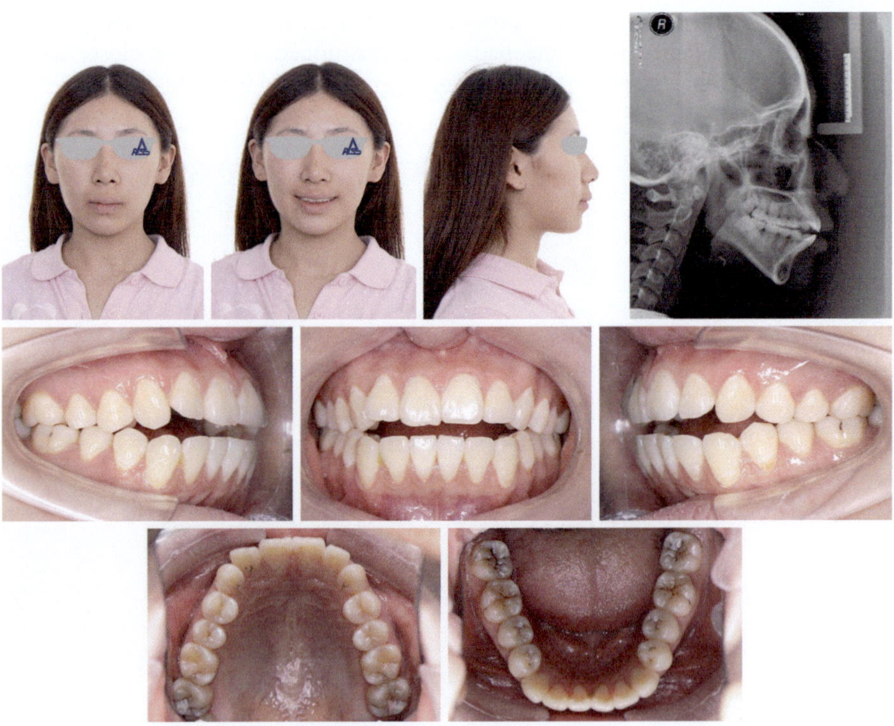

Fig. 13.3 Pretreatment facial and intraoral photographs, as well as radiograph

Table 13.1 Cephalometric analysis before and after treatment

Measurements	Norm. Mean	SD.	Pre.	Post.	Dif.
SNA (°)	82.8	4.0	86.0	85.1	−0.9
SNB (°)	80.1	3.9	78.2	79.0	0.8
ANB (°)	2.7	2.0	7.8	6.1	−1.7
Wits appraisal (mm)	−1.1	2.9	3.7	−0.2	−3.9
PP/SN (°)	9.3	2.4	10.0	10.4	0.4
MP/SN (°)	32.5	5.2	43.8	43.4	−0.4
MP/PP (°)	27.6	4.6	33.8	33.0	−0.8
FOP/PP (°)	NA	NA	−0.2	2.2	2.4
U1-AP (mm)	7.2	2.2	11.2	7.9	−3.3
L1-AP (mm)	4.9	2.1	9.8	5.7	−4.1
U1/PP (°)	115.8	5.7	120.3	108.5	−11.8
L1/MP (°)	93.9	6.2	102.4	90.0	−12.4

Her four first premolars were extracted to provide enough space for anterior retraction to improve her convex profile. The extraction space was also used to decrease the exaggerated curve of Spee in the upper arch to close the open bite. In addition, considering of her steep mandible plane and anterior open bite, TAP was prescribed to reinforce the anchorage in both vertical and sagittal direction.

During Treatment

1. Since the irregularity in the upper arch was mild and tipping angle of the malpositioned teeth was no larger than 7°, all upper brackets were bonded at the beginning of the treatment. A 0.016″ NiTi wire with normal curve of Spee was engaged through the main tube of the upper XBTs (Fig. 13.4).
2. Four months into treatment, TAP was bonded as soon as the upper teeth, especially the upper first molars, were well aligned. At the same time, all lower brackets were bonded and a 0.014″ NiTi wire was engaged to align the irregular teeth (Fig. 13.5).
3. Seven months into treatment, the archwires were changed to 0.018 × 25″ NiTi in both arches. As the curve of Spee restored gradually, the anterior open bite was almost corrected, and a stable posterior anchorage unit was established in the upper arch, which was helpful to retract the upper anterior teeth (Fig. 13.6).
4. Eight months into treatment, a 0.018 × 0.025″ SS with compensated curve of Spee plus traction hooks was used in the upper arch to close the extraction space. The open bite was closed at the early stage of space closure due to the pendulum effect of the anterior teeth and vertical control effect of the upper molars generated by TAP (Fig. 13.7).
5. Thirteen months into treatment, space closure was continued on 0.018 × 0.025″ SS in both arches. Class II elastics were used to correct the distal canine relationship. A new TAP was bonded to replace the old one, which broke under the continuous pressure of tongue (Fig. 13.8).

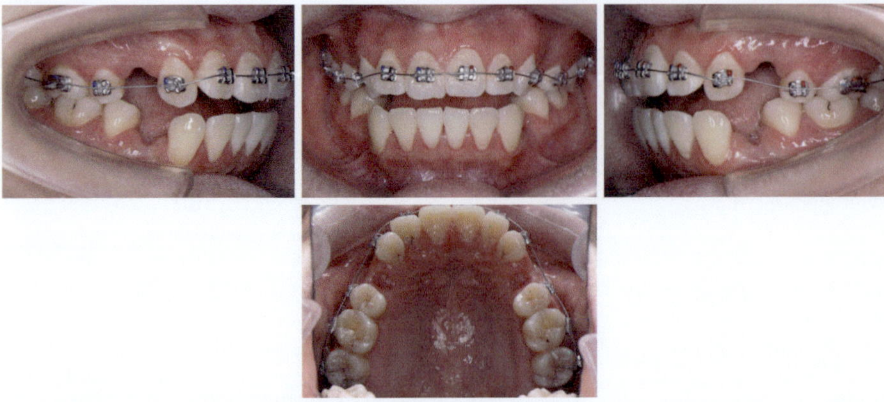

Fig. 13.4 Upper 5–5 MLF brackets and XBTs were bonded

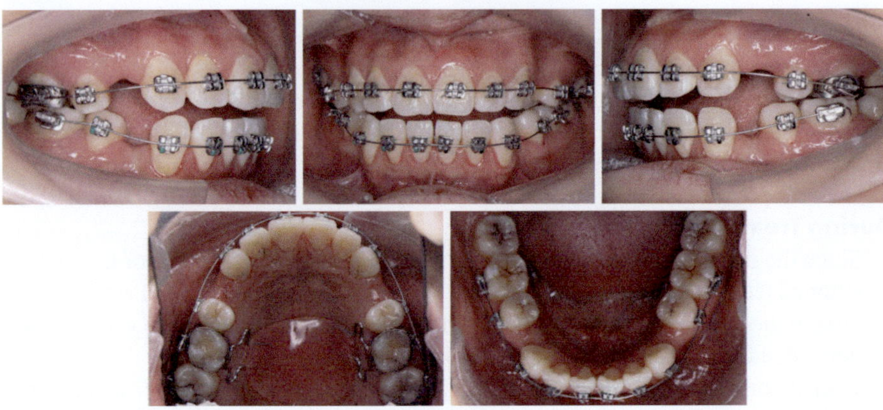

Fig. 13.5 All lower brackets and TAP were bonded

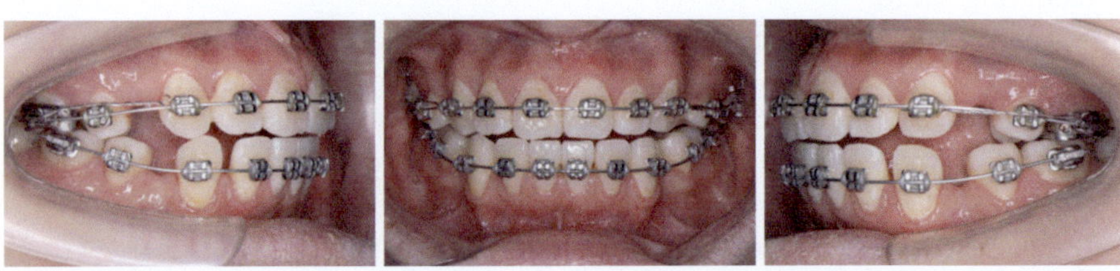

Fig. 13.6 (0.018 × 25″) NiTi wires were used to restore the curve of Spee

Due to the patient's poor compliance and several breakages of the TAP, the total treatment duration lasted for 4 years and 3 months. The final result was satisfactory. Teeth were well aligned, Class I canine and molar relationships were achieved, normal anterior OB and OJ were established and the posterior curve of Spee was

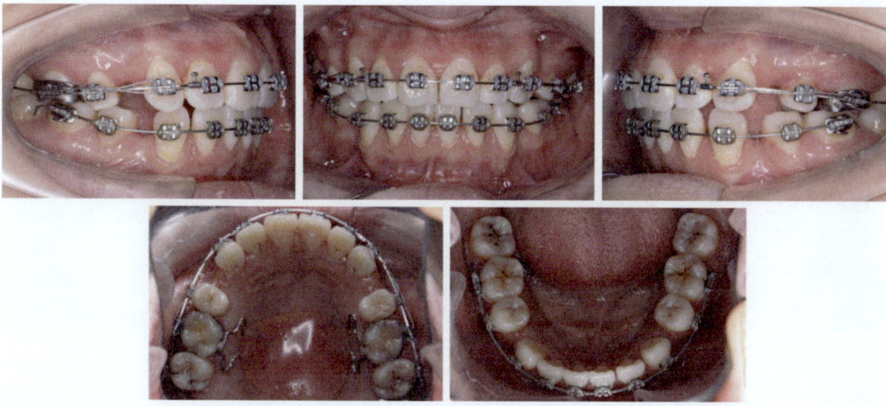

Fig. 13.7 Rectangular wire (0.018×0.025″ SS) was used to close space since the torque of the upper incisors was normal

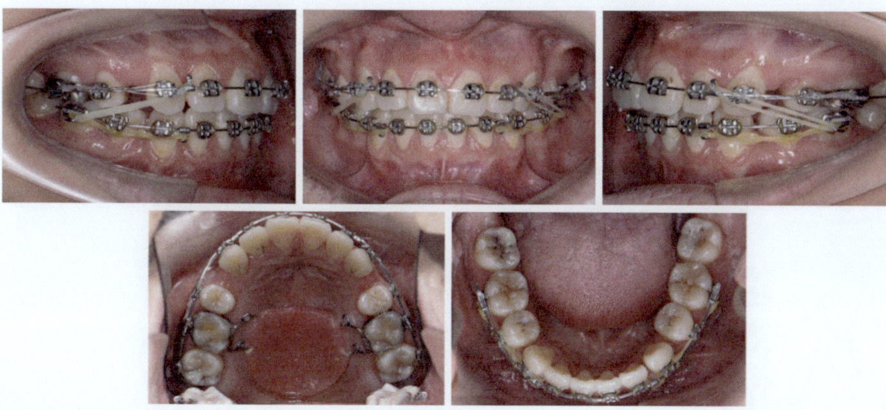

Fig. 13.8 Elastic chain was used to close space and intermaxillary elastics were used to adjust occlusion

maintained. With remarkable incisor retraction and good molar vertical control, her profile was improved. By comparing the pretreatment and posttreatment cephalograms, we surprisingly found that her chin was augmented obviously, which might indicate a mentoplasty after the orthodontic treatment to further improve her lateral contour (Fig. 13.9). Table 13.1 showed her upper incisor retroclined 11.8° and lower incisor retroclined 12.4°. Functional occlusal plane was reversed by 2.4°, while mandibular plane decreased a little bit.

Digital dental model superimposition: The maxillary digital models of pretreatment (blue) and posttreatment (red) were superimposed and analyzed (the method of digital model superimposition has been described in Chap. 7). The average intrusion of the upper first molars was 2.59 mm (Fig. 13.10).

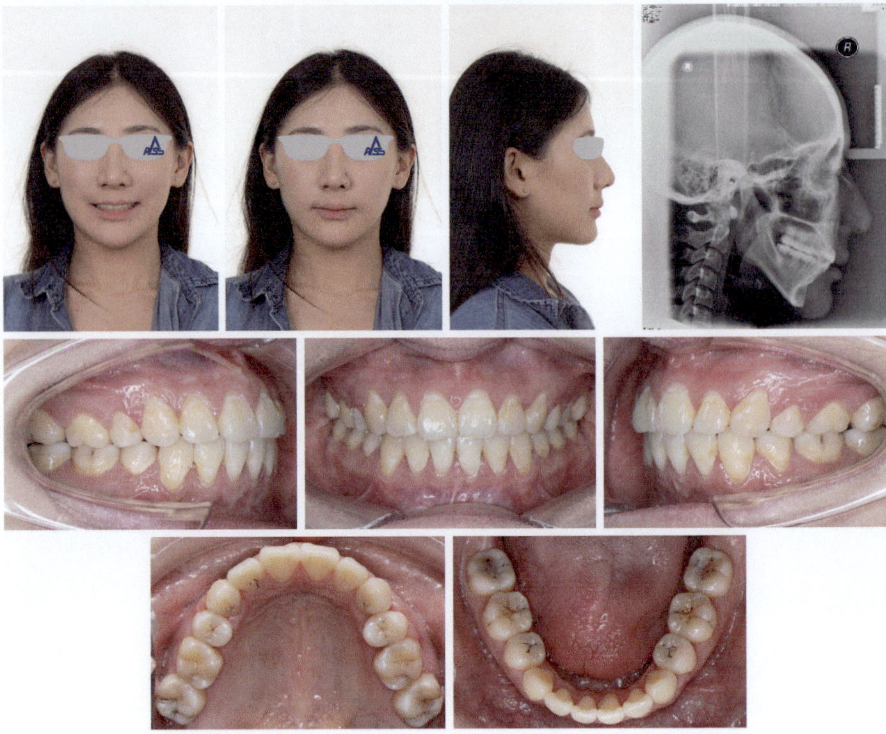

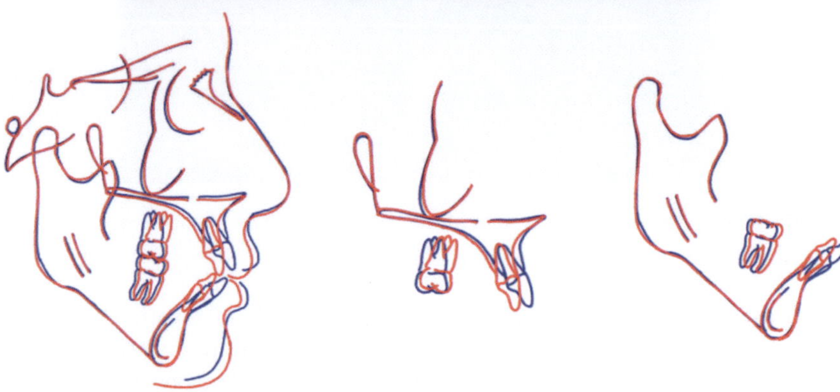

Fig. 13.9 Superimposition of pretreatment (*blue*) and posttreatment (*red*) cephalometric tracings shows good anchorage control both vertically and sagittally

Case 2. Angle's Class II^{1s} Adult Case with Severe Crowding

A 20-year-old female complained about her crooked anterior teeth. Intraoral examination showed Class I molar relationship on the right side, cusp-to-cusp Class II molar relationship on the left side, and severe crowding in both arches. A clear midline deviation was present in the lower arch because of the asymmetric crowding in

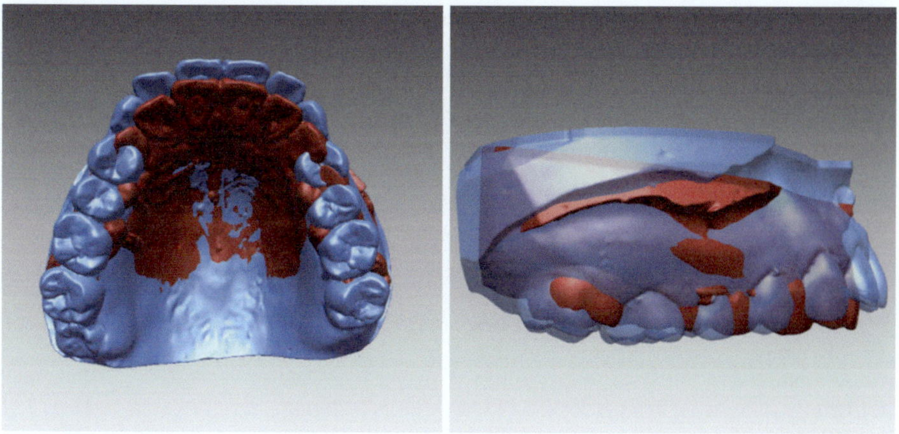

Fig. 13.10 Superimposition of pretreatment (*blue*) and posttreatment (*red*) digital model

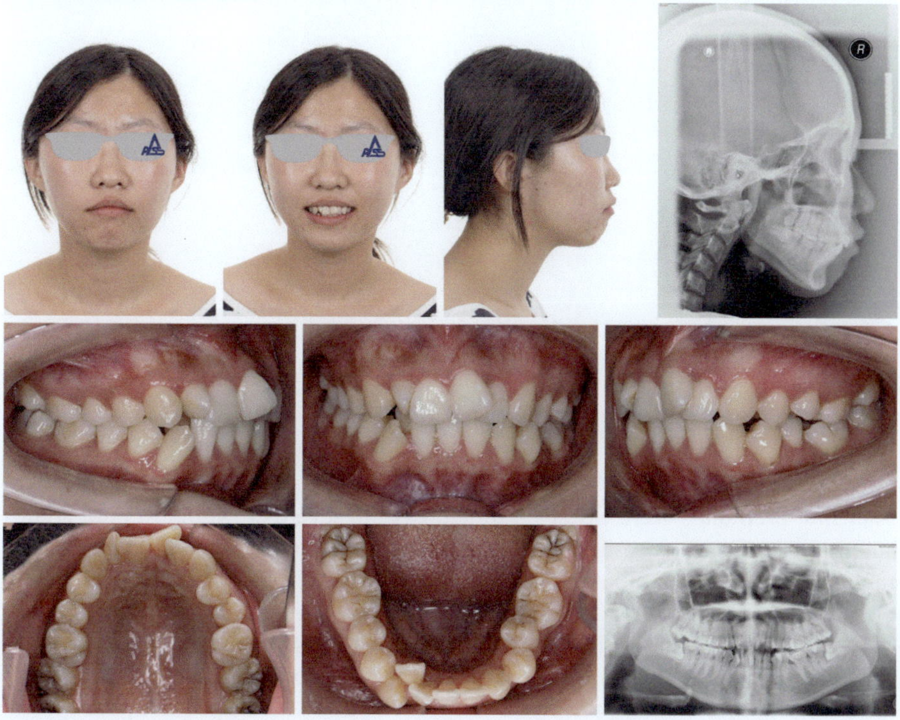

Fig. 13.11 Pretreatment facial and intraoral photographs, as well as radiographs

anterior segment. Curve of Spee was apparent in both upper and lower arch. Cephalometric analysis revealed it was a Class II (ANB 8.1°) and hyper-divergent (MP/SN 43.8°) skeletal pattern with protrusive profile (Fig. 13.11 and Table 13.2).

Table 13.2 Cephalometric analysis before and after treatment

	Norm.				
Measurements	Mean	SD.	Pre.	Post.	Dif.
SNA (°)	82.8	4.0	81.9	80.8	−1.1
SNB (°)	80.1	3.9	73.8	75.3	1.5
ANB (°)	2.7	2.0	8.1	5.5	−2.6
Wits appraisal (mm)	−1.1	2.9	10.7	−2.0	−12.7
PP/SN (°)	9.3	2.4	11.2	9.2	−2.1
MP/SN (°)	32.5	5.2	42.6	40.7	−1.9
MP/PP (°)	27.6	4.6	31.4	31.5	0.1
FOP/PP (°)	NA	NA	6.1	8.1	2.1
U1-AP (mm)	7.2	2.2	8.2	5.1	−3.0
L1-AP (mm)	4.9	2.1	2.3	3.4	1.1
U1/PP (°)	115.8	5.7	115.3	96.4	−18.9
L1/MP (°)	93.9	6.2	94.7	94.6	−0.1

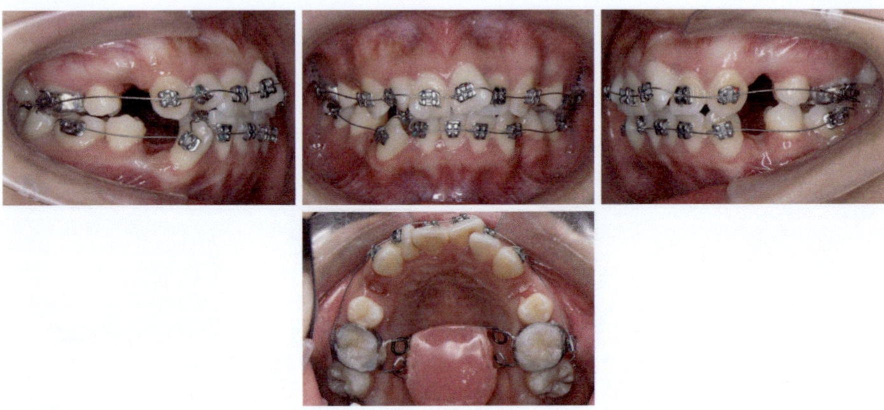

Fig. 13.12 Upper 3–3 MLF brackets, XBT tubes, and TAP were bonded at the first appointment

During Treatment

Four first premolars were extracted to address the severe crowding in both arches and retract the protrusive lips. The TAP was adopted to reinforce the vertical and sagittal anchorage. The third molars were also proposed to be extracted to relieve the posterior crowding.

In this case, we can see the most tipping teeth in the arches were upper and lower right canines. In order to place the dominant moment on anchor molars instead of the malpositioned canines, the 0.012″ NiTi archwire was engaged in tipback tubes of upper and lower first molars at the first stage. Severely rotated teeth (upper right central incisor and lower left central incisor) were ligated with 0.2 mm ligature on single wings. No canine laceback was used because it might result in forward tipping of the molars (Fig. 13.12).

Different ligating methods were used to align the irregular teeth according to the severity level. The lower right central incisor and canine were rotated and ligated

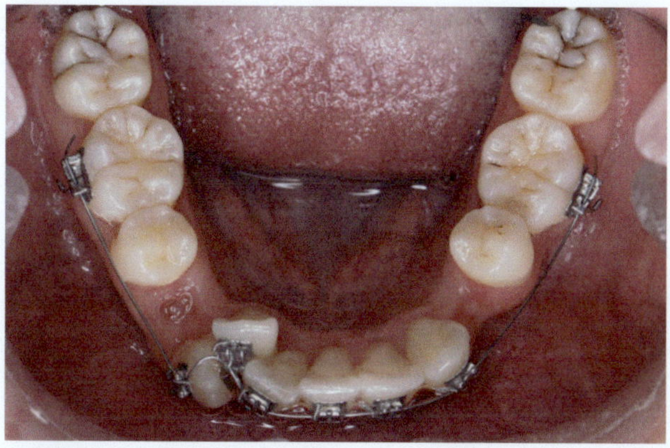

Fig. 13.13 Lower right lateral incisor, which was blocked out from the dentition, was bonded and ligated at the first appointment since PASS is of light force and low friction feature, canines usually will drift back along the archwire without elastic force on them

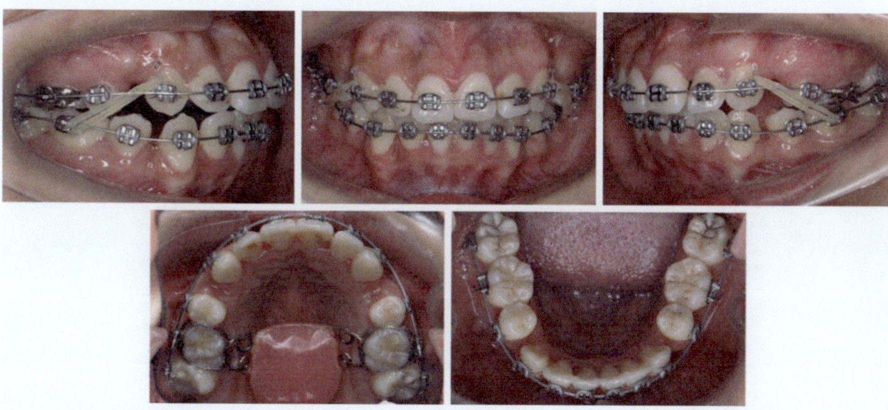

Fig. 13.14 Six months into treatment, upper first molars were intruded obviously, and steps among the upper posterior teeth were apparent as evidences of intrusion

on distal wings, while the severely malpositioned lower right lateral incisor was partially ligated. Cinchbacks were made by a NiTi cinchback plier instead of heat treating to ensure the good elasticity of NiTi wire. Only a continuous tipback moment provided by the wire in good property can stop the physiologic anchorage loss (Fig. 13.13).

Correction of the lower midline was initiated from the very beginning and finished on 0.016″ NiTi wire with canine laceback. Short Class II elastics were used on rectangular NiTi wire with curve of Spee to prevent the proclination of upper incisors (Fig. 13.14).

Space closure were conducted on 0.018 × 25″ SS with elastic chain and Class II elastics. TAP was removed at the final stage when some refinement was performed to adjust the occlusion. After 2 years and 7 months of treatment, all teeth were well aligned, the lower midline deviation was corrected, normal curve of Spee was maintained, and ideal occlusion was achieved (Fig. 13.15). Table 13.2 showed her upper incisor retracted 3 mm back and retroclined 18.9°. Functional occlusal plane was reversed by 2.1°, while MP/SN decreased 1.9°.

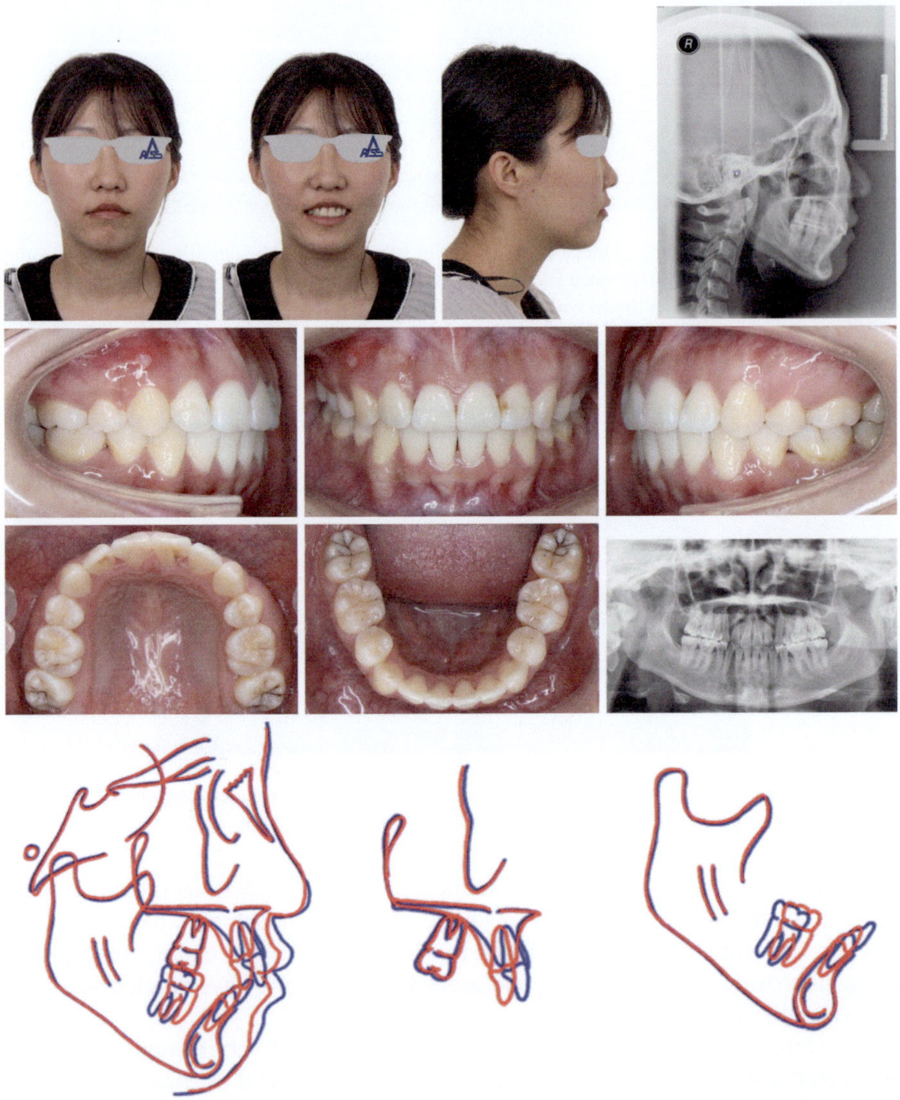

Fig. 13.15 Patient after 2 years and 7 months of treatment. Superimposition of pretreatment (*blue*) and posttreatment (*red*) cephalometric tracings shows remarkable profile improvement which should be ascribed to the retraction of the upper incisors under maximum anchorage control and maintenance of the vertical position of upper first molars, without clockwise rotation of mandible

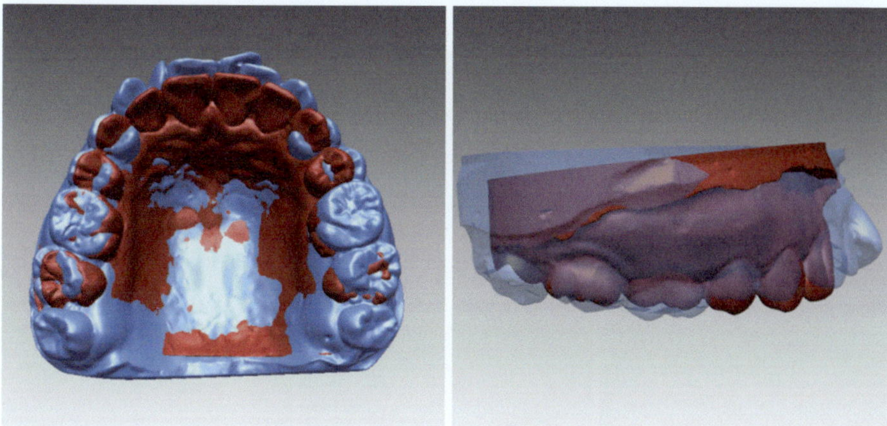

Fig. 13.16 Superimposition of pretreatment (*blue*) and posttreatment (*red*) digital model

Digital model superimposition showed the average intrusion of the upper first molar was 0.89 mm (Fig. 13.16).

Case 3. Angle's Class I Adolescent Case with Mild Crowding

A 15-year-old girl presented with the chief complaint of crooked teeth. Intraoral examination showed Class I molar relationship and mild crowding. The lower midline deviated to the left by about 1.5 mm. Curve of Spee was apparent in both upper and lower arch. Cephalometric analysis revealed it was a skeletal Class II (ANB: 5.6°) and high-angle case (MP/SN: 45.7°) (Fig. 13.17 and Table 13.3).

Considering of her mild crowding, normal molar relationship, and good profile, non-extraction method was carried out in this case. According to Chap. 7, all posterior teeth in PASS appliance are given tipback angle, which is certainly good for relieving mild crowding. The problem is if we engage all brackets with a continuous wire, anterior teeth may flare out before posterior teeth being tipped back. To prevent this unwanted change, we bonded TAP first to facilitate the backward tipping of the upper first molars.

During Treatment

1. Individual TAP was manufactured and bonded before upper fixed appliance was placed (Fig. 13.18).
2. Four months into treatment, we bonded upper 4–4 MLF brackets and engaged a 0.014″ NiTi wire in −25° tipback tube to increase the expected tooth movement and align the incisors in the meantime (Fig. 13.19).
3. Five months into treatment, with the preliminary alignment of the anterior teeth, upper second premolar MLF brackets and second molar tubes were bonded, and a 0.014″ NiTi archwire with normal curve of Spee was engaged in the −7° tube

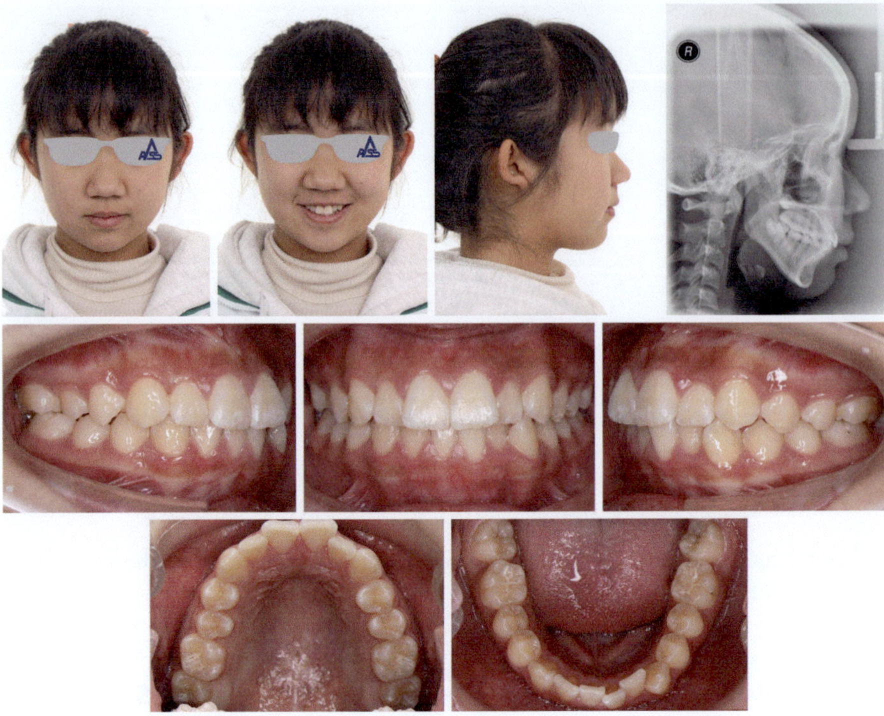

Fig. 13.17 Pretreatment facial and intraoral photographs, as well as radiograph

Table 13.3 Cephalometric analysis before and after treatment

Measurements	Norm. Mean	SD.	Pre.	Post.	Dif.
SNA (°)	82.8	4.0	81.7	81.6	−0.1
SNB (°)	80.1	3.9	76.2	76.7	0.5
ANB (°)	2.7	2.0	5.6	4.9	−0.7
Wits appraisal (mm)	−1.1	2.9	−1.6	−2.3	−0.7
PP/SN (°)	9.3	2.4	11.3	10.5	−0.8
MP/SN (°)	32.5	5.2	45.0	46.4	1.4
MP/PP (°)	27.6	4.6	33.7	35.9	2.2
FOP/PP (°)	NA	NA	3.9	6.0	2.1
U1-AP (mm)	7.2	2.2	8.8	9.0	0.2
L1-AP (mm)	4.9	2.1	4.7	6.5	1.8
U1/PP (°)	115.8	5.7	118.5	113.0	−5.5
L1/MP (°)	93.9	6.2	90.8	92.1	1.3

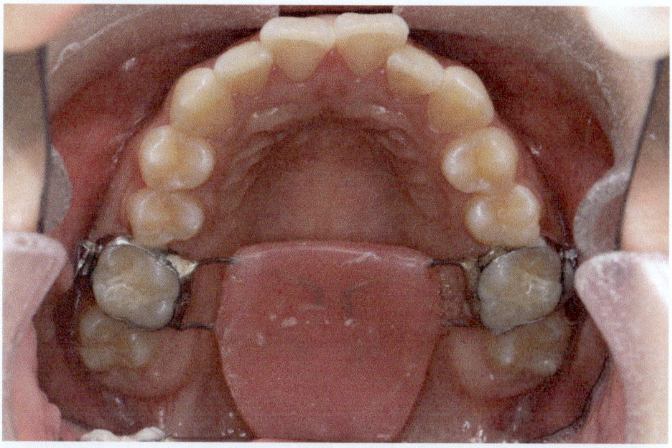

Fig. 13.18 TAP was bonded alone at the first appointment

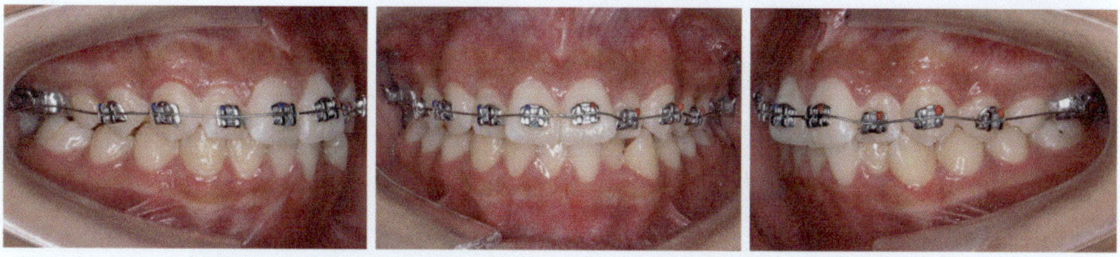

Fig. 13.19 Four months into treatment, upper 4–4 MLF brackets were bonded

of upper first molars, −9° tube of upper second molars, and −3° slot of second premolars to tip all these teeth back under the help of TAP which received backward force from tongue (Fig. 13.20).

4. Since the most tipping tooth in the lower arch was the left canine, lower 4–3 MLF brackets and lower first molar XBT tubes were bonded, also with the 0.014″ NiTi wire engaged in the tipback tube (Fig. 13.21).
5. Nine months into treatment, the midline of lower arch was corrected when the arch form got better. The remaining lower brackets were placed and a 0.014″ NiTi wire was engaged in the main tube following the initial alignment (Fig. 13.22).

Finally, the case was accomplished with satisfactory result after 18-month active treatment. The crooked teeth were well aligned and the lower midline was corrected. Meanwhile, the Class I molar relationship, the curve of Spee, the inclination of the incisors, and the good profile were well maintained (Fig. 13.23). Table 13.3 showed well vertical control of the upper molar. The SN/MP increased 0.3° due to more lower molar vertical growth than condylar growth. By tipping posterior teeth back, we reversed her functional occlusal plane by 2.1°.

The pretreatment and posttreatment digital model superimposition was applied to analyze the teeth movement in three dimensions (Fig. 13.24).

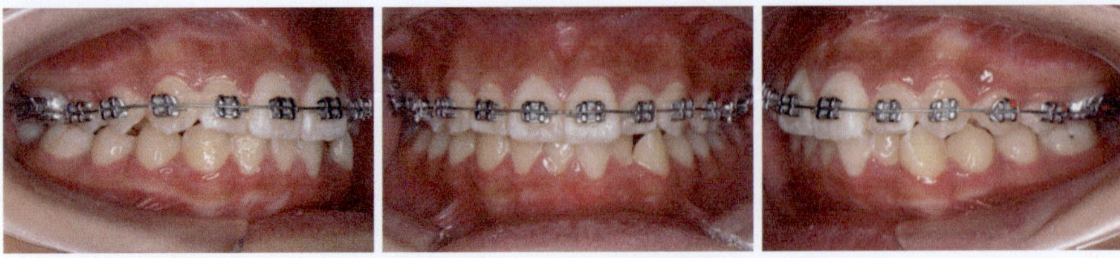

Fig. 13.20 Upper second premolar MLF brackets and second molar tubes were bonded

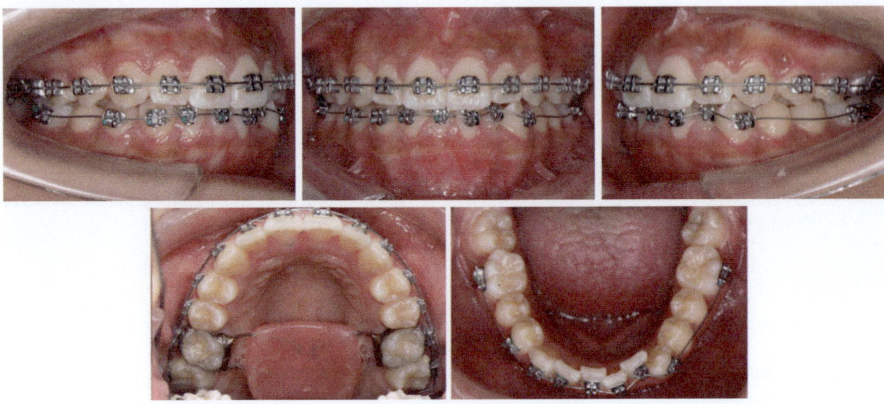

Fig. 13.21 Seven months into treatment, lower teeth were bonded selectively

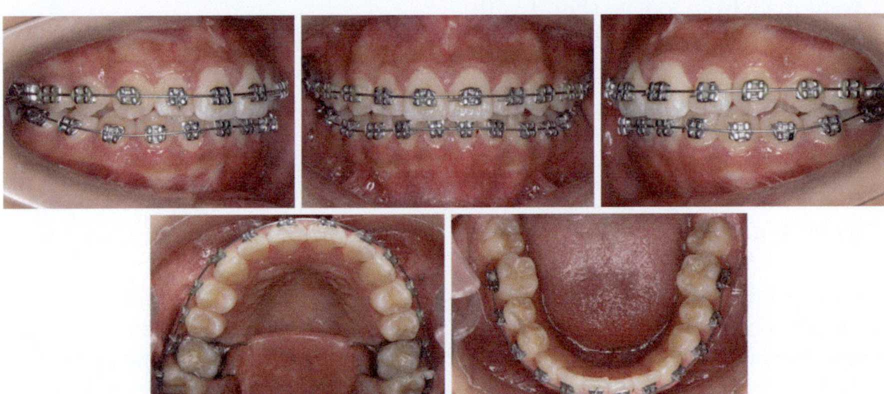

Fig. 13.22 The anterior crowding had been relieved

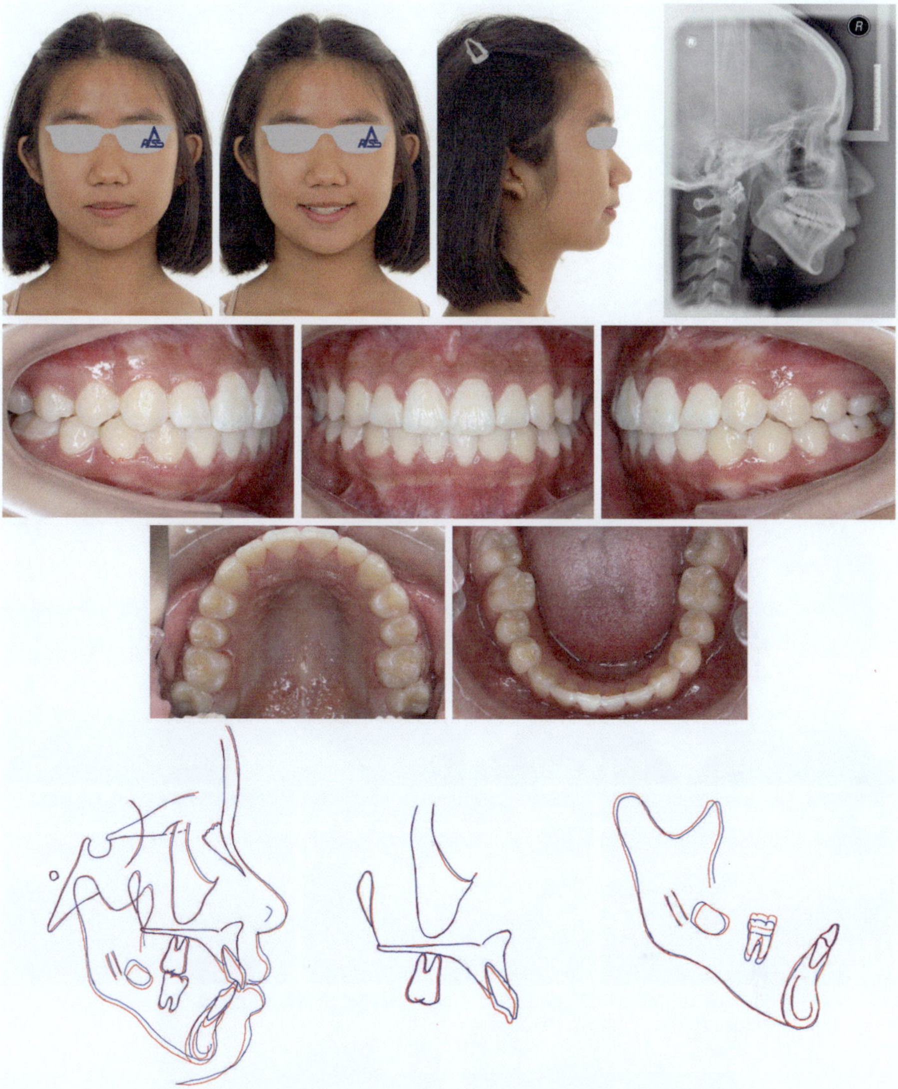

Fig. 13.23 Patient after 18 months of treatment. Superimposition of pretreatment (*blue*) and post-treatment (*red*) cephalometric tracings shows the mild improvement of profile

Case 4. Angle's Class II[1] Adolescent Case with Large Overjet

A 12-year-old male presented with the chief complaint of crooked teeth and protrusive lips. The intraoral examination showed cusp-to-cusp Class II molar relationship, moderate deep overbite, 6 mm overjet, and mild crowding in both arches. Cephalometric analysis revealed it was skeletal Class II (ANB 7.1°) with mild high-angle (MP/PP 29.8°) and protrusive profile (Fig. 13.25 and Table 13.4).

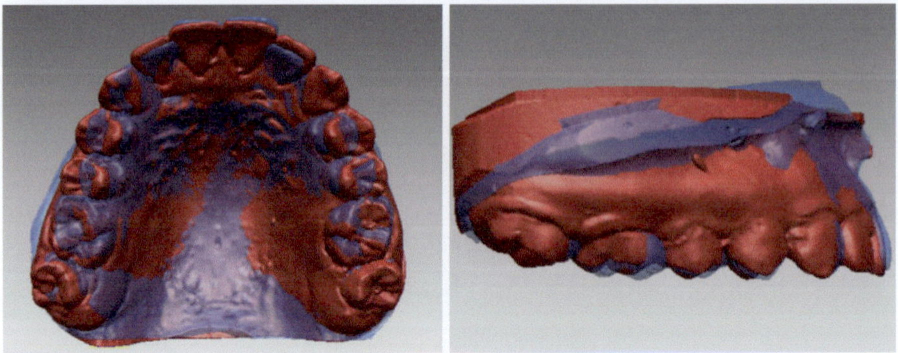

Fig. 13.24 3D digital model superimpositions show upper first molars were tipped back and intruded a little bit, and the upper arch was expanded in premolar area

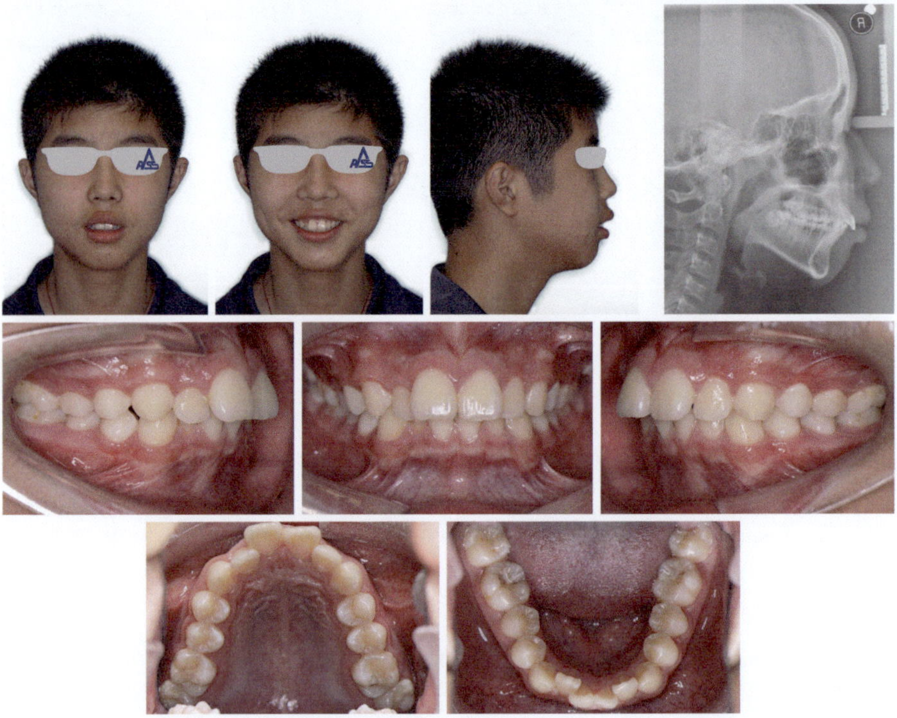

Fig. 13.25 Pretreatment facial and intraoral photographs, as well as radiograph

Since this was a growing patient (skeletal age CS3), Class II molar relationship would be improved with the potential mandibular growth; four first premolars were extracted to ensure the maximum anchorage for incisor retraction in both arches. High-pull headgear was applied for both sagittal and vertical anchorage control.

Table 13.4 Cephalometric analysis before and after treatment

Measurements	Norm. Mean	SD.	Pre.	Post.	Dif.
SNA (°)	82.8	4.0	85.1	84.9	−0.2
SNB (°)	80.1	3.9	78.0	79.2	1.2
ANB (°)	2.7	2.0	7.1	5.7	−1.4
Wits appraisal (mm)	−1.1	2.9	3.9	−1.3	−5.2
PP/SN (°)	9.3	2.4	4.8	4.8	0.0
MP/SN (°)	32.5	5.2	32.4	32.6	0.2
MP/PP (°)	27.6	4.6	27.6	27.8	0.2
FOP/PP (°)	NA	NA	12.6	15.3	2.7
U1-AP (mm)	7.2	2.2	9.8	1.8	−8.0
L1-AP (mm)	4.9	2.1	3.7	0.0	−3.7
U1/PP (°)	115.8	5.7	117.1	103.1	−14.0
L1/MP (°)	93.9	6.2	106.0	98.0	−8.0

During Treatment

1. Upper 3–3 MLF brackets and upper first molar bands with headgear tube and XBT were bonded, and 0.014″ NiTi wire was engaged in the backward tipping tube (Fig. 13.26). The lower brackets were not bonded considering of the possible occlusal interference.

High-pull headgear with 2.0–3.0 N of force per side had been worn to hold the upper molar from the beginning of treatment (Fig. 13.27).

2. Five months into treatment, with the alignment of anterior teeth, its proclination decreased simultaneously under both physiologic and orthopedic forces. Then an upper piggy back arch (0.018″ Australian wire) was utilized to intrude the incisors to correct the deep overbite and improve the lip-teeth relationship (Fig. 13.28). The extrusive reaction force on the anchor molar was resisted by the headgear.

Free physiologic drift of teeth in the lower dentition was allowed in this Class II case. The mesial drift of molars benefited the correction of molar relationship and the distal drift of the canines helped with the relieving of lower anterior crowding. Five months later, the crowding of the lower arch was alleviated automatically (Fig. 13.29).

3. After the anterior overbite was improved, lower 3–3 MLF brackets and lower first molar XBTs were able to be bonded on the appropriate position. A 0.016″ NiTi wire was ligated initially. At this moment, the molar relationship became Class I (Fig. 13.30).

After 2 years and 7 months, all brackets were debonded. A remarkable improvement in patient's smile and profile was achieved. The teeth were well aligned and occlusion was excellent (Fig. 13.31). Table 13.4 showed his upper and lower incisors were retracted apparently. FOP was reversed by 2.7° while MP/SN remained unchanged.

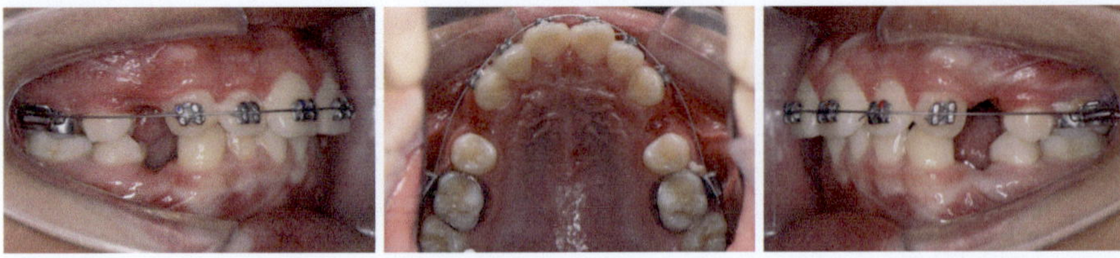

Fig. 13.26 Upper appliance was bonded first

Fig. 13.27 High-pull headgear was instructed

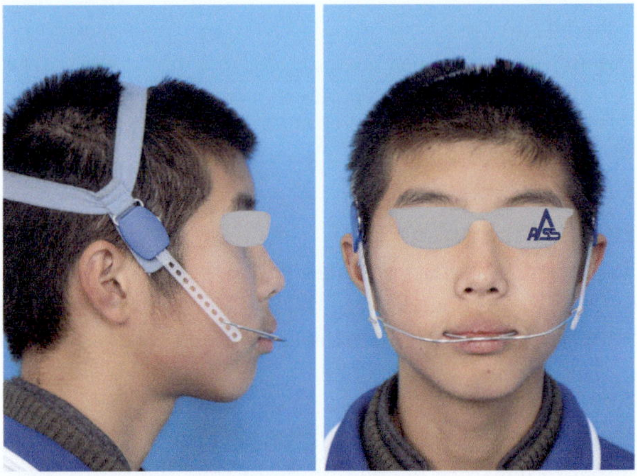

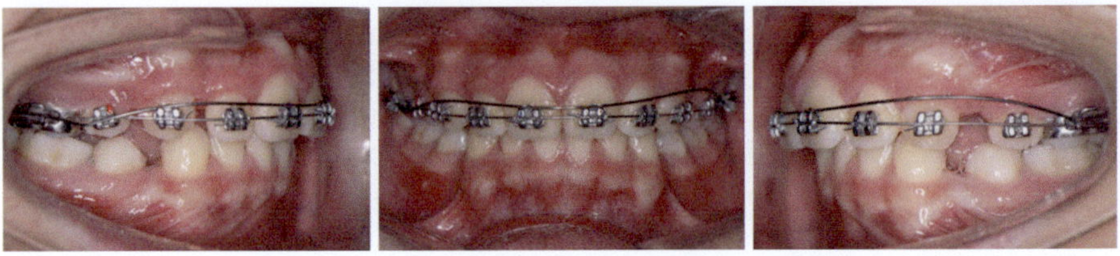

Fig. 13.28 An upper piggy back arch was utilized to intrude the incisors

Fig. 13.29 The extraction space decreased in both sides

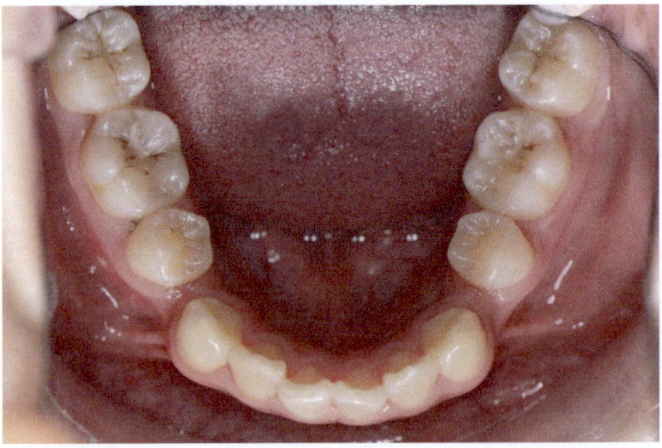

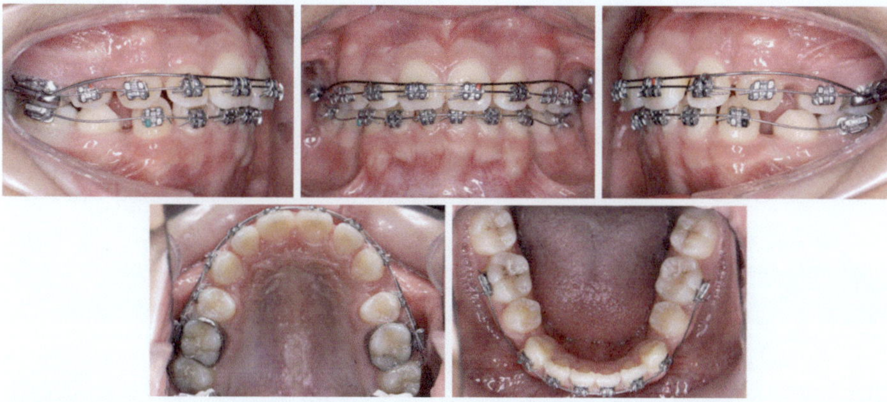

Fig. 13.30 Lower 3–3 MLF brackets and first molar XBTs were bonded after the anterior overbite was improved

Summary

Individuals with a steep mandibular angle constitute a group of clinically challenging patients in the treatment of malocclusions, especially adult patients who show no capacity of condylar growth which could aid to compensate for the inevitable molar extrusion in conventional fixed orthodontic treatment. In three of the above cases, an auxiliary TAP was applied to transmit the continuous tongue pressure both in rest and functional state to intrude the upper molars, which was substantiated by digital model superimposition or cephalometric superimposition. And subsequently, even with the eruption of the lower counterparts, the MP/SN was maintained at least as well as in case 4 with high-pull headgear.

Besides the vertical dimension, high-angle patient is also more susceptible to sagittal anchorage loss out of both physiologic (more remarkable in growing patient) and mechanical factors. Since the lingual surface of TAP was made in accordance with the functional morphologic feature of the tongue, the tongue pressure exerted on it consisted of both vertical and sagittal component, with the latter one contributing to the maximum anchorage control along with other principles in PASS technique.

The upper molars were prevented from forward tipping or even tipped back in the above four cases with the help of XBT and TAP/high-pull headgear. The upper posterior curves of Spee were maintained or restored with the help of tipback angles in upper tubes or brackets. The functional occlusal planes therefore were prevented from forward rotation or even reversed to backward rotation. These changes are certainly good for anchorage control and reducing dental protrusion, as well as the biting efficiency when the direction between posterior teeth axis and masticatory muscles is concerned.

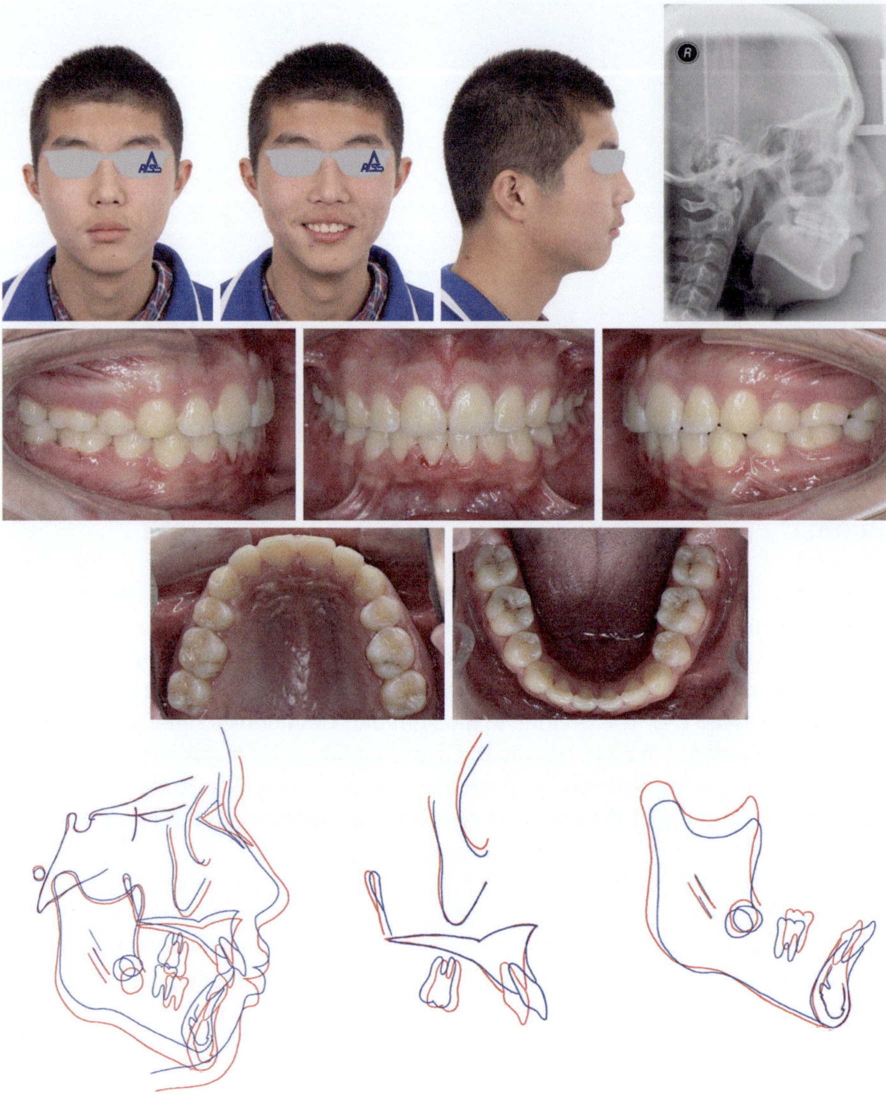

Fig. 13.31 Patient after 2 years and 7 months of treatment. Superimposition of pretreatment (*blue*) and posttreatment (*red*) cephalometric tracings shows maximum anchorage control and fabulous profile improvement. The vertical growth of the upper first molar exceeded the effect of high-pull headgear, and the vertical growth of the lower first molar was almost equal to condyle

References

1. Su H, Han B, Li S et al (2014) Compensation trends of the angulation of first molars: retrospective study of 1403 malocclusion cases. Int J Oral Sci 6(3):175–181
2. Björk A (1955) Facial growth in man, studied with the aid of metallic implants. Acta Odontol Scand 13(1):9–34

3. Schudy F (1965) The rotation of the mandible resulting from growth:its implications in orthodontic treatment. Angle Orthod 35:36–50
4. Chhibber A, Upadhyay M, Shetty VS et al (2011) Cephalometric comparison of vertical changes between Begg and preadjusted edgewise appliances. Eur J Orthod 33(6):712–720
5. Xu TM, Zhang X, Oh HS et al (2010) Randomized clinical trial comparing control of maxillary anchorage with 2 retraction techniques. Am J Orthod Dentofacial Orthop 138(5):544 e1–9
6. Bayirli B, Vaden JL, Johnston LE Jr (2013) Long-term mandibular skeletal and dental effects of standard edgewise treatment. Am J Orthod Dentofac Orthop 144(5):682–690
7. Lee J, Miyazawa K, Tabuchi M et al (2013) Midpalatal miniscrews and high-pull headgear for anteroposterior and vertical anchorage control: cephalometric comparisons of treatment changes. Am J Orthod Dentofac Orthop 144(2):238–250
8. Scheffler NR, Proffit WR, Phillips C (2014) Outcomes and stability in patients with anterior open bite and long anterior face height treated with temporary anchorage devices and a maxillary intrusion splint. Am J Orthod Dentofac Orthop 146(5):594–602
9. Xu KF, Zeng JJ, Xu TM (2016) Effect of an intraoral appliance on tongue pressure measured by force exerted during swallowing. Am J Orthod Dentofac Orthop 149(1):55–61
10. Zeng JJ, Xu KF, Gao XM (2015) Tongue resting pressure of the tongue anchorage pad in different body positions: a pilot study. J Oral Rehabil 42(6):414–419

Atypical Extraction Cases

14

Guangying Song, Tian Min Xu, Si Chen, and Fanfan Dai

Abstract

In comparison with the typical four first premolar extraction for protrusive and severe crowding cases, atypical extraction was more frequently used in borderline cases and cases with tooth size asymmetry, unfavorable tooth impaction, tooth dysplasia, premature tooth missing, severe malpositioned tooth, periodontal problems, etc. When atypical extraction happened, which teeth will we put the XBT on? Should first premolar be bonded or not? This chapter will introduce the flexible application of PASS technique in complicated atypical extraction cases.

Borderline cases often show slight facial convexity and mild crowding before treatment. Though molar distalization, arch expansion, or extraction of the second premolars can all be treatment options for this kind of cases, in patients who address more in profile or combined with thin attached gingival tissue, extraction of the second premolars might be a better choice to achieve the treatment goals. Besides second premolar extraction, molar, incisor, and even canine might be an extraction option in some times when the following situations were presented: tooth size asymmetry, unfavorable tooth impaction, tooth dysplasia, premature tooth missing, severe malpositioned tooth, periodontal problems, etc. In this section, five atypical extraction cases treated by PASS technique were discussed. Two of them were borderline cases which extracted second premolars. Another three illustrated the flexible application of PASS technique in various extraction conditions.

G. Song (✉) • T.M. Xu • S. Chen
Department of Orthodontics, Peking University School and Hospital of Stomatology, Beijing, China
e-mail: songguangying@gmail.com; tmxuortho@163.com; elisa02chen@gmail.com

F. Dai
Second Dental Center, Peking University School and Hospital of Stomatology, Beijing, China
e-mail: daifanfannihao@163.com

T.M. Xu (ed.), *Physiologic Anchorage Control*,
DOI 10.1007/978-3-319-48333-7_14

Case 1. Second Premolar Extraction in Adolescent Case

An 11year-old female presented with the chief complaint of crowding. Intraoral examination showed Class I molar relationship, mild to moderate crowding in the upper and lower arch, and lower midline shifting to the right for 2 mm (Fig. 14.1). Cephalometric analysis (Table 14.1) revealed it was a skeletal Class I (ANB, 3.9°). Lateral photograph showed slightly convex profile (Fig. 14.1). Extraction of 4 s premolars was planned. The treatment aimed to deliver moderate anchorage to relieve the crowding, to maintain Class I molar relationship, and to improve the profile.

During Treatment

1. MLF brackets were placed on upper 3–3 (Fig. 14.2). XBT tubes were bonded on upper first molars. A 0.014″ NiTi wire was engaged in the tipback tube to align anterior teeth.
2. One month into treatment (Fig. 14.3), crowding in upper anterior teeth has been alleviated. MLF brackets were placed on lower 4–4 and XBT tubes were bonded

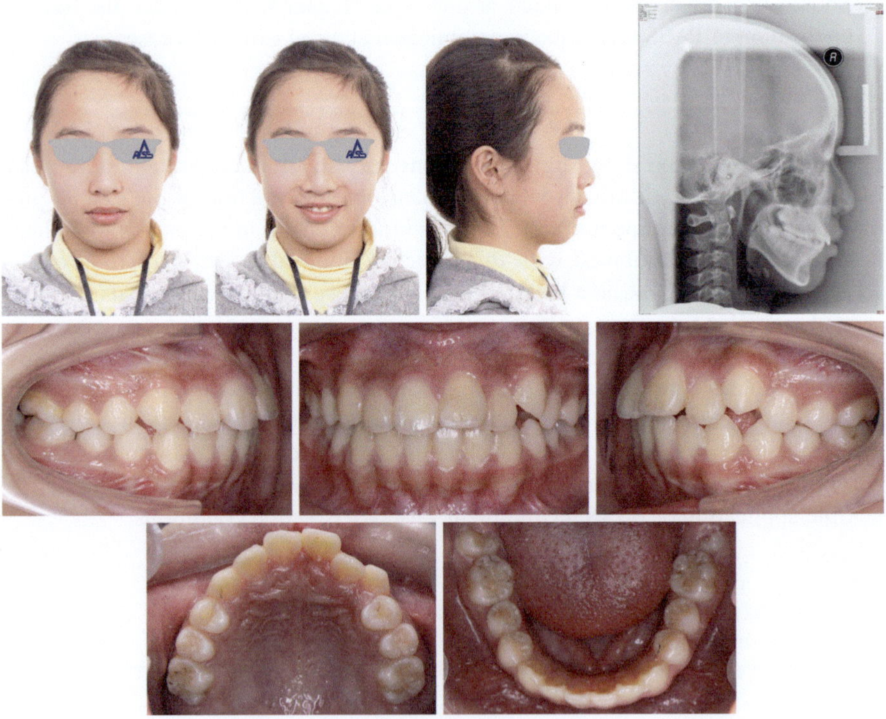

Fig. 14.1 Pretreatment facial and intraoral photographs and cephalometric radiograph

on lower first molars. A 0.014″ NiTi wire was engaged in the main tube since there were no apparent inclined teeth in lower dentition.

3. Three months into treatment (Fig. 14.4), small spacing appeared mesial to right upper first premolar and lower first premolars by drifting. MLF brackets were placed on upper first premolars. A 0.014″ NiTi wire was engaged in the main tube. Upper second molars have erupted more than 1/2.
4. Seven months into treatment (Fig. 14.5), crowding in the upper arch has been relieved. A piggyback arch was used to tie on upper canines to tip upper first molars back in order to decrease the step between the upper first molar and upper second molar. Class II elastics was used to enhance canine anchorage. Lower second molars were bonded.
5. Ten months into treatment (Fig. 14.6), upper second molars were fully erupted. XBT tubes were bonded on upper second molars. A 0.018 × 0.025″ NiTi wire

Table 14.1 Cephalometric analysis before and after treatment

	Norm.				
Measurements	Mean	SD.	Pre.	Post.	Dif.
SNA (°)	82.8	4.0	77.4	76.2	−1.3
SNB (°)	80.1	3.9	73.6	73.9	0.4
ANB (°)	2.7	2.0	3.9	2.3	−1.6
Wits appraisal (mm)	−1.1	2.9	0.1	−4.8	−4.9
PP/SN (°)	9.3	2.4	8.6	10.1	1.5
MP/SN (°)	32.5	5.2	40.5	41.1	0.7
MP/PP (°)	27.6	4.6	31.8	31.0	−0.8
FOP/PP (°)	NA	NA	3.7	5.8	2.1
U1-AP (mm)	7.2	2.2	9.0	5.6	−3.4
L1-AP (mm)	4.9	2.1	4.5	2.4	−2.1
U1/PP (°)	115.8	5.7	119.1	111.5	−7.6
L1/MP (°)	93.9	6.2	97.1	88.4	−8.8

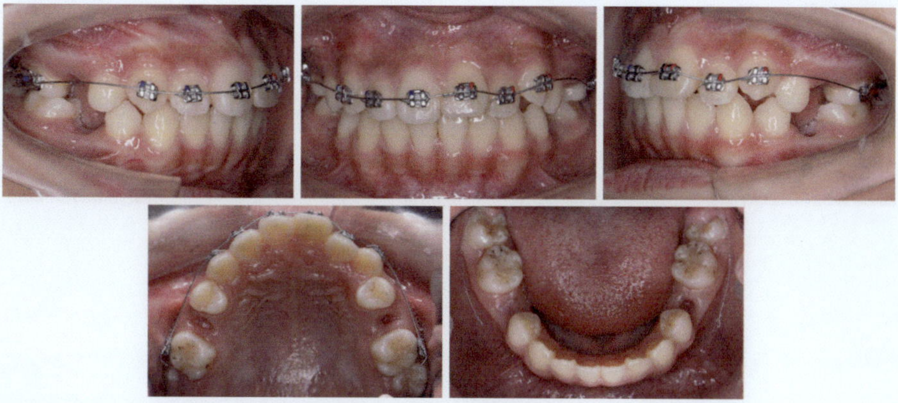

Fig. 14.2 Initial bonding of the upper appliance

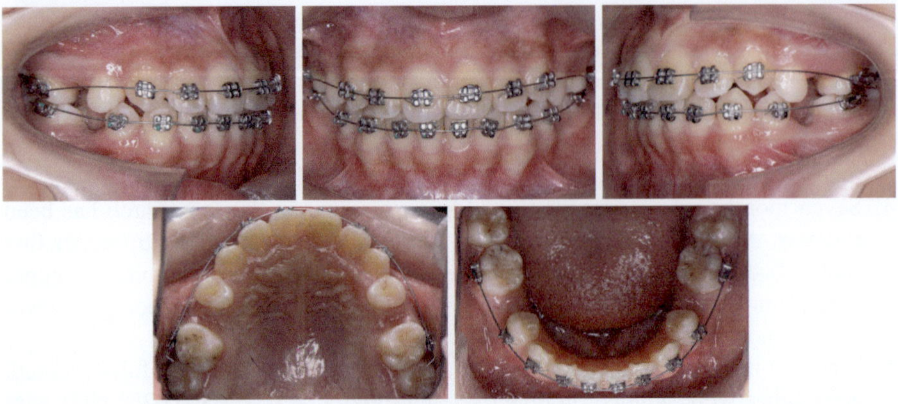

Fig. 14.3 Initial placement of the lower appliance

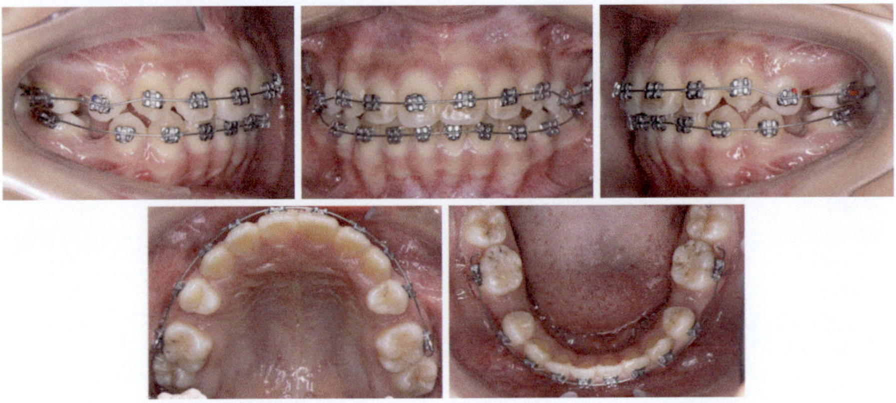

Fig. 14.4 Three months into treatment

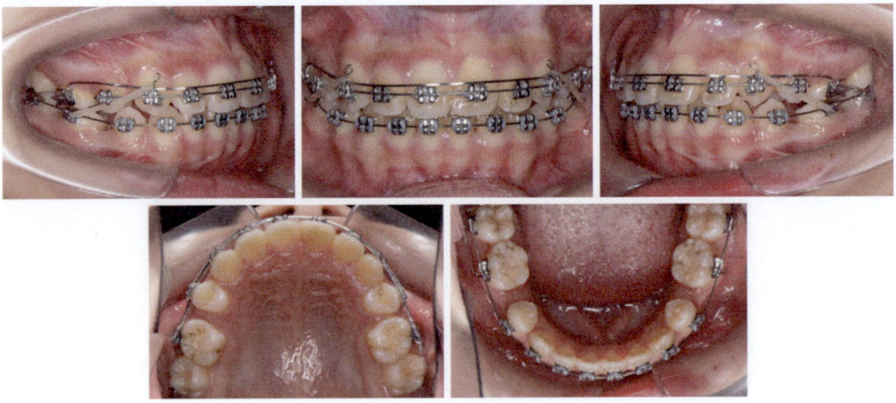

Fig. 14.5 Seven months into treatment

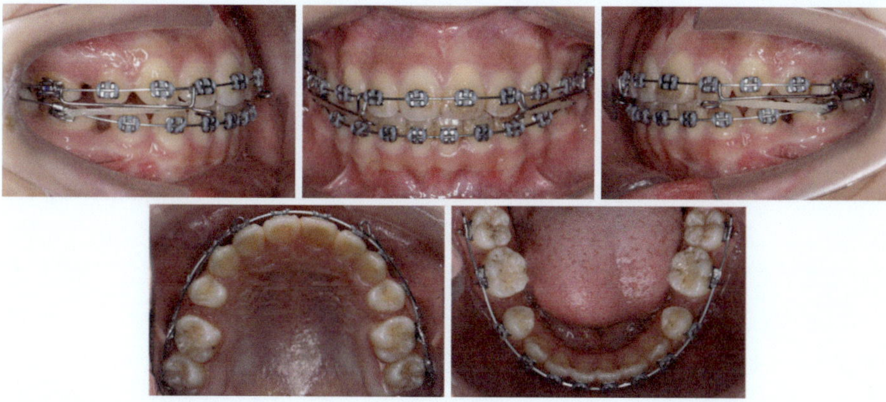

Fig. 14.6 Ten months into treatment

with normal curve of Spee was engaged in upper arch. Sliding jags were used to push upper first molars to facilitate the establishment of normal curve of Spee. A 0.018 × 0.025″ NiTi wire with reverse curve of Spee was engaged in lower arch.

6. Twelve months into treatment (Fig. 14.7), two 0.018 × 0.025″ stainless steel wires were engaged in the upper and lower arch respectively with Class II elastics.
7. Active treatment time was 26 months (Fig. 14.8).

Lateral head films show reserved curve of Spee in the upper arch. Superimposition of pretreatment and posttreatment cephalometric tracings (Fig. 14.9) showed moderate molar anchorage and remarkable lip retraction. The cephalometric analysis (Table 14.1) demonstrated 2.1° clockwise rotation of FOP referring to PP plane, indicating PAC technique could successfully prevent molar from tipping forward and reverse the FOP compensation direction in adolescent patients extracting four second premolars even if second molars were erupting.

In PASS technique, although bonding first molars with XBT tube and 3–3 with MLF brackets is a conventional method, it doesn't mean that first premolar can't be bonded in the second premolar extraction case at the initial bonding. For a case like in Fig. 14.10, since the right upper first premolar and right lower second premolar were in crossbite, upper first premolars were bonded so that the intrusive force from the NiTi wire engaged in the tipback tube could be used to relieve the crossbite. Figure 14.11 shows the intrusive effect on upper first premolar to correct the crossbite in 2 months and spacing appeared before right upper first premolar, left upper canine, and left lower first premolar showing drifting. So bonding 3–3 or 4–4 depends on whether premolar correction is needed. The mission of −25° tipback tube is to correct any malpositioned teeth until wire-slot angle of all teeth in anterior segment becomes less than 7° so that when changing to −7° rectangular tube, dominant moment is still on anchor molar.

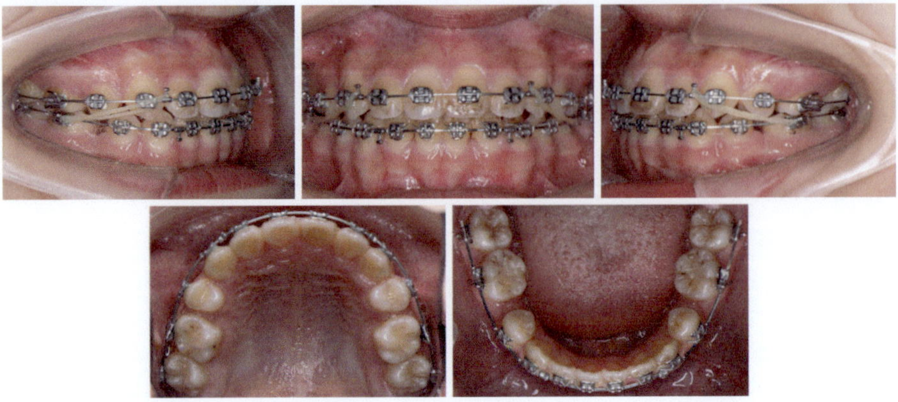

Fig. 14.7 Twelve months into treatment

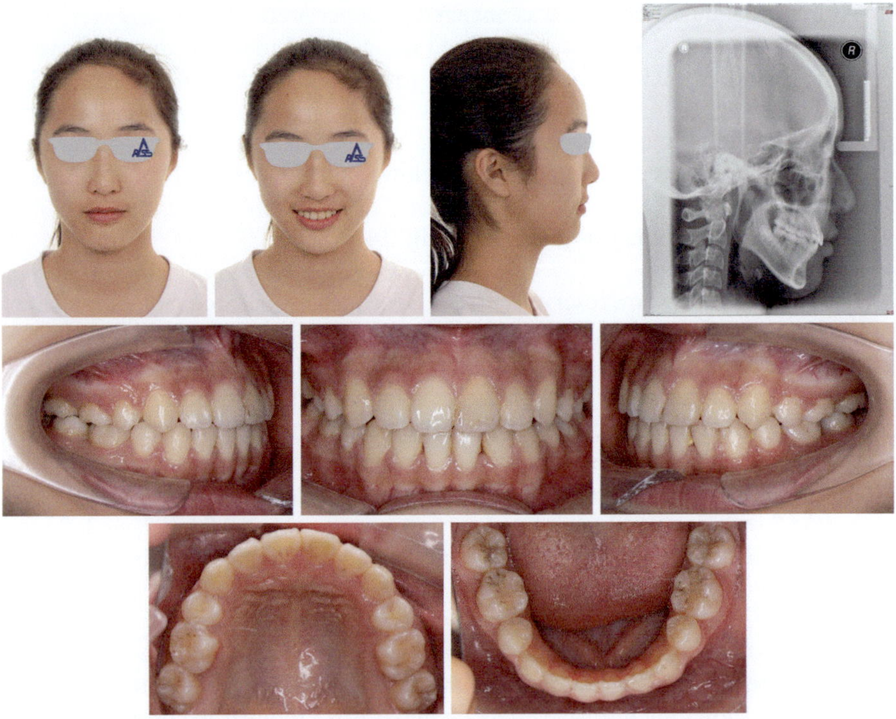

Fig. 14.8 Posttreatment facial and intraoral photographs and cephalometric radiograph

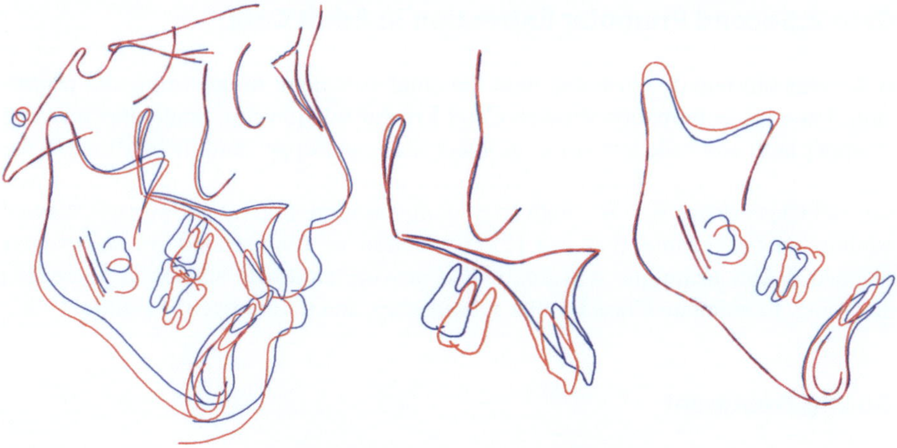

Fig. 14.9 Superimposition of pretreatment (*blue*) and posttreatment (*red*) cephalometric tracings

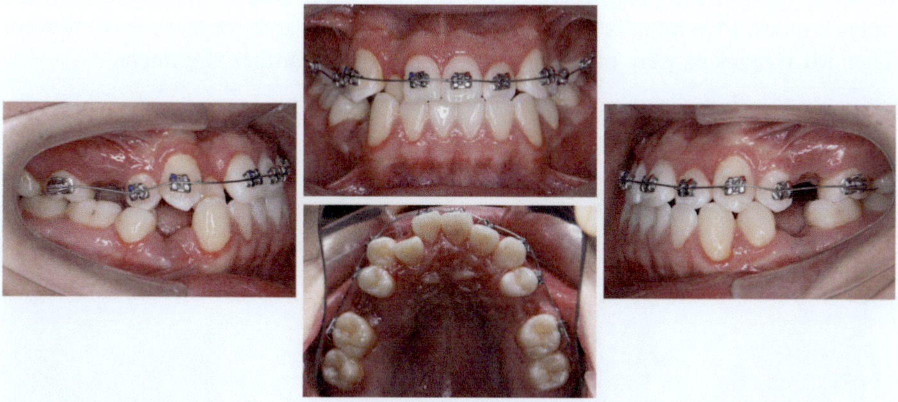

Fig. 14.10 Initial bonding of upper appliance

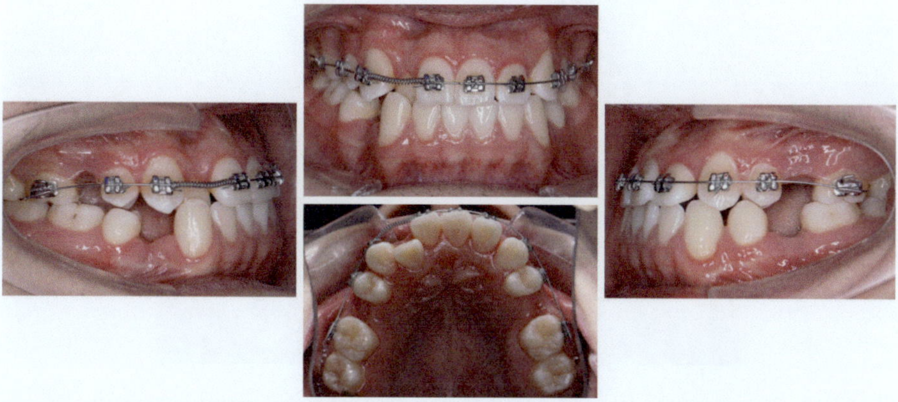

Fig. 14.11 Three months into treatment

Case 2. Second Premolar Extraction in Adult Case

A 24 year-old female presented with the chief complaint of crowding and protrusion. Intraoral examination showed Class I molar relationship, moderate crowding in upper arch and mild crowding in lower arch, and upper midline shifting to the right for 1.5 mm (Fig. 14.12). Cephalometric analysis (Table 14.2) revealed it was a skeletal Class II (ANB, 7.9°) with teeth compensation. Lateral photograph showed slightly convex profile (Fig. 14.12). Extraction of four second premolars was planned. PASS technique was applied to provide moderate anchorage to relieve crowding, to maintain Class I molar relationship, and to improve the profile.

During Treatment

MLF brackets were first placed on upper and lower 3–3. XBT tubes were bonded on first molars. Two 0.014″ NiTi wires were engaged in the tipback tubes at the initial bonding. Two months into treatment, two 0.016″ NiTi wires were engaged in the tipback tubes. Five months into treatment, crowding in anterior teeth was relieved. Then MLF brackets were placed on first premolars for further alignment.

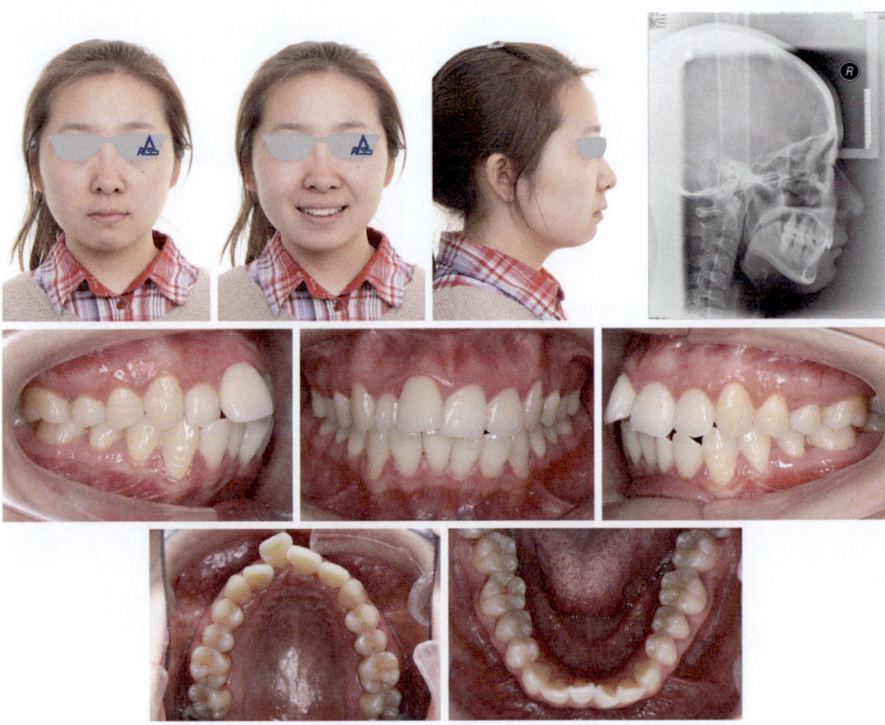

Fig. 14.12 Pretreatment facial and intraoral photographs and cephalometric radiograph

Table 14.2 Cephalometric analysis before and after treatment

Measurements	Norm. Mean	Norm. SD.	Pre.	Post.	Dif.
SNA (°)	82.8	4.0	80.3	79.5	−0.8
SNB (°)	80.1	3.9	72.4	73.0	0.6
ANB (°)	2.7	2.0	7.9	6.5	−1.4
Wits appraisal (mm)	−1.1	2.9	4.1	0.6	−3.5
PP/SN (°)	9.3	2.4	12.4	12.2	−0.2
MP/SN (°)	32.5	5.2	43.2	43.3	0.1
MP/PP (°)	27.6	4.6	30.8	31.1	0.3
FOP/PP (°)	NA	NA	14.7	17.7	3.0
U1-AP (mm)	7.2	2.2	10.4	2.9	−7.4
L1-AP (mm)	4.9	2.1	5.7	0.6	−5.1
U1/PP (°)	115.8	5.7	119.1	86.8	−32.3
L1/MP (°)	93.9	6.2	104.0	87.4	−16.7

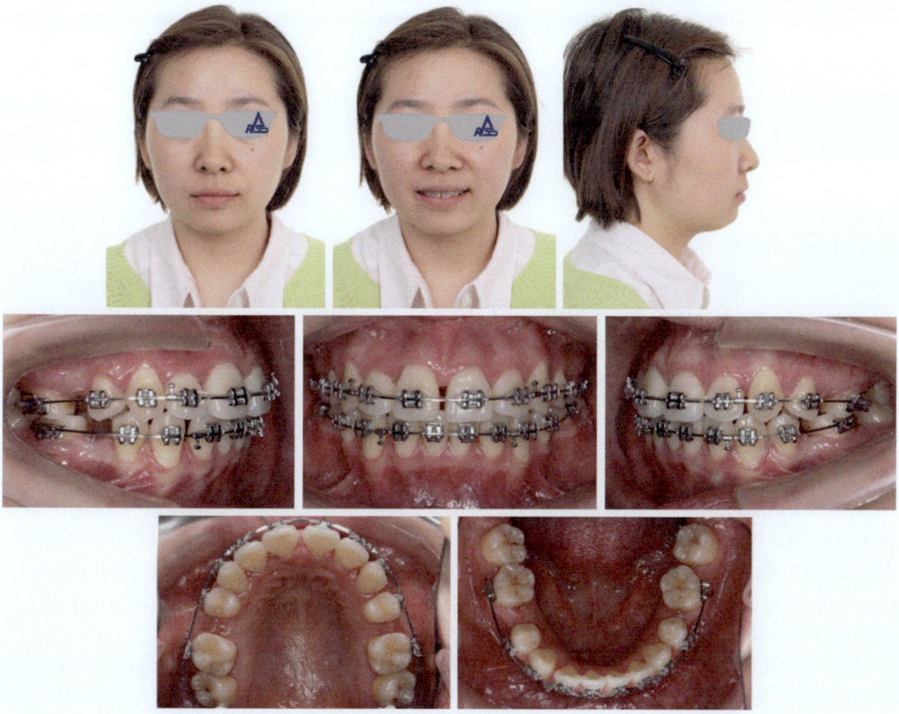

Fig. 14.13 Thirteen months into treatment

1. Thirteen months into treatment (Fig. 14.13), upper 0.018 × 0.025″ SS with curve of Spee plus traction hooks and lower 0.018 × 0.025″ SS with slight reverse curve of Spee plus traction hooks were engaged. Elastic chain was used to close space between upper incisors. Upper canines and lower first premolars automatically drifted distally. The profile became better.

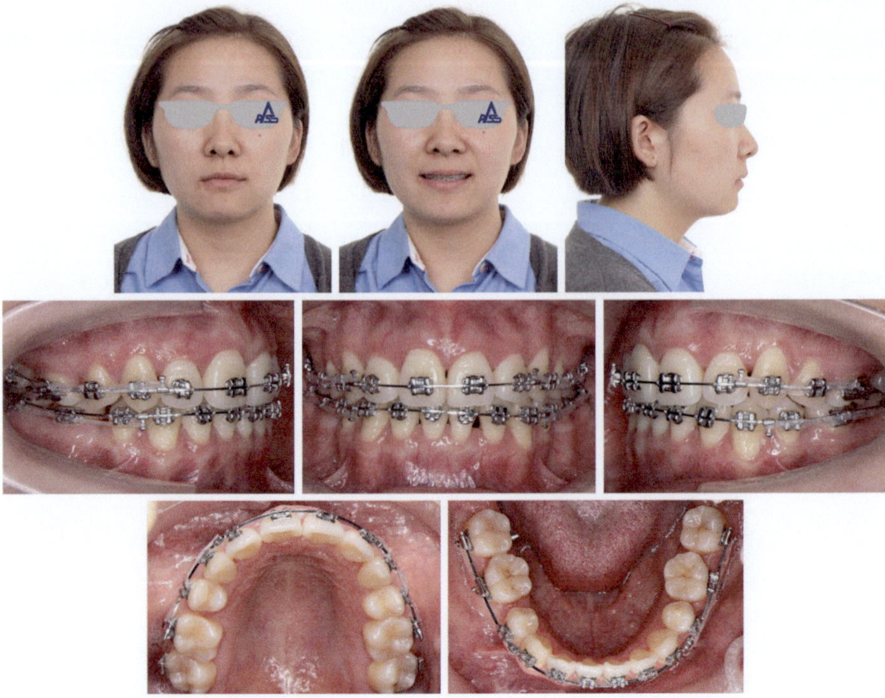

Fig. 14.14 Twenty months into treatment

2. Twenty months into treatment (Fig. 14.14), the upper midline deviation has been corrected by intermaxillary elastics. XBT tubes were bonded on second molars. Elastic chain was used to close the residual space. Her profile was apparently improved.
3. Active treatment was for 28 months (Fig. 14.15).

Superimposition of tracings (Fig. 14.16) showed good anchorage control and remarkable incisors and lower lip retraction. The cephalometric analysis (Table. 14.2) demonstrated 3.0° clockwise rotation of FOP revealing that the treatment successfully prevented forward tipping of molar and reversed FOP compensation direction in the second premolar extraction case.

The cephalometric tracing superimposition showed different strengths of molar anchorage between case 1 and case 2 (Figs. 14.9 and 14.16), which reflects the physiologic anchorage loss in adolescence. In addition, according to Chap. 7, the drifting of the first molar was greater for the second premolar extraction group than for the first premolar extraction group. It alerts that the patients with second premolar extraction should be bonded as soon as possible, in order to avoid unwanted anchor molar drifting.

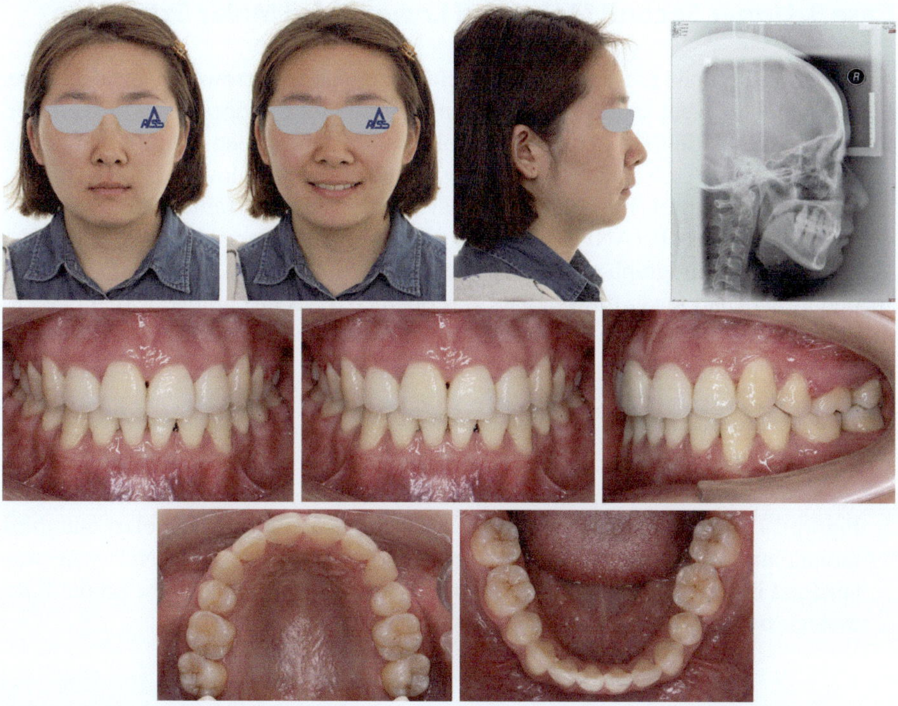

Fig. 14.15 Posttreatment facial and intraoral photographs and cephalometric radiograph

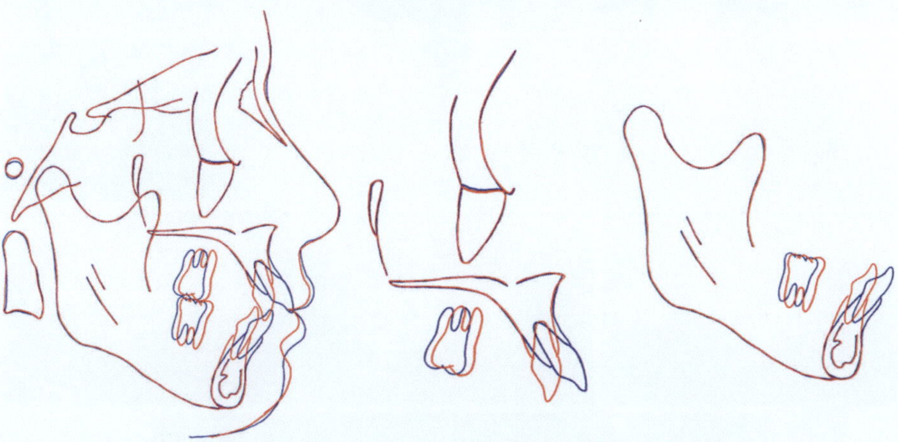

Fig. 14.16 Superimposition of pretreatment (*blue*) and posttreatment (*red*) cephalometric tracings

Case 3. Upper Second Molar and Lower Third Molar Extraction

A 27-year-old female presented with the chief complaint of crowding and deep bite. Four premolars were extracted in her first orthodontic treatment as a teenager. Intraoral examination showed Class I molar relationship, deep overbite, moderate crowding in lower arch and mild crowding in upper arch, and lower midline shifting to the right for 0.5 mm (Fig. 14.17). Cephalometric analysis (Table 14.3) revealed it was a skeletal Class II (ANB, 6.6°) with a steep mandibular plane angel (MP/SN, 44.6°). Lateral photograph showed convex profile (Fig. 14.17). Extraction of upper second molars and lower third molars was planned. PASS technique was applied to reinforce the anchorage when opening the deep overbite, to relieve crowding, and to improve the profile.

During Treatment

1. Figure 14.18 showed XBT tubes were bonded on the upper first molars and third molars and MLF brackets were placed on other teeth. A 0.014″ NiTi wire was engaged in the main tube on the first molars and in the tipback tube on the third molars to restore the normal curve of Spee.

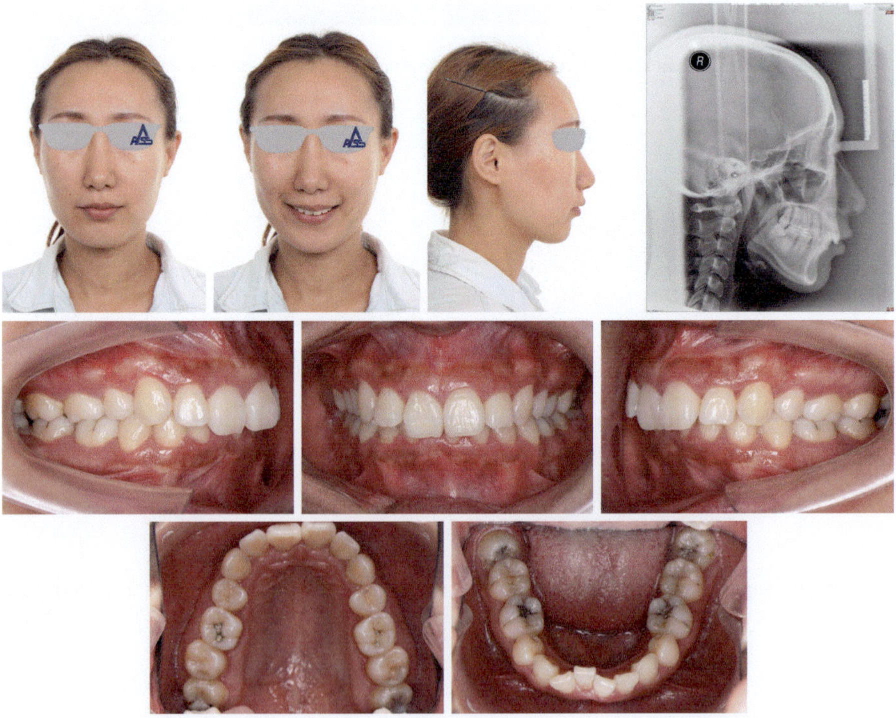

Fig. 14.17 Pretreatment facial and intraoral photographs and cephalometric radiograph

2. Two months into treatment (Fig. 14.19), upper first molars were upright distally under the effects of −7° moment on it and −25° dominant moment from upper third molar, along with the alignment of upper dentition. Then lower first molars were bonded with XBT and 3–3with MLF brackets. A 0.014 in. NiTi wire was engaged in the backward tipping tube.
3. Six months into treatment (Fig. 14.20), upper first molars keep moving backward under the tipback moments. We then changed to 0.018 × 0.025″ NiTi archwire with normal curve of Spee in the upper arch in the main tube with premolars tied back to close the space in front of first molars and bonded lower premolars and lower second molars. A 0.014″ NiTi wire was engaged in the main tube for further alignment.
4. Twelve months into treatment (Fig. 14.21), upper lateral incisors automatically drifted distally along with canines tied back. Elastic chain was used to close space between upper incisors. A piggyback arch was used to tie on

Table 14.3 Cephalometric analysis before and after treatment

	Norm.				
Measurements	Mean	SD.	Pre.	Post.	Dif.
SNA (°)	82.8	4.0	79.4	79.9	0.6
SNB (°)	80.1	3.9	72.8	74.5	1.7
ANB (°)	2.7	2.0	6.6	5.4	−1.2
Wits appraisal (mm)	−1.1	2.9	4.6	2.3	−2.3
PP/SN (°)	9.3	2.4	15.8	16.6	0.8
MP/SN (°)	32.5	5.2	44.6	42.9	−1.7
MP/PP (°)	27.6	4.6	28.8	26.3	−2.5
FOP/PP (°)	NA	NA	0.5	0.8	0.3
U1-AP (mm)	7.2	2.2	7.3	8.1	0.8
L1-AP (mm)	4.9	2.1	0.2	5.3	5.0
U1/PP (°)	115.8	5.7	102.9	120.9	18.0
L1/MP (°)	93.9	6.2	80.3	98.7	18.4

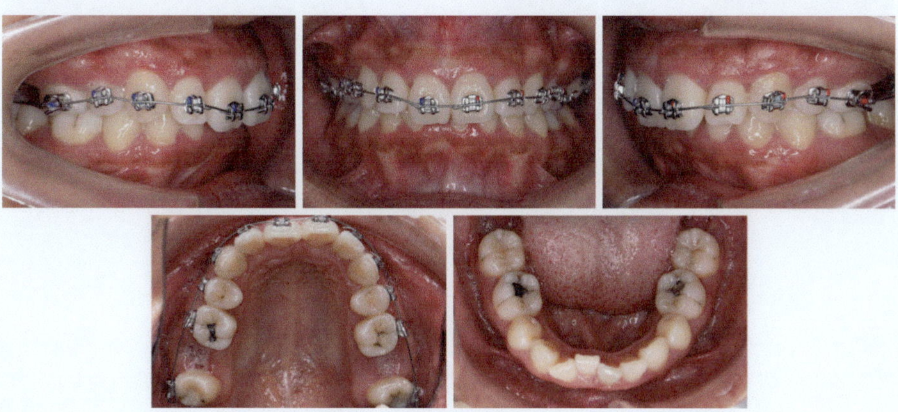

Fig. 14.18 Initial bonding of the upper appliance

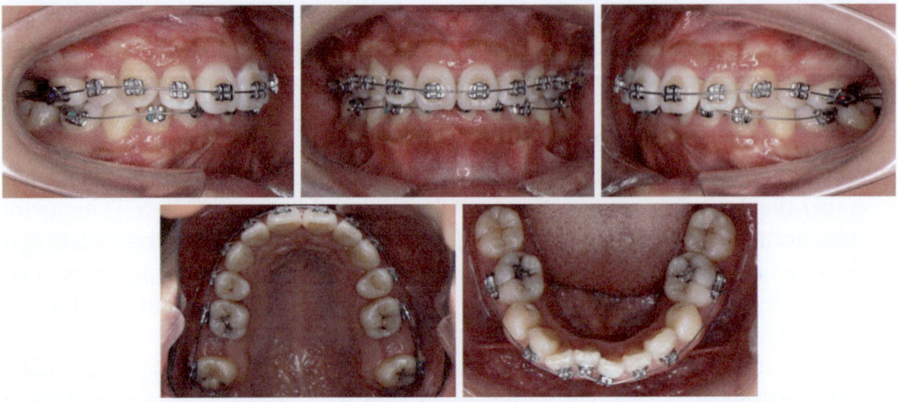

Fig. 14.19 Initial placement of lower appliance

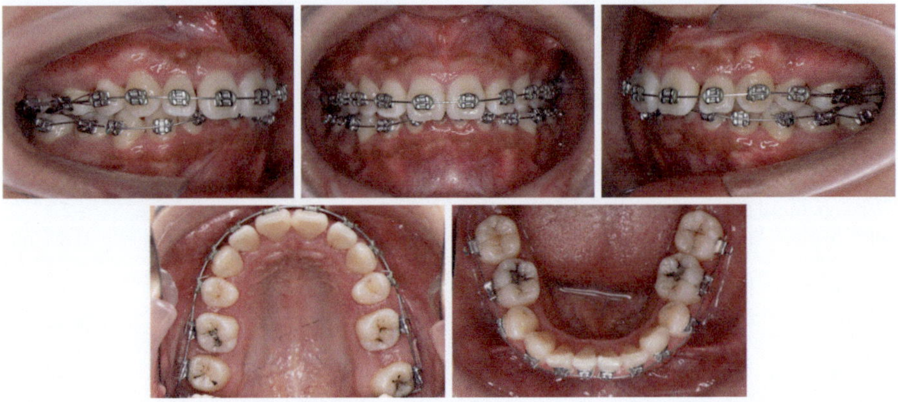

Fig. 14.20 Six months into treatment

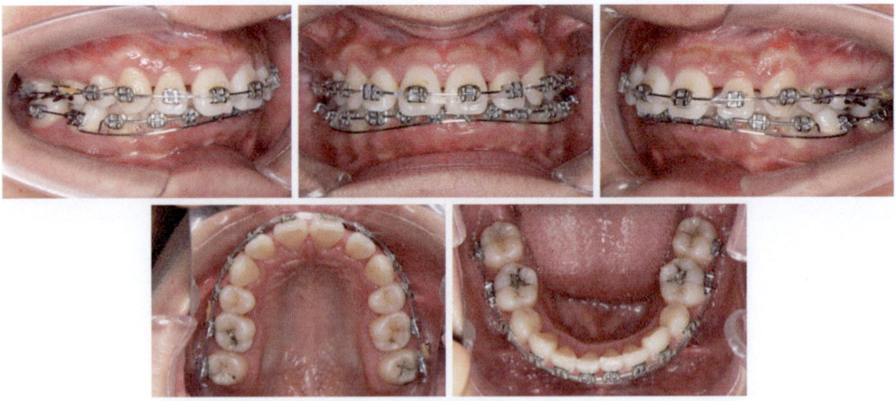

Fig. 14.21 Twelve months into treatment

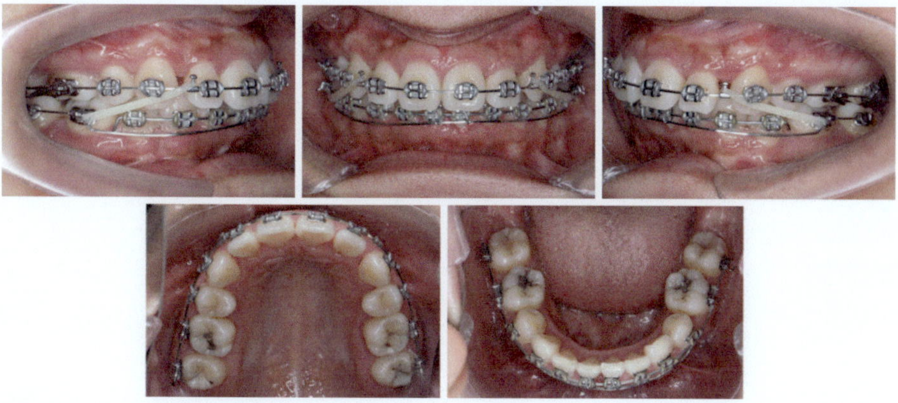

Fig. 14.22 Fifteen months into treatment

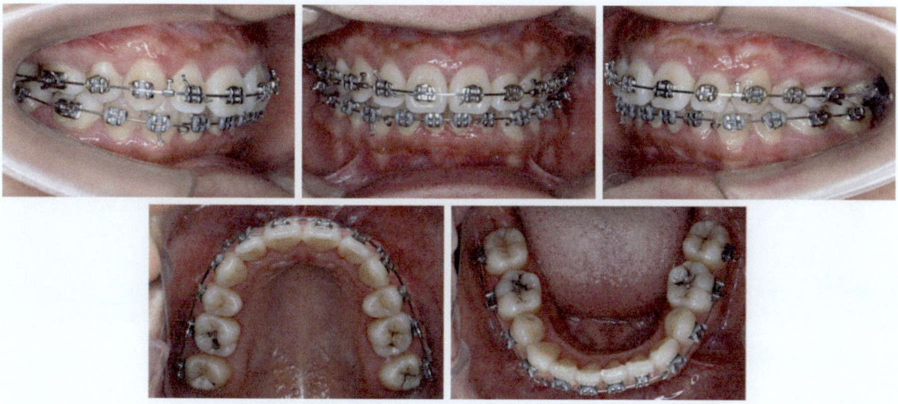

Fig. 14.23 Eighteen months into treatment

lower central incisors to open the deep overbite. The piggyback arch went through lower first molars and second molars to reinforce the lower molar anchorage.

5. Fifteen months into treatment (Fig. 14.22), deep overbite was apparently opened. A 0.018 × 0.025″ stainless steel wire with traction hooks and normal curve of Spee was engaged in the upper arch. The treatment went on with Class II elastics to correct anterior teeth inclinations.
6. Eighteen months into treatment (Fig. 14.23), deep overbite was further opened. A 0.018″ stainless steel wire with helical loop and reverse curve of Spee was engaged in lower arch.
7. Twenty-three months into treatment (Fig. 14.24), deep overbite was fully opened. Elastic chain was used to close the residual space in upper dentition.
8. Active treatment time was 24 months (Fig. 14.25).

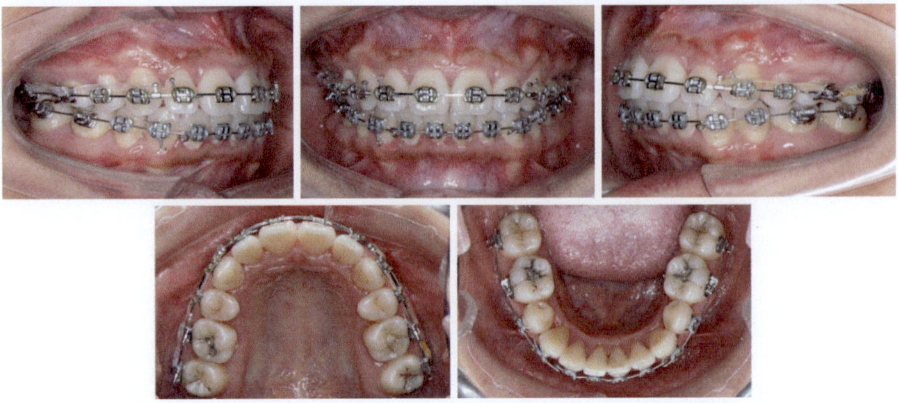

Fig. 14.24 Twenty-three months into treatment

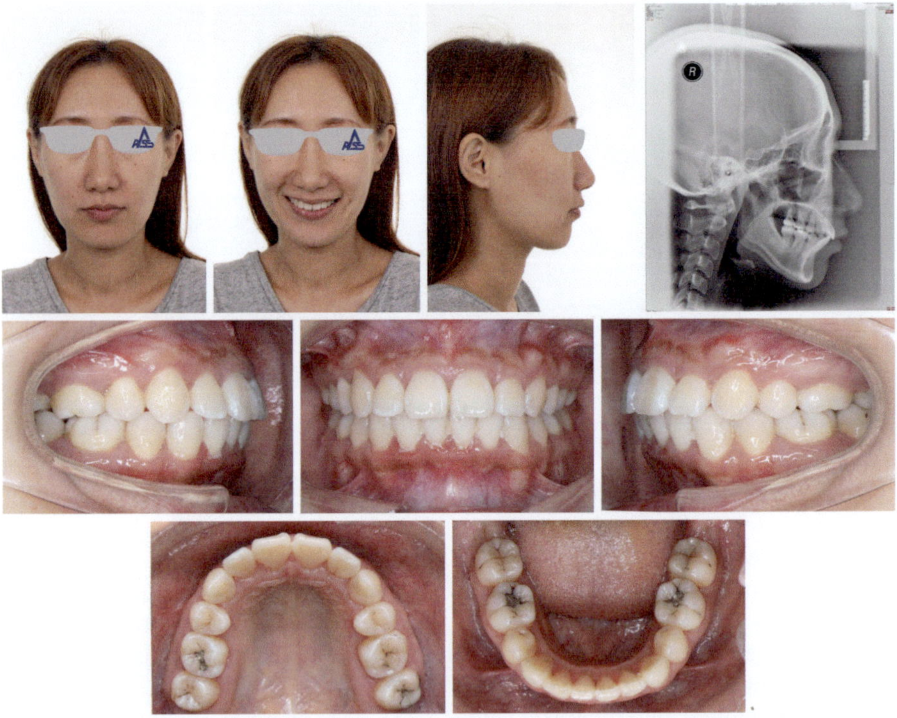

Fig. 14.25 Posttreatment facial and intraoral photographs and cephalometric radiograph

Superimposition of tracings (Fig. 14.26) showed distalization with backward tipping of upper molars and intrusion of upper incisors. It also showed backward tipping of lower molars and intrusion with proclination of lower incisors. The cephalometric analysis (Table 14.3) showed only 0.3° clockwise rotation of FOP,

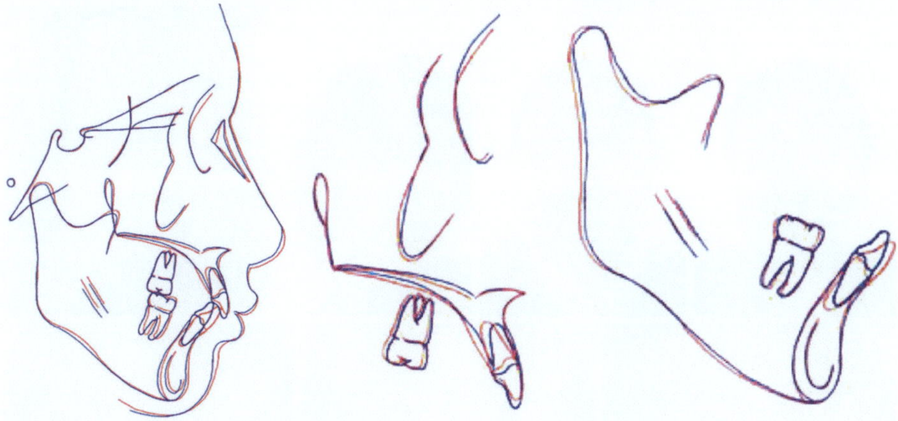

Fig. 14.26 Superimposition of pretreatment (*blue*) and posttreatment (*red*) cephalometric tracings

indicating the treatment successfully prevented forward rotation of FOP that is supposed to worsen Class II molar relationship. MP/SN was reduced from a pretreatment angle of 44.6° to a posttreatment angle of 42.9°, so was MP/PP reduced from a pretreatment angle of 28.8° to a posttreatment angle of 26.3°, which may be related with molar extraction.

Case 4. Upper Lateral Incisor Extraction Case

An 11-year-old female presented with the chief complaint of crowding. Intraoral examination showed Class II molar relationship, proclination of maxillary incisors, crowding, congenital missing of 22, retention of 63, microdontia of 12, and midline off (Fig. 14.27). Cephalometric analysis (Table. 14.4) revealed it was a skeletal Class II (ANB, 5.1°). Lateral photograph showed slightly convex profile (Fig. 14.27). Extraction of right upper lateral, left upper deciduous canine, left lower second premolar, and right lower first premolar was planned. The treatment aimed to deliver moderate anchorage to relieve the crowding, to retract the upper incisors, to achieve Class I molar relationship, and to improve the profile.

During Treatment

1. Figure 14.28 showed that in maxillary dentition, there was no severe tipping tooth, i.e., no wire-slot angle on any tooth is larger than 7°. So MLF brackets were placed on upper 5–5 at the initial bonding. XBT tubes were bonded on the first molars, using a 0.014″ NiTi wire to align upper arch.
2. Three months into treatment (Fig. 14.29), left upper canine "drifted" distally without elastic force. MLF brackets were then placed on lower 3–3. XBT tubes

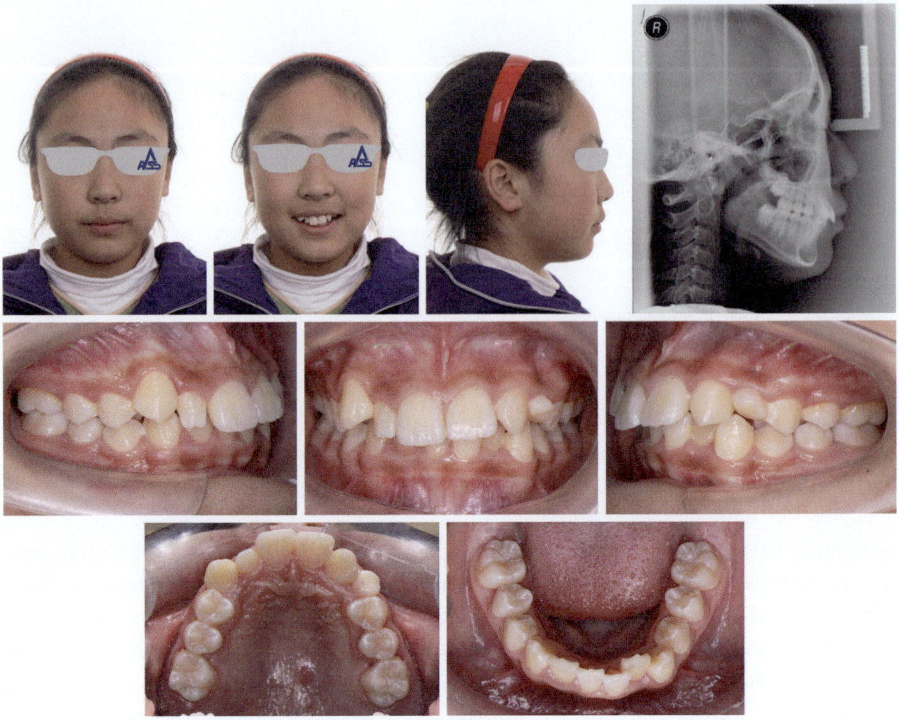

Fig. 14.27 Pretreatment facial and intraoral photographs and cephalometric radiograph

Table 14.4 Cephalometric analysis before and after treatment

Measurements	Norm. Mean	Norm. SD.	Pre.	Post.	Dif.
SNA (°)	82.8	4.0	82.6	81.6	−1.1
SNB (°)	80.1	3.9	77.6	78.1	0.5
ANB (°)	2.7	2.0	5.1	3.5	−1.6
Wits appraisal (mm)	−1.1	2.9	−0.9	−1.9	−1.0
PP/SN (°)	9.3	2.4	8.0	6.5	−1.5
MP/SN (°)	32.5	5.2	37.0	36.6	−0.3
MP/PP (°)	27.6	4.6	29.0	30.1	1.1
FOP/PP (°)	NA	NA	8.3	8.9	0.6
U1-AP (mm)	7.2	2.2	7.8	3.2	−4.7
L1-AP (mm)	4.9	2.1	1.4	0.1	−1.3
U1/PP (°)	115.8	5.7	113.4	104.9	−8.4
L1/MP (°)	93.9	6.2	93.1	89.5	−3.6

were boned on lower first molars. A 0.014″ NiTi wire was engaged in the tipback tube. Lower second molars were erupting.

3. Five months into treatment (Fig. 14.30), crowding in lower dentition was relieved. A piggyback arch was used to tie on lower central incisors to open the deep bite.

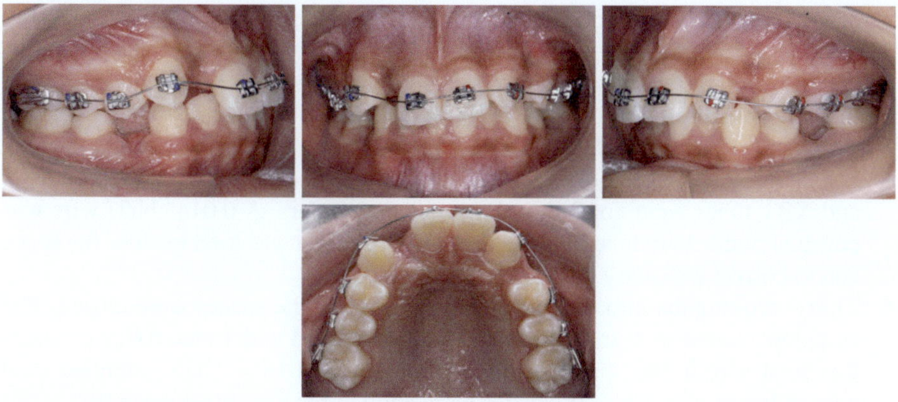

Fig. 14.28 Initial setting of the upper appliance

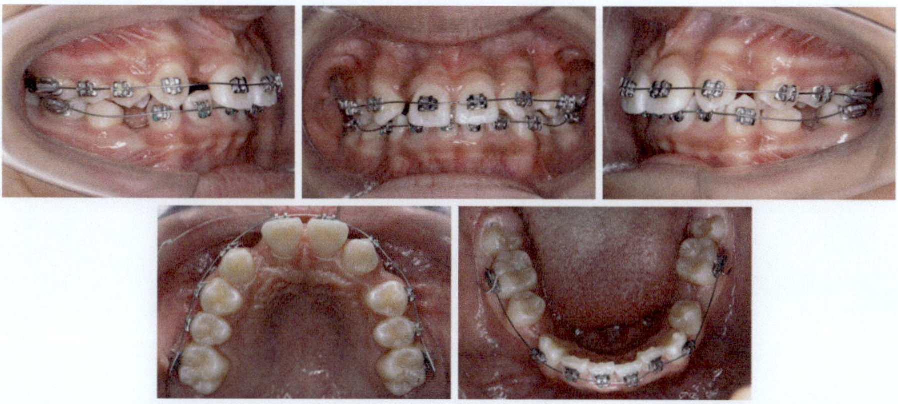

Fig. 14.29 Initial bonding of lower appliance

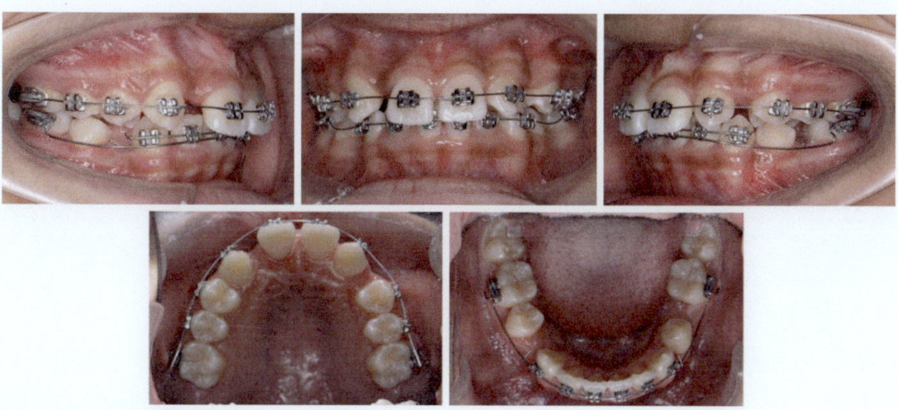

Fig. 14.30 Five months into treatment

4. Eleven months into treatment (Fig. 14.31), deep overbite was opened a little bit. A 0.018″ stainless steel wire with helical loop and normal curve of Spee was engaged in the upper arch. Class II elastics were used to correct anterior teeth inclinations. Elastic chain was used to correct upper midline.
5. Twelve months into treatment (Fig. 14.32), deep overbite was apparently opened. Upper midline was improved. MLF brackets were placed on lower premolars and XBT tubes were bonded on lower second molars. A 0.014″ NiTi wire was engaged in the main tube in lower arch. Elastic chain was used to close the space and to correct maxillary incisors inclinations.
6. Thirty-two months into treatment (Fig. 14.33), all the spaces were closed. The complete closure of extraction spaces was performed with round 0.018 in. stainless steel wire in the upper arch and rectangular 0.018 × 0.025″ stainless steel wire in lower arch. Class II elastics were applied for further refinement.
7. Active treatment time was 35 months (Fig. 14.34).

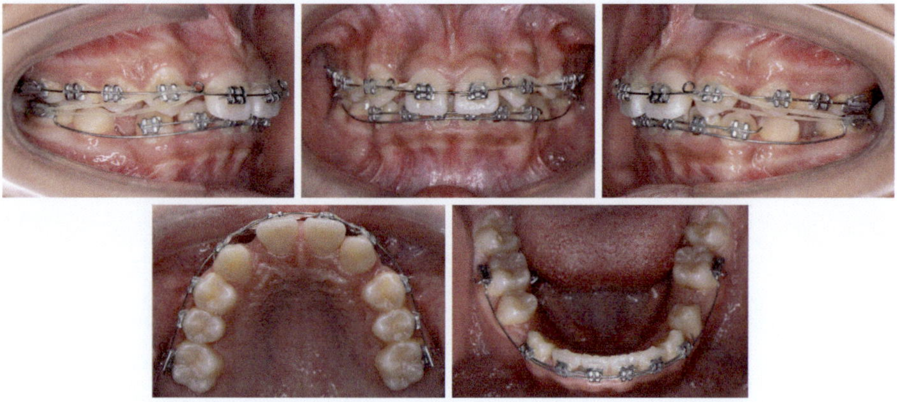

Fig. 14.31 Eleven months into treatment

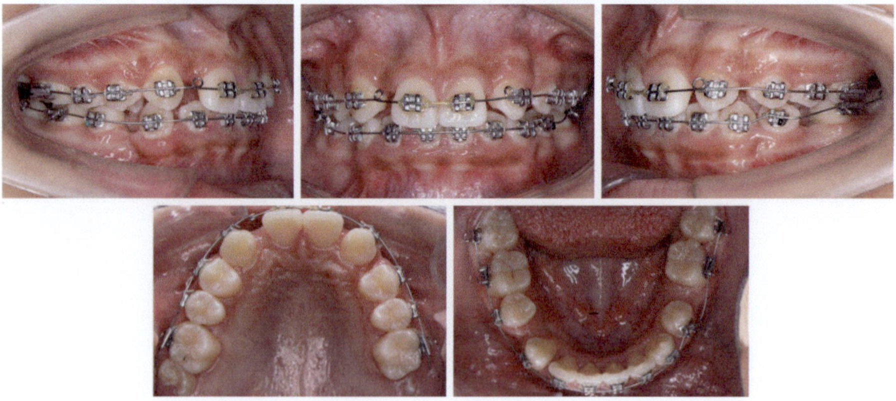

Fig. 14.32 Twelve months into treatment

Her profile was dramatically improved after the treatment. Superimposition of tracings (Fig. 14.35) showed remarkable incisor retraction and good anchorage control in both upper and lower arches considering her apparent growth during treatment. The cephalometric analysis (Table. 14.4) demonstrated a 0.6° clockwise rotation of FOP referring to PP plane indicating molars are prevented from tipping forward and the counterclockwise rotation of occlusal plane was resisted.

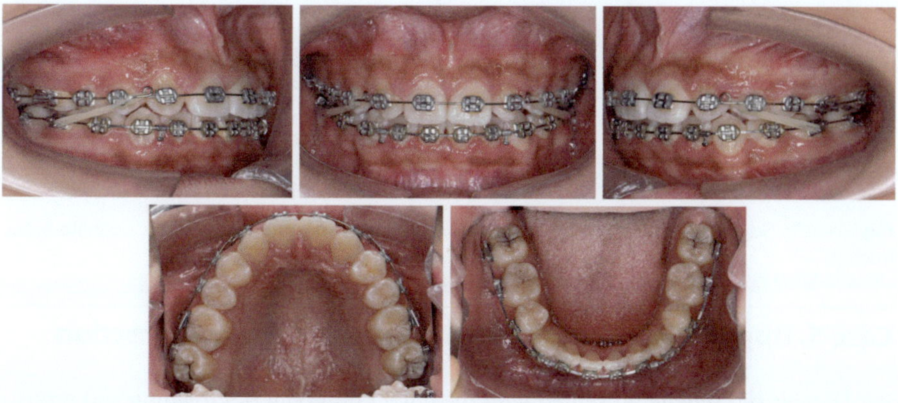

Fig. 14.33 Thirty-two months into treatment

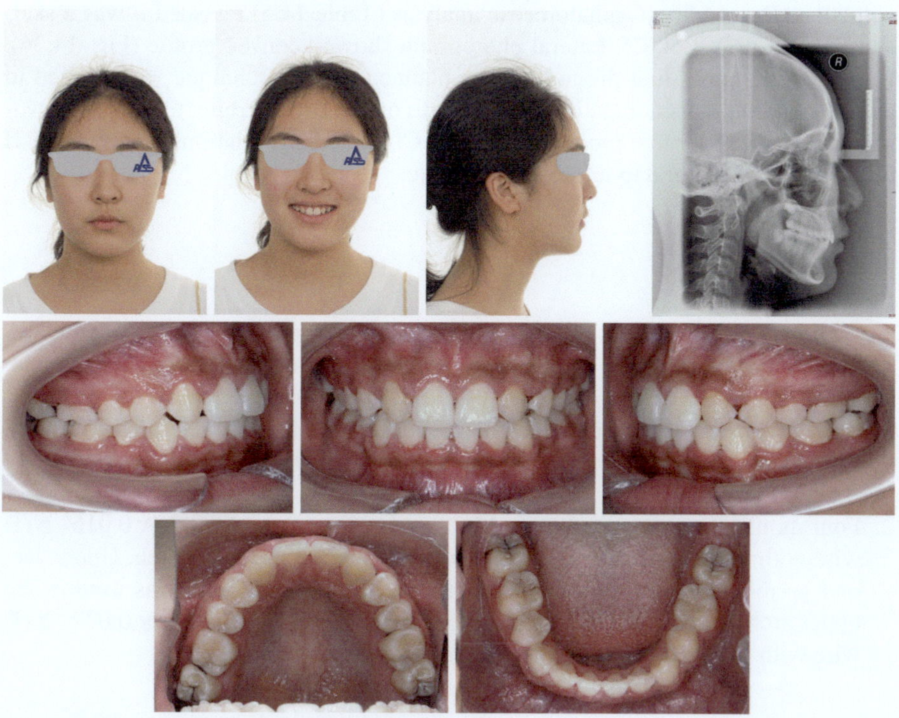

Fig. 14.34 Posttreatment facial and intraoral photographs and cephalometric radiograph

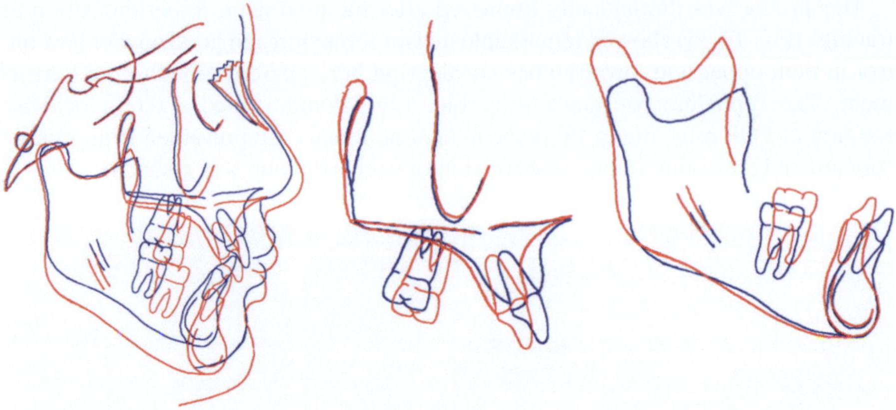

Fig. 14.35 Superimposition of pretreatment (*blue*) and posttreatment (*red*) cephalometric tracings

Case 5. Upper First Premolar and Lower First Molar Extraction

An 18-year-old female presented with the chief complaint of crowding and protrusion. Intraoral examination showed Class II canine relationship, crowding, deep overbite and overjet, and premature loss of lower first molars and upper first molar extrusion (Fig. 14.36). Cephalometric analysis (Table 14.5) revealed it was a skeletal Class II (ANB, 4.8°). Lateral photograph showed convex profile (Fig. 14.36). Extraction of upper first premolars was planned. PASS technique was applied to deliver maximum anchorage in upper arch, to open deep overbite, to relieve crowding, to intrude upper first molars, to achieve Class I canine relationship and Class II molar relationship, and to improve the profile.

During Treatment

1. Figure 14.37 shows XBT tubes were bonded on upper first molars and lower second and third molars. MLF brackets were placed on all the teeth. Since upper incisors were severely rotated, a 0.014″ NiTi wire was engaged in the −25° tip-back tube in the upper arch with upper second premolars unligated. There was no severe malposition in the lower arch, so a 0.014″ NiTi wire was engaged in the −4° main tube.
2. Four months into treatment (Fig. 14.38), crowding was relieved. A 0.016″ NiTi wire with physiologic curve of Spee was engaged in the upper arch. Upper second premolars were ligated for alignment. A piggyback arch was used in the upper arch to tie on upper laterals to open the deep bite. A 0.016 × 0.022″ NiTi wire with reverse curve of Spee was engaged in lower arch.

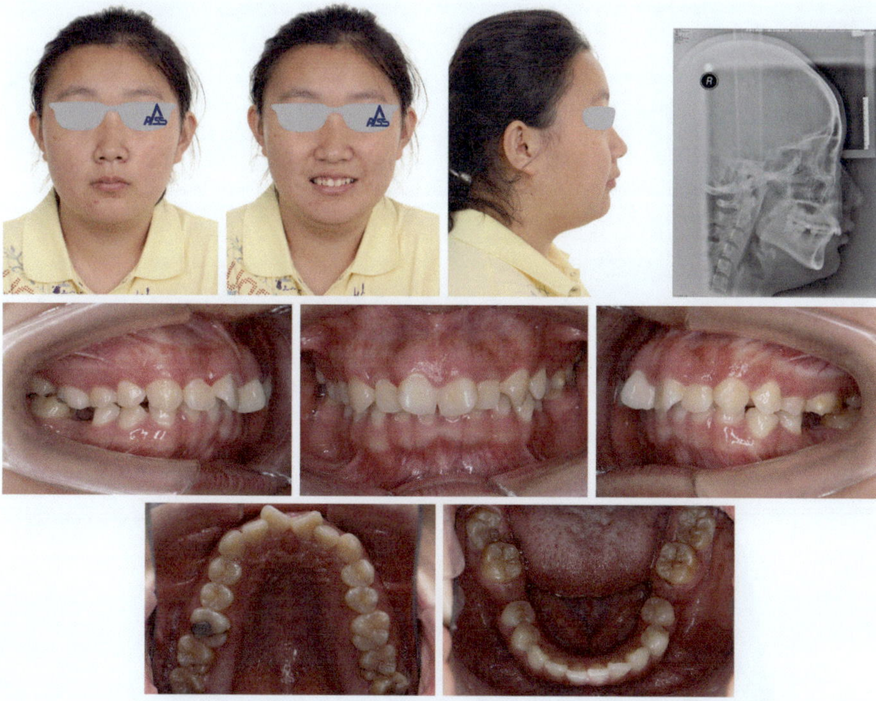

Fig. 14.36 Pretreatment facial and intraoral photographs and cephalometric radiograph

Table 14.5 Cephalometric analysis before and after treatment

Measurements	Norm. Mean	SD.	Pre.	Post.	Dif.
SNA (°)	82.8	4.0	80.6	77.2	−3.4
SNB (°)	80.1	3.9	76.3	73.2	−3.1
ANB (°)	2.7	2.0	4.2	4.0	−0.3
Wits appraisal (mm)	−1.1	2.9	1.4	−1.4	−2.9
PP/SN (°)	9.3	2.4	10.4	9.7	−0.7
MP/SN (°)	32.5	5.2	36.2	37.2	1.0
MP/PP (°)	27.6	4.6	25.8	27.5	1.7
FOP/PP (°)	NA	NA	8.3	13.6	5.3
U1-AP (mm)	7.2	2.2	9.9	5.5	−4.4
L1-AP (mm)	4.9	2.1	3.0	3.5	0.5
U1/PP (°)	115.8	5.7	117.3	103.2	−14.1
L1/MP (°)	93.9	6.2	93.5	104.7	11.2

3. Fifteen months into treatment (Fig. 14.39), the spaces were almost closed. Deep overbite has been opened. Upper first molars were obviously intruded after upper second molars were included into treatment. Physiologic curve of Spee has been

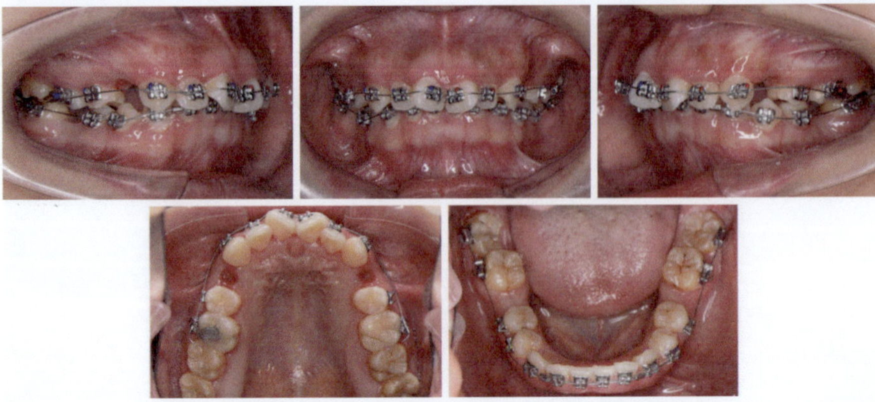

Fig. 14.37 Initial bonding of upper and lower appliances

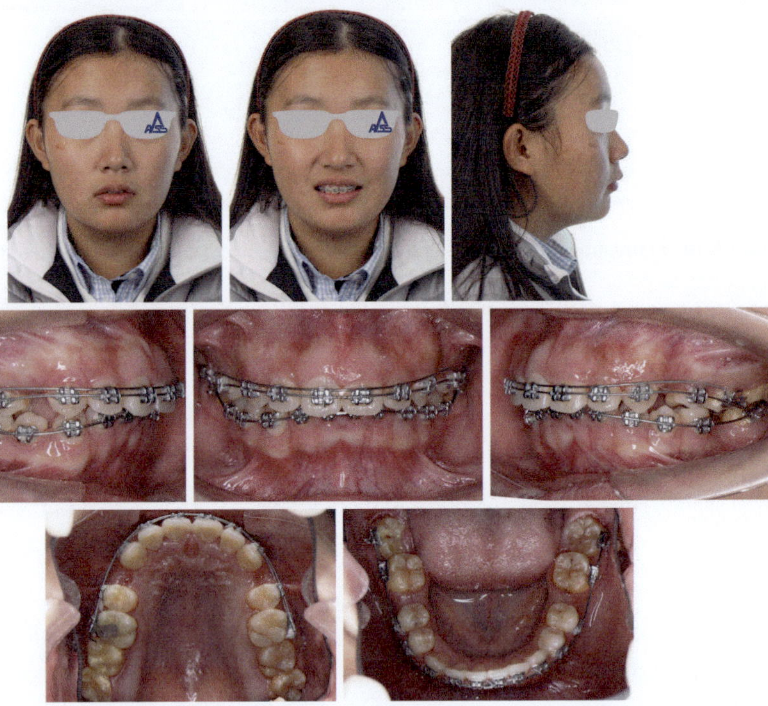

Fig. 14.38 Four months into treatment

restored in upper dentition. XBT tubes were bonded on upper third molars for the aligning of upper second molars.

4. Active treatment time was 21 months (Fig. 14.40).

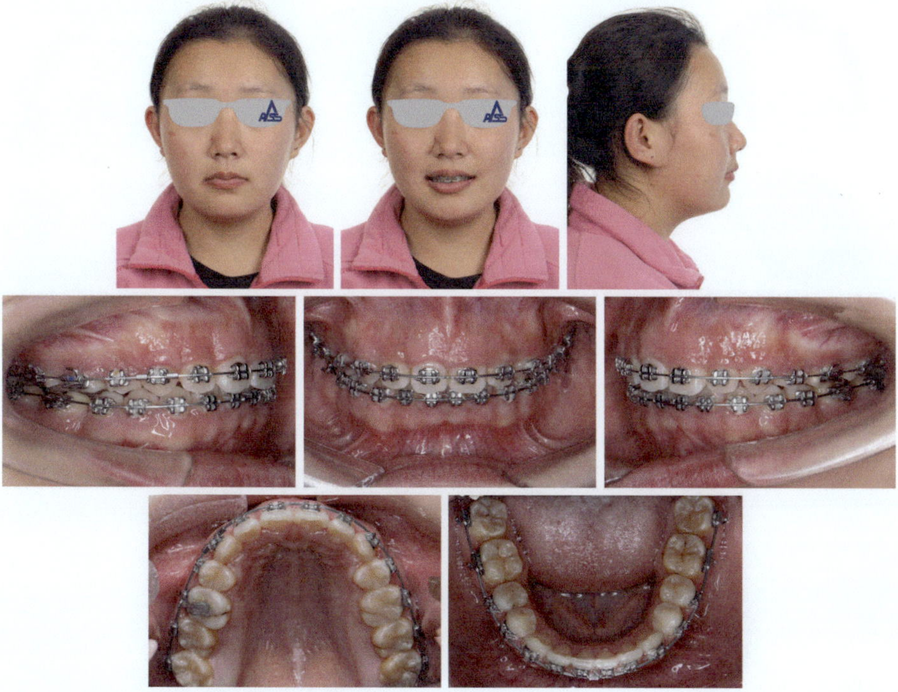

Fig. 14.39 Fifteen months into treatment

Her profile was greatly improved after treatment (Fig. 14.40). Superimposition of tracings (Fig. 14.41) showed maximum anchorage in upper arch, and lower second molars moved mesially without forward tipping as planned. Due to the successful intrusion of upper first molars, the cephalometric analysis (Table 14.5) demonstrated 5.3° clockwise rotation of FOP.

Summary

The physiologic anchorage loss in second premolar extraction cases is more prominent than in first premolar extraction cases because the drifting of the first molars is greater comparing to first premolar extraction cases according to Chap. 7. It alerts that the patients with second premolar extraction should be bonded as soon as possible, in order to avoid unwanted anchor molar forward tipping and migration.

Thanks to the well maintenance or effective restoration of upper curves of Spee, the cephalometric analysis in the above five cases all showed clockwise rotation of FOP. It indicates that molars were prevented from forward tipping and the

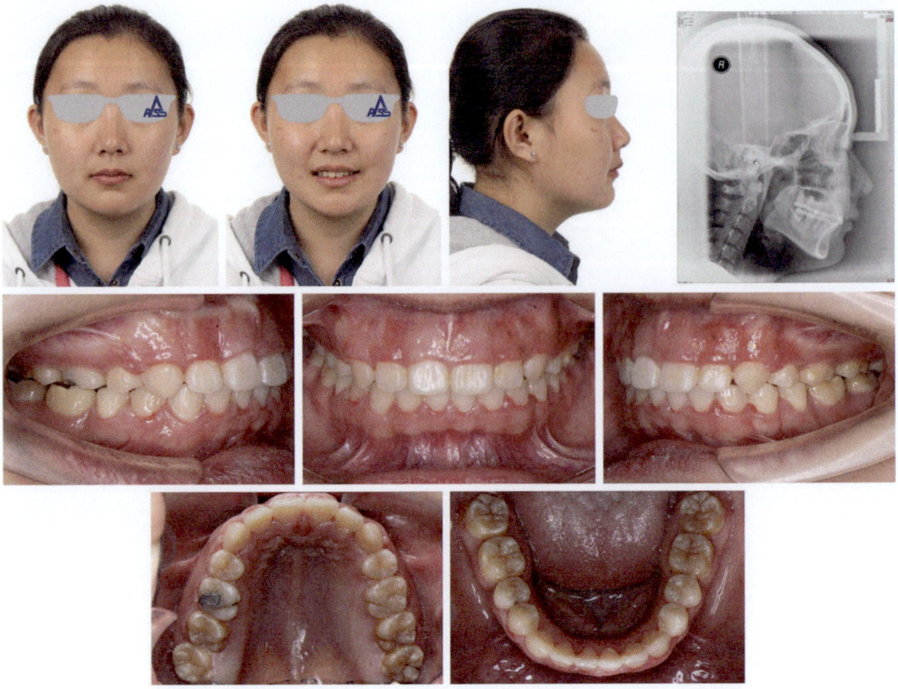

Fig. 14.40 Posttreatment facial and intraoral photographs and cephalometric radiograph

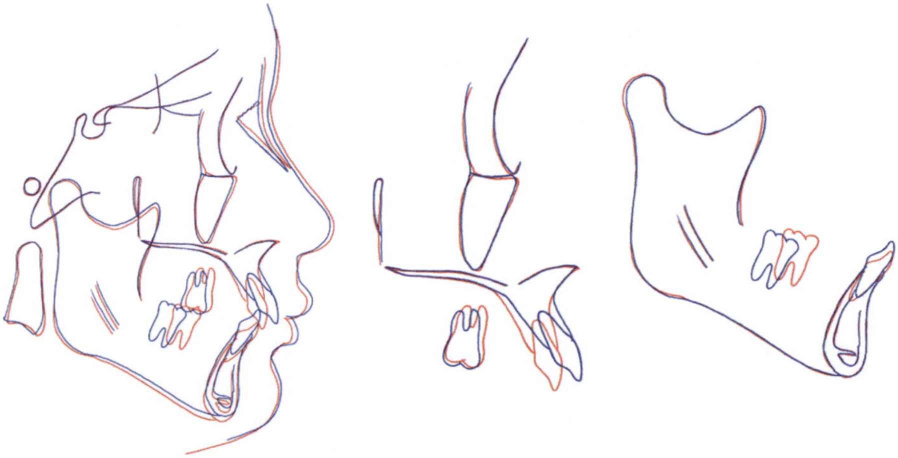

Fig. 14.41 Superimposition of pretreatment (*blue*) and posttreatment (*red*) cephalometric tracings

counterclockwise rotation of functional occlusal plane as the physiologic compensation to excessive mandible growth was resisted or reversed, which presents the typical feature of dentoalveolar compensation treatment advocated by Prof. Johnston in Chap. 3.

Index

T.M. Xu (ed.), *Physiologic Anchorage Control*,
DOI 10.1007/978-3-319-48333-7

MIX
Papier aus verantwortungsvollen Quellen
Paper from responsible sources
FSC® C105338

If you have any concerns about our products,
you can contact us on
ProductSafety@springernature.com

In case Publisher is established outside the EU,
the EU authorized representative is:
Springer Nature Customer Service Center GmbH
Europaplatz 3, 69115 Heidelberg, Germany

Printed by Libri Plureos GmbH
in Hamburg, Germany